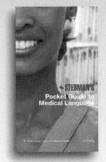

Stedman's Pocket Guide to Medical Language

ISBN: 978-0-7817-9981-2 • 2008 • 352 pages • 25 illustrations • Bonus CD-ROM

This convenient pocket guide provides students and health professionals with a quick reference to key medical terminology and related information. It covers the building blocks of medical terminology such as how to form medical terms, common prefixes, suffixes, combining forms and vowels, and pronunciation guidelines. A bound-in CD-ROM is available including audio English and Spanish pronunciations and an image bank for easy reference.

Stedman's Medical Terminology Flash Cards, Second Edition

ISBN: 978-1-60831-178-1 • 2009 • 800 cards • 455 illustrations

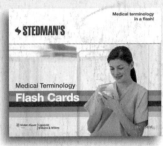

This helpful resource contains 800 flash cards made up of prefixes, suffixes, and root words to help you learn the building blocks of medical terminology. Each form is presented on the front of the card, and the definition and word building samples appear on the back. This edition features a new full-color design with specialties color-coded and illustrations added to cards. A companion website is also available offering an audio pronunciation glossary and a question bank.

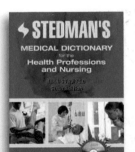

Stedman's Medical Dictionary for the Health Professions and Nursing, Sixth Edition

ISBN: 978-0-7817-7618-9 • 2008 • 2,432 pages • 1,000 illustrations • Bonus CD-ROM

This valuable reference contains over 54,000 entries and 1,000 enriched color images and photographs, including key medical terminology used in over 30 of today's fastest growing health profession areas—plus comprehensive inclusion of entries suited for the nursing field. The bonus CD-ROM includes complete book content in a searchable format and over 48,000 audio pronunciations. Plus *Stedman's Plus Medical/Pharmaceutical Spellchecker* is included for free on CD-ROM – $99 value!

Student Success for Health Professionals Made Incredibly Easy – Nancy Olrech, MSHP, BSN, RN

ISBN: 978-0-7817-8061-2 • 2007 • 281 pages • 137 illustrations

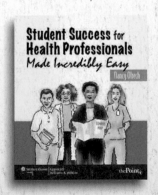

This unique guide shows health professions and nursing students how to "win at the game of school." Working with content that is fun and easy to learn, you'll gain the skills needed to succeed in your studies and in your career as a health professional. This book introduces you to four main characters: three students and one health professional. You'll easily identify with the challenges these characters face in trying to manage their time, discover their personal learning styles, make the most of their studying, and prepare for tests. By mimicking their actions, you can overcome any obstacle that stands in your way to success.

A Short Course in Medical Terminology

SECOND EDITION

C. Edward Collins
Adjunct Professor and Curriculum Consultant
Lambton College
Sarnia, Ontario

Ann DePetris, RN, BSN, MSA
Adjunct Professor
Oakland Community College
Program Manager, Cardiology Research
William Beaumont Hospital
Royal Oak, Michigan

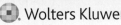
. Wolters Kluwer | Lippincott Williams & Wilkins
Health

Philadelphia • Baltimore • New York • London
Buenos Aires • Hong Kong • Sydney • Tokyo

Senior Publisher: Julie Stegman
Product Director: Eric Branger
Product Manager: Amy Millholen
Developmental Editor: Jennifer Ajello
Marketing Manager: Allison Powell
Compositor: Absolute Service Inc /MDC
Printer: C&C Offset Printing

351 West Camden Street   530 Walnut Street
Baltimore, Maryland 21201   Philadelphia, Pennsylvania 19106

Printed in the People's Republic of China

Library of Congress Cataloging-in-Publication Data

Collins, C. Edward.
  A short course in medical terminology / C. Edward Collins, Ann DePetris. – 2nd ed.
      p. ; cm.
  Includes bibliographical references and index.
  ISBN 978-0-7817-9883-9 (alk. paper)
  1. Medicine–Terminology. 2. Medical sciences–Terminology. I. DePetris, Ann. II. Title.
  [DNLM: 1. Terminology as Topic–Problems and Exercises. W 15 C712s 2011]

  R123.C594 2011
  610.1'4–dc22

                        2009044804

To purchase additional copies of this book, call our customer service department at **(800) 638-3030** or fax orders to **(301) 824-7390**. International customers should call **(301) 714-2324**.

Visit Lippincott Williams & Wilkins on the Internet: *http://www.LWW.com*. Lippincott Williams & Wilkins customer service representatives are available from 8:30 am to 6:00 pm, EST.

                                                                    11
                                                        1 2 3 4 5 6 7 8 9 10

PREFACE

Welcome to *A Short Course in Medical Terminology, Second Edition*. The goals for this edition were to ensure that the text remains concise and appropriate for a one-semester or continuing education medical terminology course, to enhance the format and chapter structure, and to provide additional tools and resources to help students learn medical language. This edition is suitable for use in the classroom or self-directed study.

New to This Edition

With this new edition, it was our intention to build upon the foundation established with the first edition. We reviewed our chapter organization and fine-tuned each chapter, and also introduced pharmacology terms into each chapter. In addition to this, we expanded our chapter exercise sections to include additional exercises of crosswords and labeling exercises. We paid special attention to students' different learning style preferences and made sure to represent a variety of exercises which appeal to each preference: visual, kinesthetic (hands on), and auditory. And finally, we expanded our content by adding more full-color illustrations and additional appendices: a Glossary of Prefixes, Suffixes, and Combining Forms and Glossary of Medical Abbreviations, along with the ISMP's List of Error-Prone Abbreviations, Symbols, and Dose Designations.

We hope that you will be pleased with our changes and that the changes ensure that, after using this book, you have strong foundation in medical language.

Approach and Content Organization

Learning to use many different combinations of word elements to form new terms yields rich rewards. Therefore, the text is divided into two parts: Part One Introduction to Medical Terminology reveals the basics of word building and sets the foundation for learning words relative to the body systems and beyond. Part Two Body Systems offers an overview of each system, briefly describes and identifies the structure and function of that system, and introduces terms naming common abnormal conditions, along with those related to their diagnosis and treatment.

- Part One Introduction to Medical Terminology consists of Chapters 1 and 2, which identify the foundations of term formation, including singular and plural endings and pronunciations.
- Part Two Body Systems begins with Chapter 3, which introduces the human body and briefly discusses terms related to the body's organization—from cells to organs—as well as the terms needed to locate specific points in the body: positioning, body planes, and body cavities. The systems chapters are rearranged in this edition to yield fewer chapters and a consistent format. Body systems chapters are structured in the following way:
  - *Learning Objectives* open each chapter and identify the terms you can expect to learn.
  - *Word Elements* specific to each body system are presented in a table.
  - An *Overview of the System* offers an introduction to the system and its main purpose.
  - *Structure/Function* helps students understand the basic anatomy and physiology of each body system, along with the terms related to it.
  - *Disorders and Treatments* presents terms relating to diseases and diagnostic and treatment procedures of the various body systems.
  - *Pharmacology*, a new section in each system chapter, helps students learn drug classification terms that relate to the body system discussed.

- *Abbreviations* lists various abbreviations for terms commonly abbreviated.
- A *Study Table*, a popular feature carried over from the previous edition, is placed at the end of each chapter. It gives a phonetic pronunciation, etymological analysis, and definition for each term.
- *Chapter Exercises* are incorporated to reinforce learning. They include matching, crosswords, case studies, and anatomical labeling.
- A *Chapter Quiz* concludes each chapter to test comprehension of the chapter contents. Answers to chapter quizzes are included in an appendix.

Additional Resources

The chapters in *A Short Course in Medical Terminology, Second Edition* are designed to support the diverse learning styles of students. In addition to the text content, ancillary materials complement the text and also appeal to various student learning styles.

Student Resources:
- Question Bank with a variety of exercise types to reinforce chapter material
- Educational Games, such as crossword puzzles, Hangman, and word building challenges
- Audio Glossary
- Flash Cards, including Flash Card Generator
- Chapter Quizzes
- Final Exam

Instructor Resources:
- PowerPoint slides and Lesson Plans include useful information to facilitate presentation of material by instructors.
- Test Generator with more than 500 questions to test students' knowledge of terms, their meanings, and abbreviations.
- Handouts include additional puzzles and games for additional student practice.

TO THE STUDENT

In order to learn the language of the health professions, you need to have a plan. You should think of what methods of learning suit you best. Some students are "audio" learners while others are "visual" or "tactile." You may be good at memorizing terms as you see them in the text or in presentations, or you may be one who needs to repeatedly write terms down to help commit them to memory. You might prefer to record terms on tape for replay as often as needed. Use whatever technique is best for you. Below are some study tips.

Study Tips:
- Use the "2X" study rule: study twice the number of credit hours of the class each week. For example, if the class is a 3-credit course, study 6 hours each week. This number may be adjusted to meet individual needs, of course.
- Create flash cards for each chapter. Index cards make convenient flash cards to carry around, or use the flash card generator that is part of the student resources to create your own cards. You can study on breaks, while waiting in line, or before class.
- Ask a family member or peer to test you with the flashcards.
- Use mnemonic tricks, such as relating a new term to a situation in your personal life or something you are familiar with. For example, if you know the cleaning product Lysol and know that it destroys germs, you can associate it with the word element lysis, which means destruction. For example, the term neurolysis means "destruction of nerves."
- Complete all the exercises and chapter quizzes in the book. Then, work through the various exercises included in the online Student Resources. You can do this with a friend to reinforce and discuss the terms.

- Listen to and repeat ten terms at a time from the online audio glossary. Then, listen to and repeat another ten. Repeat the process until you have gone through all the chapter terms.

Learning Medical Terminology should not be intimidating. Developing a good foundation involves memorization, which is easy if you learn the word parts first. However, each student has his or her own method of learning. Identify what works for you and create a plan. You will be surprised by how quickly you acquire a working knowledge of medical terminology.

C. Edward Collins
Adjunct Professor and Curriculum Consultant
Lambton College

Ann DePetris, RN, BSN, MSA
Adjunct Professor
Oakland Community College
Program Manager, Cardiology Research
William Beaumont Hospital

USER'S GUIDE

....

A Short Course in Medical Terminology, Second Edition was developed to provide you with an easy, efficient, and effective way to study medical terminology. The tools and features in the text and ancillaries will help you work through the material presented. This User's Guide will introduce you to the features of the book that will enhance your learning experience.

A **logical organization** guides you through the basics of medical terminology, word elements, and word analysis.

Part One: Introduction to Medial Terminology introduces the basics of word building and sets the foundation for learning words relative to the body systems and beyond.

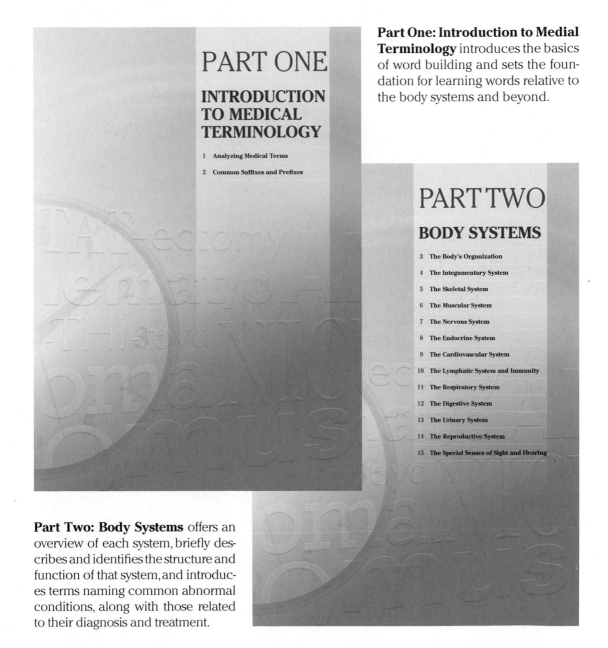

PART ONE

INTRODUCTION TO MEDICAL TERMINOLOGY

1 Analyzing Medical Terms

2 Common Suffixes and Prefixes

PART TWO

BODY SYSTEMS

3   The Body's Organization

4   The Integumentary System

5   The Skeletal System

6   The Muscular System

7   The Nervous System

8   The Endocrine System

9   The Cardiovascular System

10 The Lymphatic System and Immunity

11 The Respiratory System

12 The Digestive System

13 The Urinary System

14 The Reproductive System

15 The Special Senses of Sight and Hearing

Part Two: Body Systems offers an overview of each system, briefly describes and identifies the structure and function of that system, and introduces terms naming common abnormal conditions, along with those related to their diagnosis and treatment.

LEARNING OBJECTIVES

Upon completion of this chapter, you should be able to:

- Distinguish among the three elements of medical terms: **root**, **suffix**, and **prefix**.
- Describe how medical terms are divided into word elements.
- Explain what the phrase **combining form** means.
- State the rules for determining singular and plural endings.
- Recognize the importance of proper spelling and pronunciation of medical terms.
- Define the commonly used roots, suffixes, and prefixes introduced in this chapter.

Learning Objectives open each chapter and identify the points that you can expect to learn and understand by the end of the chapter.

Word Elements • Integumentary System

WORD ELEMENT	MEANING	EXAMPLE
albin/o	white	albinism
cirrh/o, jaund/o, xanth/o	yellow	cirrhosis, jaundice, xanthoderma
cutane/o	skin	cutaneous
cyan/o	blue	cyanosis
-cyte, cyt/o	cell	melanocyte
derm/o, dermat/o	skin	dermatitis
epi-	upon	epidermal
erythr/o	red	erythema
ichthy/o	dry, scaly (fish-like)	ichthyosis
kerat/o	horn-like	keratosis
leuk/o	white	leukoderma
melan/o	black	melanoma
myc/o	fungus	dermatomycosis
onych/o	nail	onychophagia
pil/o	hair	pilonidal
scler/o	hardening	scleroderma
seb/o	sebum	seborrhea
sub-	below	subcutaneous
sudor/i	sweat	sudoriferous
xer/o	dry	xeroderma

Word Elements specific to each body system are presented in table format early in the chapter.

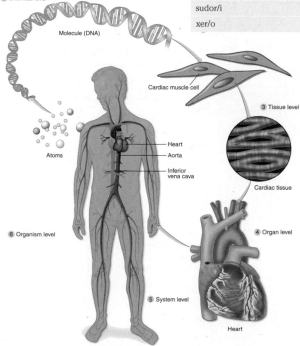

Full-color Illustrations throughout the book help to illustrate harder subject areas and aid the visual learner.

Word Sense feature highlights facts about medical terms.

>|< *The medical phrase for floating ribs is* **costae fluctuantes**. *Since rib pairs 8, 9, and 10, together with the "floating ribs" 11 and 12, are sometimes collectively called* **false ribs** *or* **costae spuriae**, *it follows that the first seven pairs of ribs are* **costae verae** *("true ribs"). If you know the English words* fluctuate, spurious, *and* verify, *you can associate them with the three terms above as a help in remembering them. If you are unfamiliar with those English words, you might want to look them up in a good dictionary and make them part of your general vocabulary.*

Abbreviation Table • The Skeletal System

ABBREVIATION	MEANING
ACL	anterior cruciate ligament
C (C1, C2, etc.)	cervical
CT	computed tomography
CTS	carpal tunnel syndrome
Fx	fracture
L (L1, L2, etc.)	lumbar
LE	lower extremity
RA	rheumatoid arthritis
ROM	range of motion
S	sacral
T	thoracic
THR	total hip replacement
TKA	total knee arthroplasty
TKR	total knee replacement
Tx	traction

Abbreviations Tables include the most common abbreviations and their meanings for each body system.

Study Table • Common Suffixes

SUFFIX	MEANING	EXAMPLE
-ac, -al, -an, -aneous, -ar, -ary, -eal, -eous, -iac, -iatric, -ic, -ical, -oid, -otic, -ous, -tic, -ular	converts a root or a noun term to an adjective atrial, cardiac, ureteral	geriatric, orthopedic, ocular, dental, cutaneous, cyanotic,
-cele	protrusion, hernia	rectocele
-centesis	surgical puncture	thoracentesis
-cyte	cell	leukocyte
-desis	surgical binding	arthrodesis
-dynia, -algia	pain	arthrodynia
-ectasis, -ectasia	expansion or dilation	angiectasis
-ectomy	surgical removal	appendectomy
-edema	excessive fluid in intracellular tissues	angioedema
-emesis	vomiting	hematemesis
-emia	blood	uremia
-gen, -genic, -genesis	origin, producing	osteogenic
-gram	written or pictorial record	electrocardiogram
-graph	device for graphic or pictorial recording	electrocardiograph
-graphy	act of graphic or pictorial recording	electrocardiography
-ian, -iatrist, -ist, -logist, -logy, -ics, -iatry, -iatrics	specialty of, study of, practice of	geriatrist, pediatrician, gynecology
-iasis	a suffix used to convert a verb to a noun indicating a condition	cholelithiasis
-ism	a condition of; a process; or a state of	dwarfism, gigantism
-itis	inflammation	appendicitis
-lith	stone, calculus, calcification	pneumolith
-lysis	disintegration	hemolysis
-malacia	softening	osteomalacia
-megaly	enlargement	gastromegaly

Study Tables provide a summary of chapter terms for reinforcement of the material in an easy-to-reference format.

Chapter Exercises, including matching, crossword puzzles, word building, fill-in-the-blank, spelling, true/false, case studies, and figure labeling, help reinforce the content you've learned and help you retain the chapter's most important information.

---

10   PART ONE • INTRODUCTION TO MEDICAL TERMINOLOGY

EXERCISE 1-2   Combining Roots and Suffixes

Combine the suffixes *-logy*, *-itis*, *-algia*, *-dynia*, *-path/y*, and *-derm* with as many of the roots below as you can. Try to find at least one appropriate root for each suffix and write the resulting words in the "Word" column. Then write a brief definition in the "Meaning" column for each of your choices. You may use as many combinations as you think are appropriate.

ROOT	SUFFIX	WORD
1. psych/o	____	_____
2. path/o	____	_____
3. cardi/o	____	_____
4. hem/o, hemat/o	____	_____
5. derm/o, dermat/o	____	_____
6. arthr/o	____	_____
7. neur/o	____	_____
8. oste/o	____	_____

EXERCISE 1-3   Matching Word Elements with Meanings

Match the numbers in Column 1 with the letters in Column 2 according to the corresponding terms and definitions they designate.

1. ____ -itis
2. ____ neur/o
3. ____ -algia
4. ____ -logy
5. ____ hemat/o
6. ____ gastr/o
7. ____ psych/o
8. ____ dermat/o
9. ____ path/o
10. ____ oste/o

A. A suffix meaning "pain"
B. A root meaning "stomach"
C. A root meaning "skin"
D. A suffix meaning "the study of"
E. A root referring to the mind
F. A suffix meaning "inflammation"
G. A root referring to the nervous system
H. A root meaning "blood"
I. A root meaning "bone"
J. A word root that can also be a suffix

CHAPTER 1 QUIZ

Write the answers to the following questions using the spaces provided.

1. Name the three word elements of a medical term.
   _____ , _____ , _____

2. What is dermatitis?
   _____

3. A cardiologist treats diseases of what body organ?
   _____

4. What is a neuroma?
   _____

5. The plural for nucleus is _____.

6. What is the term for study of the elderly?
   _____

7. A combining form is composed of what two word parts?
   _____ and _____

Complete the sentences below using a medical term.

8. Judy injured her knee, and the doctor wants to use an instrument to view her knee joint. This instrument is called a(n) _____.

9. Tom has a history of bleeding stomach ulcers. He needs to have his stomach removed. This procedure is called a(n) _____.

10. Amy was told that she has an enlarged liver. The medical term for this is _____.

Chapter Quizzes at the end of each chapter test your comprehension of the material. Answers to the chapter quizzes are provided in the appendix.

Student Resources

All new, enhanced student resources provide additional opportunity to practice and assess your mastery of the content. Student Resources include:

- Question Bank: Multiple Choice, True/False, Fill-in-the-Blank, Spelling Bee, Word Building, Figure Labeling, Image Matching, Medical Record Exercises
- Games: Crossword Puzzles, Get the Picture (Hangman), Raise the Roof Word Building, 60-Second Challenge Word Building
- Flash Cards with audio, including build-your-own
- Animations
- Audio Pronunciation Glossary

The student resources can be accessed online at http://thepoint.lww.com/Collins2e. See the inside front cover for more information.

REVIEWERS

The authors and publisher would like to thank the following individuals who helped to review this textbook:

Vicki Aube, AAS, CST
Instructor
Surgical Technology
Tennessee Technology Center at Knoxville
Knoxville, TN

Cynthia Carr, MS, OTR/L
Associate Professor
Master of Occupational Therapy Program
Governors State University
University Park, IL

Donna J. Catron, RN, BSN, MEd
Professional Nurse Educator
School of Nursing
Jameson Health System
New Castle, PA

Mary Fabick, MSN, MEd, RN-BC, CEN
Area of Nursing
Milligan College
Milligan College, TN

Craig Harradine, DC
Nursing Instructor
Nursing Department
Apollo College
Boise, ID

Lu Herbeck, BS
Adjunct Professor
Health Exercise Science and Medical
Minnesota School of Business
Shakopee, MN

Nancy Hislop, BSN
Online Instructor
Globe Education Network
Globe University/Minnesota School of Business
Richfield, MN

Krista Hoekstra, MA, RN
Director of Nursing
Practical Nursing Department
Hennepin Technical College
Brooklyn Park & Eden Prairie, MN

Patti Kalvelage, MS, OTR/L
Lecturer
Master of Occupational Therapy Program
Governors State University
University Park, IL

Louise Lee, MHA, PA-C
Assistant Professor of PA Studies
Physician Assistant
Physician Assistant Studies
Massachusetts College of Pharmacy & Health Sciences
Manchester, NH

Lisa Miller, RMA, EMT-B, MLT(ASCP), CPC, BBA
Medical Assistant Instructor
Allied Health Education
Coffeyville Community College
Coffeyville, KS

Melyssa Munch
Star Technical Institute
Lakewood, NJ

Catharine A. Muskus, MS, FNP-BC
Clinical Assistant Professor
Nursing Department
University of Vermont
Burlington, VT

Bernard Pegis, MD
Family Practice Physician
Skyline Family Practice
Front Royal, VA

Sharyn Shaner, RN, MSN
Professional Nurse Educator
School of Nursing
Jameson Memorial Hospital
New Castle, PA

Janis Simpson, RN, BSN, MA, EdS
Director of Nursing
Practical Nursing
Tennessee Technology Center @ Athens
Athens, TN

Lisa Smith, CMA-AAMA
Medical Instructor
Medical Program Chair
Minnesota School of Business
Waite Park, MN

Donna Williams
Tennessee Technology Center
Knoxville, TN

Brenda Willoughby, MS, BSN, RN
Professor of Nursing
Division of Nursing
Bluegrass Community and Technical College
Lexington, KY

Margaret A. Yoder, RN, MS, MHA
Associate Professor Nurse Education
Coordinator Practical Nursing Program
Quinsigamond Community College
Worcester, MA

LaTanya J. Young, MMSc, MPH, RMA, PA-C
Assistant Professor, Physician Assistant
Health Care Management
Clayton State University
Morrow, GA

ACKNOWLEDGMENTS

....

This edition would not have come into being without the talents of many people, first of whom are the members of the editorial staff of LWW. Very special thanks go to Julie Stegman for overseeing the entire project and for applying her excellent executive skills in making important decisions about content and direction, Amy Millholen for managing the program and keeping us constantly aware of requirements and guidelines, Jennifer Ajello, who as development editor is the real architect of the final product, and Teresa Exley for her diligent work during the production stage.

Thanks also to Bernard Pegis, MD, for reading the entire manuscript to make sure the many technical statements contained therein were accurate.

We wish to offer a very special thanks to Bob Henry, Dean of International Education and former Dean of the School of Health Sciences at Lambton College, for his ongoing support and encouragement. Special thanks also to David Felton, MD, PhD, Vice President and Medical Director of the Research Institute, William Beaumont Hospital, for mentoring and for sharing his vast authorship experiences. Special recognition goes to colleagues at the Research Institute, William Beaumont Hospital, and to Theresa Wangler, RN, MS Ed., Department Chairperson of Health Sciences at Oakland Community College, whose help and support are much appreciated.

TABLE OF CONTENTS

....

PART ONE   **INTRODUCTION TO MEDICAL TERMINOLOGY**

CHAPTER 1   Analyzing Medical Terms   3

CHAPTER 2   Common Suffixes and Prefixes   12

PART TWO   **BODY SYSTEMS**

CHAPTER 3   The Body's Organization   37

CHAPTER 4   The Integumentary System   53

CHAPTER 5   The Skeletal System   74

CHAPTER 6   The Muscular System   108

CHAPTER 7   The Nervous System   126

CHAPTER 8   The Endocrine System   154

CHAPTER 9   The Cardiovascular System   179

CHAPTER 10   The Lymphatic System and Immunity   211

CHAPTER 11   The Respiratory System   226

CHAPTER 12   The Digestive System   255

CHAPTER 13   The Urinary System   280

CHAPTER 14   The Reproductive System   301

CHAPTER 15   The Special Senses of Sight and Hearing   334

APPENDICES

APPENDIX A   Answers to Chapter Exercises   361

APPENDIX B   Glossary of Prefixes, Suffixes, and Combining Forms   382

APPENDIX C   Glossary of Medical Abbreviations   387

APPENDIX D   ISMP's List of Error-Prone Abbreviations, Symbols, and
Dose Designations   400

INDEX   404

PART ONE

INTRODUCTION TO MEDICAL TERMINOLOGY

1   Analyzing Medical Terms

2   Common Suffixes and Prefixes

CHAPTER 1

Analyzing
Medical Terms

LEARNING OBJECTIVES

Upon completion of this chapter, you should be able to:

- Distinguish among the four elements of medical terms: roots, suffixes, prefixes, and combining forms.
- Describe how medical terms are divided into word elements.
- Explain what the phrase combining form means.
- State the rules for determining singular and plural endings.
- Recognize the importance of proper spelling and pronunciation of medical terms.
- Define the commonly used roots, suffixes, and prefixes introduced in this chapter.

Introduction

Medical terminology might seem like a new language at first since most medical terms have a foundation in the Latin or Greek languages. However, medical terms are always part of the language that includes them. For example, the word **artery** is English; in French, it is *artère,* but it is *arteria* in Spanish and *pulsader* in German. The word element, *arteri,* is Greek and means artery. In medical terminology, we use a word root and combine it with other word elements to form medical terms. Once you understand the rules for putting medical terms together, you will find it easy to understand them. You will discover that in learning medical terminology, you are not studying a foreign language but rather increasing your English vocabulary.

Let's look at some examples. The root word **mast** is derived from the Greek word for breast. We can combine it with the suffix **-ectomy**, which means "removal of." The new word **mastectomy** means "removal of the breast." Another example is **psychology**. **Psych** (from the Greek word for "mind") coupled with **-logy** tells us that psychology is the study of mental processes and behavior.

When you look at a medical term, think of it as a whole term that can be broken up into pieces. These pieces help to define the word. As mentioned earlier, the suffix -logy means "the study of." You can add that piece to other word roots and form a number of new words. **Pathology** (study of disease), **dermatology** (study of the skin), and **gerontology** (study of the elderly) are all examples of this process. You need to learn the meanings of the word roots **path** (disease), **dermat** (skin), and **geront** (elderly). By knowing these word root definitions and the meaning of the suffix -logy, you'll have added three new medical terms to your vocabulary. Medical terms are words made up of different parts or elements. By learning the word roots and then analyzing the other word elements, you will be able to learn and understand medical terminology. The four types of word elements are discussed in the following section.

Word Elements

The four types of word elements that make up medical terms are roots, suffixes, prefixes, and combining forms. Medical terms contain one or more of these elements.

- The **word root** reveals the central meaning of the word and frequently describes a body part. It is the base element from which other related terms may be formed. In one of the examples mentioned earlier, the word root *mast* describes the breast. In another example, **periarthritis**, **arthr** (joint) is the root.
- **Suffixes** always come at the end of the word. They add meaning to the root. A few examples of suffixes are **-ectomy** (removal of), **-logy** (study of), **-itis** (inflammation of), **-algia** (pain), and **-oma** (tumor). There are numerous suffixes that can be added to various word roots. You only have to learn the suffixes once because they are used repeatedly in medical terminology. For example, once you know that **-itis** refers to "inflammation of," then you'll know **mastitis** (inflammation of the breast), **gastritis** (inflammation of the stomach), and **arthritis** (inflammation of a joint). Likewise, once you know the word roots, it is easy to learn the terms **mastectomy** (removal of a breast), **gastrectomy** (removal of the stomach), and **arthrectomy** (removal of a joint). However, not all terms have a suffix.
- **Prefixes** always come at the beginning of the word and will frequently suggest information about the number of parts, location of the organ, direction, time, or frequency. Generally, a new medical term is formed when a prefix is added to a term. **Hyper-** (over, above, excessive), **peri-** (around), **tachy-** (rapid, fast), **epi-** (upon, over), and **tri-** (three) are all examples of prefixes. These can be added to word roots and/or word roots with a suffix. **Hypergastric** (meaning above the stomach), **periarthritis** (inflammation around the joint), and **tachycardia** (a rapid heart rate) are some terms with prefixes.

Now that you've been introduced to three of the four main elements that compose medical terms, you must learn how to divide terms into their word elements—roots, suffixes, and prefixes—in order to understand their meanings. See the examples below.

EXAMPLES:	GASTR / ITIS		HYPER / GASTR / IC		
Word	gastr	-itis	hyper	gastr	-ic
	↓	↓	↓	↓	↓
Element	root	suffix	prefix	root	suffix
	↓	↓	↓	↓	↓
Element Meaning	stomach	inflammation of	excessive, above	stomach	pertaining to
Word Meaning	inflammation of the stomach		pertaining to above the stomach		

Word elements are generally classified as a root, prefix, or suffix. This is not a hard and fast rule, however. Sometimes, you will see a word root being used as a suffix. In the following example, **path/o** is used as a word root in pathology (study of disease) and then again as a suffix in **psychopath** (disease of the mind). Example: "path" = *path / o / logy* and *psych / o / path*

The fourth element to consider is the combining form, which consists of the word root plus one or more vowels, often an "o." The vowel is required to facilitate pronunciation. The "o" is called the **combining vowel**. A combining vowel is used between two word roots. It is also used between a root and a suffix when the suffix begins with a consonant.

EXAMPLE: COMBINING VOWEL: BETWEEN ROOTS	GASTR / O / ENTER / ITIS		
Word	gastr/o	enter	-itis
	↓	↓	↓
Element	combining form (root + vowel)	root	suffix
	↓	↓	↓
Element Meaning	stomach	intestines	inflammation of
Word Meaning	inflammation of the stomach and intestines		

EXAMPLE: COMBINING VOWEL: ROOT AND SUFFIX	CARD/I / O / LOGY	
Word	card/i/o	-logy
	↓	↓
Element	combining form (root + vowels)	suffix
	↓	↓
Element Meaning	heart	study of
Word Meaning	study of the heart	

WORD DIVISION MARKS

Each root introduced hereafter will include its most common accompanying vowels or vowel-consonant combinations separated by forward slant bars, as shown below:

1. psych/o = mind
2. path/o = disease
3. arthr/o = joint
4. derm/o, dermat/o = skin

Each suffix when it appears by itself is written with a preceding hyphen (e.g., -logy), indicating that one or more word elements will always come before it. Likewise, each prefix when it appears by itself is written with a following hyphen (e.g., pre-) to indicate that one or more word elements normally follow. For example1the pre- in prefix is itself a prefix meaning "before," a meaning that may help you remember the meaning of the word prefix—namely, a word element that comes before.

Analyzing Medical Terms

Now that you know how to divide a medical term into its basic elements, you can start analyzing medical terms using the following steps:

1. Separate the term into its word parts: identify root(s), suffix, and prefix.
2. Attach the meaning to each of the word elements.
3. Translate by starting at the end of the word with the suffix and moving to the prefix, if any, and then finally to the root, as in the example below.

EXAMPLE:	PERI- / ARTHR / -ITIS		
Word	peri-	arthr	-itis
	↓	↓	↓
Element	prefix	root	suffix
	↓	↓	↓
Element Meaning	around	joint	inflammation
Word Meaning	inflammation around a joint		

By following these three steps, you will be able to determine the meaning of almost any term. Try one more example: **gastroscopy**.

1. Separate the word into its elements: the combining form gastr/o and the suffix -scopy.
2. Attach a meaning to the word elements: gastr/o means stomach and -scopy means visual examination.
3. Translate by starting with the suffix and moving back to the word root: a visual examination of the stomach.

Deciphering medical terms is like a game, and once you know the rules and strategies, it can be fun.

Singular and Plural Endings

In English, we usually add an *s* or *es* to make a word plural. Since many of the medical terms have Greek and Latin origins, the plural endings sometimes follow the rules of

Table 1-1   Singular and Plural Word Endings

Singular Ending	Example	Plural Ending	Example
-a	vertebra	-ae	vertebrae
-ax	thorax	-aces	thoraces
-is	diagnosis	-es	diagnoses
-ix, -ex	appendix	-ices	appendices
-um	diverticulum	-a	diverticula
-us	bronchus	-i	bronchi
y	ovary	-ies	ovaries

these languages. Where English rules are not preferred, plurals are formed in the following ways:

- If the term ends in *a*, the plural is formed by adding an *e* to the word.
  Example: singular   **scapula**   plural   **scapulae**
- When a term ends in *ax*, change the *ax* to *aces* to form the plural.
  Example: singular   **thorax**   plural   **thoraces**
- To form the plural of a singular term ending in *is*, change the *i* to an *e*.
  Example: singular   **neurosis**   plural   **neuroses**
- If a term ends in *ix* or *ie*, change the ending to *ices* to form the plural.
  Example: singular   **cervix**   plural   **cervices**
- A term ending in *um* is made plural by changing the *um* to an *a*.
  Example: singular   **septum**   plural   **septa**
- To form the plural of words ending in *us*, change the *us* to an *i*.
  Example: singular   **calculus**   plural   **calculi**
- If a term ends in *y*, make it plural by dropping the *y* and adding *ies*.
  Example: singular   **biopsy**   plural   **biopsies**

As noted earlier, these rules will help form the plural in most cases, but there are some exceptions, as you might expect (e.g., the plural of virus is viruses, not viri). Table 1-1 includes additional examples of changing terms from singular to plural.

Pronouncing Medical Terms

A medical term is easier to understand, spell correctly, and remember when you know how to pronounce it correctly. Exercise 1-1 contains a list of 10 medical terms. Practice pronouncing these terms to a classmate.

Beginning with Chapter 4, all of the medical words introduced will include a phonetic spelling so you can begin learning how to pronounce them. Phonetic spelling indicates the sound of the word. For example, a phonetic spelling of psychology would be "sy-KOL-uh-jee." Capitalization indicates the syllable upon which the accent falls. As a further help in learning to pronounce medical terms, the online student ancillaries include an audio pronunciation glossary.

Getting Started

The roots, suffixes, and prefixes in Tables 1-2, 1-3, and 1-4 include some commonly used word elements. These refer to a variety of anatomical systems, which you will study in some depth in later chapters. They are mentioned here so that you can practice what you have learned by completing the exercises at the end of this chapter.

Table 1-2   Common Roots in Medical Terms

Root	Refers to
arthr/o	joint
bronch/o	bronchus
cardi/o	heart
derm/o, dermat/o	skin
gastr/o	stomach
ger/o, geront/o	aged
hem/o, hemat/o	blood
hep/o, hepat/o	liver
neur/o	a nerve cell, the nervous system
oste/o	bone
path/o	disease
psych/o	mind

Table 1-3   Common Suffixes in Medical Terms

gen = cause formation of

Suffix	Meaning
-ac, -al, -ar, -ia, -ic, -ory	pertaining to
-algia	pain
-centesis	surgical puncture
-cyte	cell
-ectomy	to surgically excise, remove
-graph	to write, record
-ist	one who specializes, agent
-itis	inflammation
-logy	study of, specialty of
-megaly	enlargement
-oma	tumor
-path/y	disease
-scope	an instrument to view

Table 1-4   Common Prefixes in Medical Terms

Prefix	Meaning
a-, an-	no, not, without
anti-, contra-	against
brady-	slow
cyan-	bluish
dys-	painful, difficult
en-, endo-, intra-	within, inner
epi-	above, upon
ex-, exo-	out, away from
hyper-, supra-	excessive, above
inter-	between
post-	after
pre-	before, in front of
tachy-	fast, rapid

EXERCISES

EXERCISE 1-1   Word Elements

Identify the components of each word in the appropriate box. The first word is an example that is completed for you. Not all terms have a prefix.

| | COMPONENTS OF MEDICAL WORDS | | | |
MEDICAL WORD AND MEANING	PREFIX	COMBINING FORM (ROOT + VOWEL)	WORD ROOT(S)	SUFFIX
epi / gastr / ic above stomach pertaining to	epi-	—	gastr	-ic
1. append / ectomy appendix excision ap-pen-DEK-toh-mee	—		append	ectomy
2. post / nat / al after birth pertaining to post-NAY-tal	post		nat	al
3. mast / itis breast inflammation mast-EYE-tis	—		mast	itis
4. colon / o / scope colon instrument to view ko-LON-o-skope	—	colon + o		scope
5. enter / o / col / itis intestinal colon inflammation en-ter-o-ko-LEYE-tis	—	1. entero 2. o	col	itis
6. pre / nat / al before birth pertaining to pre-NAY-tal	pre		nat	al
7. oste / o / arthr / itis bone joint inflammation os-te-oh-ar-THRY-tis	—	1. osteo 2. o	arthr	itis
8. arthr / o / tomy joint incision into ar-THROT-oh-mee	—	arthr to		tomy
9. thyroid / ectomy thyroid excision, removed thi-roy-DEKto-mee	—		thyroid	ectomy
10. amni / o / centesis amnion surgical puncture AM-ne-o-sen-TEE-sis	—	amni - o		centesis

EXERCISE 1-2   Combining Roots and Suffixes

Combine the suffixes *-logy, -itis, -algia, -dynia, -path/y*, and *-derm* with as many of the roots below as you can. Try to find at least one appropriate root for each suffix and write the resulting words in the "Word" column. Then write a brief definition in the "Meaning" column for each of your choices. You may use as many combinations as you think are appropriate.

ROOT	SUFFIX	WORD	MEANING
1. psych/o	ology	_____	_____
2. path/o	ology	_____	_____
3. cardi/o	ology	_____	_____
4. hem/o, hemat/o	____	_____	_____
5. derm/o, dermat/o	____	_____	_____
6. arthr/o	____	_____	_____
7. neur/o	____	_____	_____
8. oste/o	____	_____	_____

 EXERCISE 1-3   Matching Word Elements with Meanings

Match the numbers in Column 1 with the letters in Column 2 according to the corresponding terms and definitions they designate.

1. _____ -itis

2. _____ neur/o

3. _____ -algia

4. _____ -logy

5. _____ hemat/o

6. _____ gastr/o

7. _____ psych/o

8. _____ dermat/o

9. _____ path/o

10. _____ oste/o

A. A suffix meaning "pain"

B. A root meaning "stomach"

C. A root meaning "skin"

D. A suffix meaning "the study of"

E. A root referring to the mind

F. A suffix meaning "inflammation"

G. A root referring to the nervous system

H. A root meaning "blood"

I. A root meaning "bone"

J. A word root that can also be a suffix

CHAPTER 1 QUIZ

Write the answers to the following questions using the spaces provided.

1. Name the three word elements of a medical term.

    prefix , _root_ , _suffix_

2. What is dermatitis?

    inflammation of the skin

3. A cardiologist treats diseases of what body organ?

    heart

4. What is a neuroma?

    tumor in neural region

5. The plural for nucleus is _nuclei_ .

6. What is the term for study of the elderly?

    gerentology

7. A combining form is composed of what two word parts?

    root and _combining_ _vowel_

Complete the sentences below using a medical term.

8. Judy injured her knee, and the doctor wants to use an instrument to view her knee joint. This instrument is called a(n) _arthroscopy_ .

9. Tom has a history of bleeding stomach ulcers. He needs to have his stomach removed. This procedure is called a(n) _gastrectomy_ .

10. Amy was told that she has an enlarged liver. The medical term for this is _hepatitis_ .

CHAPTER 2

Common Suffixes
and Prefixes

LEARNING OBJECTIVES

Upon completion of this chapter, you should be able to:

- Define a suffix.
- Define a prefix.
- Identify all of the suffixes and prefixes presented in this chapter.
- Analyze and define new terms introduced in this chapter.
- Pronounce, write, and accurately spell all terms introduced in this chapter.

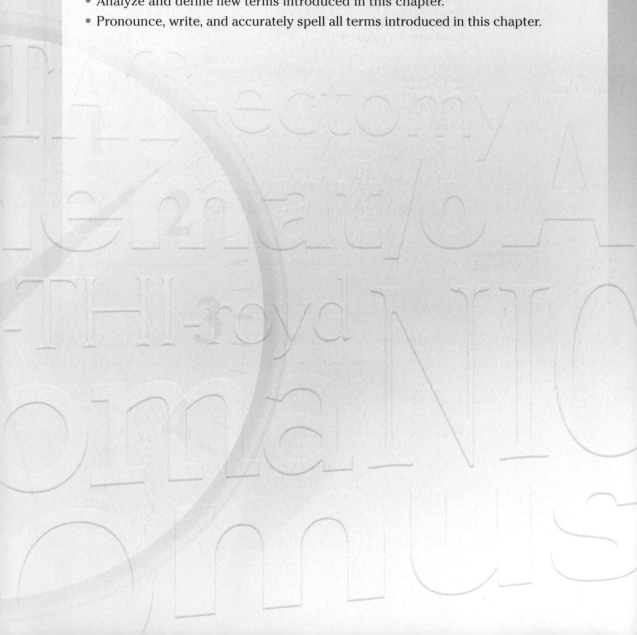

Introduction

Chapter 1 presented the four common word elements used in medical terminology: roots, suffixes, prefixes, and combining forms. This chapter will focus on suffixes and prefixes in greater detail to facilitate a better understanding and confidence in learning medical terms.

Recall in Chapter 1 that a suffix is the word part that comes at the end of a word. The word suffix comes from the Latin word *suffixum*, which may be translated as "to attach under or to the end of." Although the suffix is located last in a medical term, it most often comes first in its definition. For example, appendicitis means "inflammation (*-itis*) of the appendix." Therefore, the suffix, in this case -itis, provides us with the first word of the defining phrase. The term gastrectomy is another example. It is defined as "the removal of the stomach." The definition begins with the meaning of the suffix, -ectomy, which means "removal of." We analyzed the medical term by dividing it into its basic elements and translating it beginning with the suffix.

In Chapter 1, we also noted that a prefix is a word element that comes at the beginning of a word. Note that the word prefix itself contains a prefix, namely, pre-. The second part of the word prefix is "fix," which gives us a perfect definition of prefix: something attached (fixed) in front of or before (pre-) something else. Most of the prefixes occurring in medical terms are also found in everyday English. Although we have all used most of the prefixes contained in this chapter, we may have done so without realizing that they are prefixes. For example, when we are admitted to an anteroom, we may not stop to think that the prefix **ante-** means "before" and that an anteroom is so called because it is a room we enter before entering another room.

Categories of Suffixes

A suffix attached to the end of a word adds meaning to the root. It may modify the root to indicate a condition, diagnostic test, procedure, or specialty. For example, consider the term **arteriostenosis** by observing how it is divided into the word elements and how the suffix **-stenosis** modifies the root:

EXAMPLE: COMBINING VOWEL BETWEEN ROOTS	ARTERI / O / STENOSIS	
Word	arteri/o	-stenosis
	↓	↓
Element	combining form (root + vowel)	suffix
	↓	↓
Element Meaning	artery	narrowing
Word Meaning	narrowing of an artery	

Although not all medical terms have suffixes, when one is used, it is added to the root or combining form.

Dividing suffixes into functional categories makes them easier to learn. The four divisions are as follows:
- Suffixes that signify medical conditions
- Suffixes that signify diagnostic terms, test information, or surgical procedures
- Suffixes associated with a medical specialty or specialist
- Suffixes that convert a noun to an adjective

SUFFIXES SIGNIFYING MEDICAL CONDITIONS

Suffixes are used throughout medical terminology to convert roots or combining forms to nouns or nouns to other nouns. For example, the noun **dwarfism** is formed by adding the suffix **-ism** to the noun dwarf. The definition of dwarfism is "a medical condition characterized by being abnormally small." The suffix **-ism** means "a condition of; a process; or a state of." Another example is the noun **osteoporosis**. The suffix **-porosis** is added to the combining form **oste/o**, and the term osteoporosis is formed. The definition of osteoporosis is "a porous condition of bone" or, more completely, "a reduction in the quantity of bone or atrophy of skeletal tissue". Common suffixes that convert roots to nouns are listed in Table 2-1.

SUFFIXES SIGNIFYING DIAGNOSTIC TERMS, TEST INFORMATION, OR SURGICAL PROCEDURES

This category of suffixes is used to form terms related to test information, diagnoses, and procedures. Many of these suffixes are attached to a root to indicate a procedure or test performed on a body part. The term **appendectomy** is an example. The suffix **-ectomy** means "removal of," and **append** is the root for appendix. Thus, the term means "removal of the appendix." Table 2-2 lists common suffixes that signify diagnostic terms, test information, or procedures.

SUFFIXES ASSOCIATED WITH A MEDICAL SPECIALTY OR SPECIALIST

Some of the suffixes relating to medical specialties and specialists are derived from the Greek word *iatros*, which means "physician" or "medical treatment." This Greek word is the source of the suffixes **-iatrics** and **-iatry** (e.g., in the terms **psychiatry** [the medical specialty concerned with diagnosis and treatment of mental disorders] and **pediatrics** [the specialty relating to children]). The suffixes **-ician** and **-ist** are used when indicating a specialist. While they both refer to a specialist, the suffix -ist is more often associated with a person who practices or specializes in

TABLE 2-1   Suffixes That Signify Medical Conditions

Suffix	Refers to	Examples
-algia	pain	arthralgia
-cele	protrusion, hernia	rectocele
-dynia	pain	arthrodynia
-ectasis, -ectasia	expansion or dilation	angiectasis
-emia	blood	anemia
-iasis	presence of; formation of	cholelithiasis
-ism	a condition, a process, or a state of	dwarfism
-itis	inflammation	appendicitis
-malacia	softening	osteomalacia
-megaly	enlargement	gastromegaly
-oma	tumor	gastroma
-osis	abnormal condition	osteoporosis
-penia	reduction of size or quantity	leukopenia
-plegia	paralysis	hemiplegia
-pnea	breathing	tachypnea
-porosis	porous condition	osteoporosis
-ptosis	downward displacement	nephroptosis
-rrhage	flowing forth	hemorrhage
-rrhea	discharge	diarrhea
-rrhexis	rupture	hysterorrhexis
-spasm	muscular contraction	angiospasm

TABLE 2-2 Suffixes That Signify Diagnostic Terms, Test Information, or Surgical Procedures

Suffix	Refers to	Examples
-centesis	surgical puncture	thoracentesis
-desis	surgical binding	arthrodesis
-ectomy	surgical removal	appendectomy
-gen, -genic, -genesis	origin, producing	osteogenic
-gram	written or pictorial record	electrocardiogram
-graph	device for graphic or pictorial recording	electrocardiograph
-graphy	act of graphic or pictorial recording	electrocardiography
-meter	device for measuring	audiometer
-metry	act of measuring	audiometry
-pexy	surgical fixation	hysteropexy
-plasty	surgical repair	rhinoplasty
-rrhaphy	suture	herniorrhaphy
-scope	device for viewing	arthroscope
-scopy	act of viewing	arthroscopy
-tomy	incision	colotomy
-tripsy	crushing	lithotripsy

a particular field of medicine or health care. An example is the **gerontologist**, a physician who diagnoses and treats disorders brought on by aging.

Terms denoting a field or medical specialty may also end with the suffix **-logy**. Table 2-3 lists the suffixes for medical specialties and specialists.

TABLE 2-3 Suffixes That Signify Medical Specialties and Specialists

Suffix	Refers to	Examples
-ian	specialist	pediatrician
-iatrics	medical specialty	pediatrics
-iatry	medical specialty	psychiatry
-ics	medical specialty	orthopedics
-ist	specialist in a field of study	orthopedist
-logy	study of	gynecology

> ✳ *Please note that **gen** can be a root or a suffix and that terms formed with the suffix **-genic** are adjectives, owing to the **-ic** ending. As you will see in the discussion that follows, -ic is also a suffix by itself.*

SUFFIXES THAT DENOTE ADJECTIVES

Similar to suffixes that signify medical specialties and specialists, suffixes used to create adjective forms are not governed by a clear set of rules. Nevertheless, there are some rules that come into play (i.e., the rules of English pronunciation). For example, we replace the final letter, x, in the word appendix with a c to form the adjective appendicitis because "appendixitis" does not sound much like an English word.

In creating adjectives, we will also sometimes change noun terms that name specialties. For example, psychiatry and pediatrics are the names of specialties. Dropping the y from psychiatry and adding the adjective suffix -ic converts the specialty name to an adjective:

psychia**tric** medicine   psychia**tric** hospital

With pediatrics, on the other hand, all we need to do to form the adjective is drop the *s*:

pediatr**ic** medicine   pediatr**ic** hospital

Examples of adjective suffixes are listed in Table 2-4, along with other common suffixes.

TABLE 2-4 Suffixes That Denote Adjectives and Other Common Suffixes

Suffix	Meaning	Examples
-ac, -al, -an, -aneous, -ar, -ary, -eous, -iac, -iatric, -ic, -ical, -oid, -otic, -ous, -ular	converts a root or noun to an adjective	geriatric, orthopedic, ocular
-cyte	cell	leukocyte
-emesis	vomiting	hematemesis
-iasis	a suffix used to convert a verb to a noun indicating a condition	cholelithiasis
-lith	a stone, calculus, calcification	pneumolith
-lysis	disintegration or destruction of	hemolysis
-megaly	enlarged	gastromegaly
-opsy	visual examination	biopsy
-pathy	disease	cardiopathy
-phobia	a word meaning fear, often appearing as a suffix	claustrophobia
-poiesis	producing or formation	erythropoiesis
-ptosis	drooping	nephroptosis
-sclerosis	hardness	arteriosclerosis
-stasis	level, unchanging	hemostasis
-stenosis	narrowed, blocked	arteriostenosis
-stomy	permanent opening	colostomy
-tome	instrument for cutting	osteotome

✳ *Please note that -logy sometimes signals the study of a field and the specialty (e.g., psychology refers to both the field and the specialty). In other cases, however, the field and the specialty are differentiated, as in gerontology, which means "the study of the aging process," and **geriatrics**, which refers to the specialty of treating patients who suffer from disorders brought on by aging.*

Categories of Prefixes

Not all medical terms include a prefix, although when one is present, it is critical to the term's meaning. For example, **hyper**glycemia (high blood sugar) and **hypo**glycemia (low blood sugar) name conditions that are exact opposites.

✳ *Pay special attention to all similar-sounding prefix pairs, such as hyper- and hypo-. Hyper- means "above" or "beyond normal"; hypo- means "below" or "below normal." **Hypergastric** (above the stomach) and **hypogastric** (below the stomach) are examples of these two prefixes. Also beware of the prefixes ante- and anti-, which are pronounced alike but have different meanings. Ante- means "before," and anti- means "against." Examples are **antepartum** (before labor and delivery) and **antidepressant** (against depression).*

Let's look at an example of how to analyze a term with a prefix.

EXAMPLE: COMBINING VOWEL BETWEEN ROOTS	MICRO / SCOPE	
Word	micro- ↓	-scope ↓
Element	prefix ↓	root ↓
Element Meaning	smallness	instrument for viewing
Word Meaning	instrument that magnifies small objects	

Seeing prefixes in words we already know helps us assimilate their meanings quickly and enables us to understand medical terms we encounter later on. For that reason, we have chosen common English words as examples in some of the following paragraphs and tables.

Dividing prefixes into functional categories, just as we did with suffixes, also makes them easier to learn. There are four logical divisions:

- Prefixes of time or speed
- Prefixes of direction
- Prefixes of position
- Prefixes of size or number

PREFIXES OF TIME OR SPEED

Prefixes denoting time or speed are used in everyday English language. **Pre**historic and **post**graduate are common words with a prefix relating to time. Table 2-5 lists examples of this category of prefix.

TABLE 2-5 Prefixes of Time or Speed

Prefix	Refers to	Examples
ante-, pre-	before	antepartum, premature
brady-	abnormally slow rate of speed	bradycardia
neo-	new	neoplasm
post-	after	postsynaptic
tachy-	rapid, abnormally high rate of speed	tachycardia

PREFIXES OF DIRECTION

The word **ab**normal is an example of a word containing a prefix that signifies direction. **Ab-** means "away from," so abnormal means "away from normal." We use prefixes in our everyday communications without bothering to analyze them. For example, we normally would not take the time to think about the prefix **contra-** (against) in the word contradiction, yet we understand the meaning of the term. Prefixes relating to direction are listed in Table 2-6.

TABLE 2-6 Prefixes of Direction

Prefix	Refers to	Examples
ab-	away from, outside of, beyond	abnormal
ad-	toward, near to	addiction
con-, sym-, syn-	with	congenital, sympathetic, synarthrosis
contra-	against	contraindicate
dia-	across, through	diarrhea

PREFIXES OF POSITION

Infrastructure (infra- means "inside" or "below"), **inter**state (inter- means "between"), and **para**legal (para- means "alongside") are all words we frequently use that have prefixes of position preceding their roots. Having these prefix meanings already in our vocabularies makes it easier to learn their medical uses. Prefixes of position are commonly used during diagnostic and treatment procedures. Table 2-7 lists the prefixes related to position.

TABLE 2-7   Prefixes of Position

Prefix	Refers to	Examples
ec-, ecto-, ex-, exo-	outside	ectopy
en-	inside	encephalopathy
endo-	within	endoscopy
epi-	upon, subsequent to	epigastric
extra-	beyond	extrasystole
hyper-	above, beyond normal	hypergastric
hypo-	below, below normal	hypogastric
infra-	inside or below	infrastructure
inter-	between	intercostal
intra-	inside, within	intracerebral
meso-	middle	mesothelium
meta-	beyond	metacarpal
pan-	all or everywhere	pancarditis
para-	alongside, like	paraplegia
retro-	backward, behind	retroperitoneal

PREFIXES OF SIZE AND NUMBER

A **semi**annual (semi- means "half"; annual means "yearly") sale is one that occurs every six months. The **uni**corn (uni- means "one") is a fictitious creature that has one horn. Prefixes of size and number are very common. Table 2-8 lists prefixes of size and number; many are easily recognizable.

TABLE 2-8   Prefixes of Size and Number

Prefix	Refers to	Examples
bi-	two	biannual
di-, dipl-	two, twice	diplopia
hemi-, semi-	half	hemiplegia
macro-	big	macrocyte
micro-	small	microscope
mono-	one	monocyte
olig-, oligo-	a few	oliguria
pan-	all or everywhere	pancarditis
poly-	many	polydactyly
quadri-	four	quadriplegia
semi-	half, partial	semiannual
tetra-	four	tetradactyl
tri-	three	triceps
uni-	one	unicellular

Suffixes and prefixes as presented in this chapter will become familiar as we progress through the chapters on body systems. Review the study tables and perform the exercises for self-testing.

Study Table • Common Suffixes

SUFFIX	MEANING	EXAMPLE
-ac, -al, -an, -aneous, -ar, -ary, -eal, -eous, -iac, -iatric, -ic, -ical, -oid, -otic, -ous, -tic, -ular	converts a root or a noun term to an adjective atrial, cardiac, ureteral	geriatric, orthopedic, ocular, dental, cutaneous, cyanotic,
-cele	protrusion, hernia	rectocele
-centesis	surgical puncture	thoracentesis
-cyte	cell	leukocyte
-desis	surgical binding	arthrodesis
-dynia, -algia	pain	arthrodynia
-ectasis, -ectasia	expansion or dilation	angiectasis
-ectomy	surgical removal	appendectomy
-edema	excessive fluid in intracellular tissues	angioedema
-emesis	vomiting	hematemesis
-emia	blood	uremia
-gen, -genic, -genesis	origin, producing	osteogenic
-gram	written or pictorial record	electrocardiogram
-graph	device for graphic or pictorial recording	electrocardiograph
-graphy	act of graphic or pictorial recording	electrocardiography
-ian, -iatrist, -ist, -logist, -logy, -ics, -iatry, -iatrics	specialty of, study of, practice of	geriatrist, pediatrician, gynecology
-iasis	a suffix used to convert a verb to a noun indicating a condition	cholelithiasis
-ism	a condition of; a process; or a state of	dwarfism, gigantism
-itis	inflammation	appendicitis
-lith	stone, calculus, calcification	pneumolith
-lysis	disintegration	hemolysis
-malacia	softening	osteomalacia
-megaly	enlargement	gastromegaly

(continued)

SUFFIX	MEANING	EXAMPLE
-meter	device for measuring	audiometer
-metry	act of measuring	audiometry
-oid	resembling or like	android
-oma	tumor	gastroma
-opsy	visual examination	biopsy
-osis	abnormal condition	osteoporosis, arthrosis
-pathy	disease	cardiopathy
-penia	reduction of size or quantity	leukopenia
-pexy	surgical fixation	hysteropexy
-phobia	fear, appears mainly as a suffix	claustrophobia
-plasia	abnormal formation	chondroplasia
-plasty	surgical repair	rhinoplasty
-plegia	paralysis	hemiplegia
-pnea	breath, respiration	tachypnea
-poiesis	producing	erythropoiesis
-porosis	porous condition	osteoporosis
-ptosis	downward displacement	nephroptosis
-rrhage	flowing forth	hemorrhage
-rrhaphy	suture	herniorrhaphy
-rrhea	discharge	diarrhea
-rrhexis	rupture	hysterorrhexis
-sclerosis	hardness	arteriosclerosis
-scope	device for viewing	arthroscope
-scopy	act of viewing	arthroscopy
-spasm	muscular contraction	arteriospasm
-stasis	level; unchanging	hemostasis
-stenosis	narrowed; blocked	arteriostenosis
-stomy	permanent opening	colostomy
-tome	instrument for cutting	osteotome
-tomy	incision	osteotomy
-tripsy	crushing	lithotripsy

Study Table • Common Prefixes

PREFIX	MEANING	EXAMPLE
ab-	away from, outside of, beyond	abnormal
ad-	toward, near to	addiction
ante-, pre-	before	antepartum, premature
anti-	against, opposed	antibiotic
bi-	two	biannual
brady-	abnormally slow rate of speed	bradycardia
con-, sym-, syn-	with	congenital, sympathetic, synarthrosis
contra-	against	contraindicate
dia-	across, through	diarrhea
dys-	painful, bad, difficult	dyspnea
ec-, ecto-	outside, away from	ectopy
en-, endo-	inside	endoscopy
epi-	upon, subsequent to	epigastric
ex-, exo-	outside	exoskeleton
extra-	beyond	extrasystole
hemi-, semi-	half	hemiplegia
hyper-	above, beyond normal	hypergastric
hypo-	below, below normal	hypogastric
infra-	inside or below	infrastructure
inter-	between	intercostal
intra-	inside	intracerebral
macro-	big	macrocyte
meso-	middle	mesothelium
meta-	beyond	metacarpal
micro-	small	microscope
mono-, uni-	one	monocyte
neo-	new	neoplasm
olig-, oligo-	a few	oliguria
pan-	everywhere	pancarditis

(continued)

PREFIX	MEANING	EXAMPLE
para-	alongside, like	paraplegia
post-	after	postsynaptic
quadri-	four	quadriceps
retro-	backward, behind	retroperitoneal
tachy-	abnormally high rate of speed	tachycardia
tri-	three	tricep

EXERCISES

EXERCISE 2-1   Combining Roots and Suffixes That Signify Medical Conditions

NOTE: Since the object of this chapter section is to introduce suffixes, not whole terms, these particular roots were selected for use only because they combine easily with more than one suffix. Additional roots will be introduced within the various anatomic system chapters.

Build terms by combining the correct form of each of the roots below with the suffixes appearing next to it. Suffixes and their definitions may be found in the Study Table on suffixes for this chapter. Write a definition for each term in the space to the right. Use a medical dictionary for definitions if needed.

ROOT	SUFFIX	WORD	MEANING
1. card/i/o	-cele	_____	_____
	-dynia	_____	_____
	-ectasia	_____	_____
	-itis	_____	_____
	-malacia	_____	_____
	-megaly	_____	_____
	-ptosis	_____	_____
	-plegia	_____	_____
	-rrhexis	_____	_____
	-spasm	_____	_____
2. dermat/o	-itis	_____	_____
	-oma	_____	_____
	-megaly	_____	_____
	-osis	_____	_____
3. hem/o, hemat/o	-lysis	_____	_____
	-genesis	_____	_____
	-oma	_____	_____
	-osis	_____	_____

4. neur/o   -algia   _____   _____

-ectasis   _____   _____

-itis   _____   _____

-oma   _____   _____

5. oste/o   -dynia   _____   _____

-oma   _____   _____

-malacia   _____   _____

-penia   _____   _____

-porosis   _____   _____

-itis   _____   _____

6. psych/o   -osis   _____   _____

EXERCISE 2-2   Combining Roots and Suffixes That Signify Diagnostic Terms, Test Information, or Surgical Procedures

Build terms by combining the correct form of each of the roots below with the suffixes appearing next to it. Suffixes and their definitions may be found in the Study Table on suffixes for this chapter. Write a definition for each term in the space to the right. Use a medical dictionary for definitions if needed.

ROOT	SUFFIX	WORD	MEANING
1. card/i/o	-genic	_____	_____
	-gram	_____	_____
	-graph	_____	_____
	-graphy	_____	_____
	-pathy	_____	_____
	-rrhaphy	_____	_____
2. dermat/o	-plasty	_____	_____
3. hemat/o	-genesis	_____	_____
	-metry	_____	_____

4. neur/o   -ectomy   _____   _____

           -genic   _____   _____

           -genesis   _____   _____

5. oste/o ·   -rrhaphy   _____   _____

           -plasty   _____   _____

           -genesis   _____   _____

           -ectomy   _____   _____

           -tomy   _____   _____

6. path/o   -gen   _____   _____

           -genic   _____   _____

           -genesis   _____   _____

7. psych/o   -genic   _____   _____

           -genesis   _____   _____

           -metry   _____   _____

           -path/o   _____   _____

EXERCISE 2-3   Combining Roots and Suffixes Associated with a Medical Specialist or Specialty

Build terms by combining the correct form of each of the roots below with the suffixes appearing next to it. Suffixes and their definitions may be found in the Study Table on suffixes for this chapter. Write a definition for each term in the space to the right. Use a medical dictionary for definitions if needed.

ROOT   **SUFFIX**   **WORD**   **MEANING**

1. card/i/o   -logy   _____   _____

               -logist   _____   _____

2. derm/o, dermat/o   -logy   _____   _____

               -logist   _____   _____

3. ger/o/nt/o   -iatrics   _____   _____

                     -logy   _____   _____

                     -logist   _____   _____

4. hem/o, hemat/o   -logy   _____   _____

                     -logist   _____   _____

5. neur/o   -logy   _____   _____

                     -logist   _____   _____

6. oste/o   -logy   _____   _____

                     -logist   _____   _____

7. path/o   -logy   _____   _____

                     -logist   _____   _____

8. ped/o, pedi/o   -atrics   _____   _____

   pedia/o, pediatr/o -ician   _____   _____

9. psych/o   -logy   _____   _____

                     -iatry   _____   _____

                     -iatrist   _____   _____

EXERCISE 2-4   Combining Roots and Suffixes That Denote Adjectives

Build terms by combining the correct form of each of the roots below with the suffixes appearing next to it. Suffixes and their definitions may be found in the Study Table on suffixes for this chapter. Write a definition for each term in the space to the right. Use a medical dictionary for definitions if needed.

ROOT	SUFFIX	WORD	MEANING
1. card/i/o	-ac	_____	_____
2. hem/o, hemat/o	-ic	_____	_____

3. derm/o, dermat/o   -al   _____   _____

                           -ic   _____   _____

4. ger/o/, geront/o   -iatric   _____   _____

                           -al   _____   _____

5. neur/o   -al   _____   _____

                           -ic   _____   _____

6. spin/o   -al   _____   _____

                           -ous   _____   _____

7. oste/o   -al   _____   _____

                           -oid   _____   _____

EXERCISE 2-5   Matching Suffixes with Meanings

Choose the letter next to the Column 2 definition corresponding to each suffix in Column 1 and write it in the space provided. Suffixes and their definitions may be found in the Study Table on suffixes for this chapter.

COLUMN 1   COLUMN 2

1. _____ -cyte   A. a morbid impulse toward a specific object or thought

2. _____ -edema   B. vomiting

3. _____ -emesis   C. a stone, calculus, calcification

4. _____ -sclerosis   D. a condition, a process or state of

5. _____ -tome   E. disease

6. _____ -ism   F. visual examination

7. _____ -lith   G. cell

8. _____ -lysis   H. disintegration

9. _____ -opsy   I. excessive fluid in intracellular tissues

10. _____ -pathy   J. instrument for cutting

11. _____ -phobia   K. level; unchanging

12. _____ -poiesis   L. narrowed; blocked

13. _____ -stomy   M. hardness

14. _____ -stasis   N. permanent opening

15. _____ -stenosis   O. producing

 EXERCISE 2-6   Adding Prefixes of Time or Speed

Add each prefix in the list below to the word or word part appearing next to it and write the definition of the word thus formed in the space to the right. Refer to a standard English dictionary as needed.

PREFIX	WORD	WORD FORMED	MEANING
1. ante-	room	_____	_____
2. neo-	classic	_____	_____
3. post-	glacial	_____	_____
4. pre-	dominant	_____	_____
5. tachy-	meter	_____	_____

 EXERCISE 2-7   Adding Prefixes of Direction

Add each prefix in the list below to the word or word part appearing next to it and write the definition of the word thus formed in the space to the right. Refer to a standard English dictionary as needed.

PREFIX	WORD	WORD FORMED	MEANING
1. ab-	normal	_____	_____
2. ad-	joining	_____	_____
3. con-	centric	_____	_____
4. contra-	lateral	_____	_____
5. dia-	gram	_____	_____
6. sym-	pathetic	_____	_____
7. syn-	thesis	_____	_____

EXERCISE 2-8   Adding Prefixes of Position

Add each prefix in the list below to the word or word part appearing next to it and write the definition of the word thus formed in the space to the right. Refer to a standard English dictionary as needed.

PREFIX	WORD	WORD FORMED	MEANING
1. ec-	centric	_____	_____
2. ecto-	morph	_____	_____
3. en-	slave	_____	_____
4. endo-	cardial	_____	_____
5. epi-	demic	_____	_____
6. ex-	change	_____	_____
7. exo-	sphere	_____	_____
8. extra-	terrestrial	_____	_____
9. hyper-	sensitive	_____	_____
10. hypo-	thesis	_____	_____
11. infra-	structure	_____	_____
12. inter-	collegiate	_____	_____
13. intra-	mural	_____	_____
14. meso-	sphere	_____	_____
15. meta-	physics	_____	_____
16. pan-	orama	_____	_____
17. para-	legal	_____	_____
18. retro-	rocket	_____	_____

EXERCISE 2-9 Adding Prefixes of Size or Number

Add each prefix in the list below to the word or word part appearing next to it and write the definition of the word thus formed in the space to the right. Refer to a standard English dictionary as needed. The prefixes may all be found in the Study Table on prefixes or in the text.

PREFIX	WORD	WORD FORMED	MEANING
1. bi-	annual	_____	_____
2. hemi-	sphere	_____	_____
3. macro-	cosm	_____	_____
4. micro-	scope	_____	_____
5. mono-	rail	_____	_____
6. olig-	archy	_____	_____
7. quadri-	lateral	_____	_____
8. semi-	annual	_____	_____
9. tri-	angle	_____	_____
10. uni-	cycle	_____	_____

EXERCISE 2-10 Crossword Puzzle: Suffixes and Prefixes

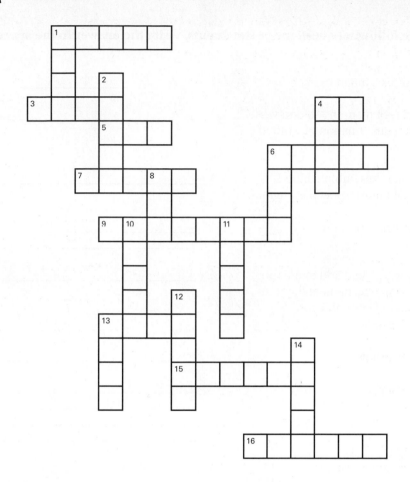

ACROSS
1. prefix, big
3. suffix, study of
4. prefix, away from
5. prefix, total or everywhere
6. prefix, between or across
7. suffix, pictorial recording device
9. suffix, narrowing
13. suffix, cell
15. suffix, removal of
16. prefix, four

DOWN
1. prefix, one
2. prefix, above or beyond normal
4. prefix, against
6. suffix, inflammation
8. prefix, before
10. prefix, abnormally fast
11. suffix, act of viewing
12. suffix, device for measuring
13. suffix, protrusion
14. suffix, pain

CHAPTER 2 QUIZ

Suffixes

For each of the following questions or statements, write the answer in the space to the right.

1. What two suffixes mean "pain"?

    1. _dynia, algia_

2. *Ang/i/o* is a root meaning "blood vessel." What term means "dilation of a blood vessel"?

    2. _angiectasis_

3. Angioid means "resembling blood vessels." What part of speech is angioid?

    3. _adjective_

4. Define *angiorrhaphy*.

    4. _structure of a blood vessel_

5. What suffix would you add to the root *ang/i/o* to form a term meaning "the act of making a pictorial record of blood vessels"?

    5. _-graphy_

6. What is an angioma?

    6. _tumor of blood vessel_

7. What does *-plasty* mean?

    7. _surgical repair_

8. What term denotes a skin specialist?

    8. _dermatologist_

9. A gerontologist treats what age of patients, young or old?

    9. _old_

10. What is the difference in meaning between *gerontology* and *geriatrics*?

    10. _ology - noun_
        atrics - adjective

Prefixes

For each of the following questions or statements, write the answer in the space to the right.

1. The prefixes *ab-* and *ad-* are opposites; which one means "toward"?

   1. _____ad_____

2. The prefix *pre-* means "before"; what other prefix means the same thing?

   2. _____ante_____

3. Write a brief definition of bradycardia.

   3. _abnormally slow_ _heartbeat_

4. What does the prefix *extra-* mean in the word extrasensory?

   4. _____beyond_____

5. What prefix would you use in a term that means "high blood pressure"?

   5. _____hyper_____

6. Given the meaning of *anti-*, what would be the purpose of an anticollision radar?

   6. _radar used to prevent_ _collision_

7. Given the meaning of the prefix *tri-*, how many engines does a trijet have?

   7. _____3_____

8. Does the prefix *micro-* refer to the physical size of a microscope? If not, what does its presence in the word tell us?

   8. _no - instrument makes_ _visible objects too_ _small to see_

9. Write a medical term by combining the prefix *endo-* with the root *card/i/o*, meaning "heart," and the suffix that means "inflammation." Using only your knowledge of these three word elements, write the best definition you can for the term.

   9. _endocarditis - inflammation_ _of the inside of_ _the heart_

10. The suffix *-pnea*, meaning "breathing" or "respiration," can follow both *tachy-* and *dys-*. Define the terms *tachypnea* and *dyspnea*.

    10. _tachy - rapid_ _dys - difficulty or_ _painful breathing_

PART TWO

BODY SYSTEMS

3 **The Body's Organization**

4 **The Integumentary System**

5 **The Skeletal System**

6 **The Muscular System**

7 **The Nervous System**

8 **The Endocrine System**

9 **The Cardiovascular System**

10 **The Lymphatic System and Immunity**

11 **The Respiratory System**

12 **The Digestive System**

13 **The Urinary System**

14 **The Reproductive System**

15 **The Special Senses of Sight and Hearing**

CHAPTER 3

The Body's Organization

LEARNING OBJECTIVES

Upon completion of this chapter, you should be able to:

- Discuss the levels of body organization.
- Name the body systems.
- Define anatomical position and the directional terms used in relation to the body.
- Describe what is meant by thc planes of the body.
- Identify the body cavities.
- Name the divisions of the abdomen and back.
- Analyze, define, and pronounce the new terms introduced in this chapter.

Introduction

To begin building medical terms, we must first come to understand how the human body is constructed and how it works. The first distinction to be made is between the terms anatomy and physiology. Briefly, anatomy (Greek word *anatome* means "dissection"; ana- means "apart" and -tome means "to cut") is the study of body structure, and physiology (physio means "physical" and -logy means "the study of") is the study of the body's functions.

The human body has a chemical basis, and the chemicals act together to form cells. The cells, which power the biologic "machinery" contained within them, process the food we eat and the air we breathe. The human body also removes unwanted substances and enables cells to reproduce themselves, each cell according to the DNA code it contains.

Word Elements • *Body Organization*

ROOT	MEANING
anter/o	front, anterior
cerv/o	neck
chondr/o	cartilage
cyt/o, -cyte	cell
dors/o	back
inguin/o	groin
my/o	muscle
myel/o	spinal cord
neur/o	nerve, neuron
poster/o	posterior, back
proxim/o	near
super/o	superior
trans/o	across

Levels of Organization

The body consists of four structural levels of organization: cellular, tissue, organ, and system, which are discussed in the following sections. The levels act together to form the human organism. Although the body begins at the chemical level, we will start by discussing the cellular level (Fig. 3-1).

CELLULAR LEVEL

The body consists of millions of cells that work individually and together to maintain life. Each cell, the basic unit of all living organisms, has an individual structure and shape, which enables it to perform specific functions (Fig. 3-2). Although cells consist of different components, they have common elements:

- Cell membrane: Surrounds the cell and allows certain substances to come in and out of the cell.

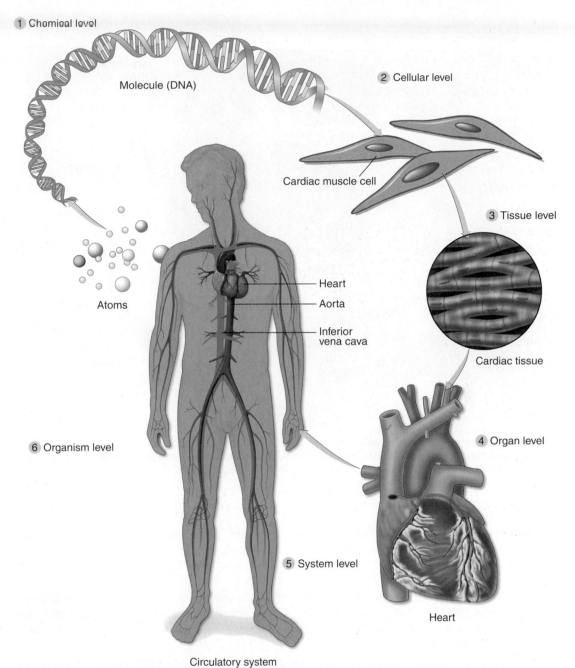

FIGURE 3-1 Body organization. The six levels of the body's organization can be seen here: 1. chemical level, 2. cellular level, 3. tissue level, 4. organ level, 5. system level, and finally 6. organism level, the human body. From Premkumar K. The Massage Connection Anatomy and Physiology. Baltimore: Lippincott Williams & Wilkins, 2004.

- Nucleus: Powerhouse of the cell; directs activities within the cell. The nucleus also contains the chromosomes that house the genetic code of the body. Note: Mature red blood cells are the only cells in the human body that do not have a nucleus.
- Cytoplasm: A watery fluid that fills the cell from the nuclear membrane to the cell membrane. It provides the work area in which cell activities occur.

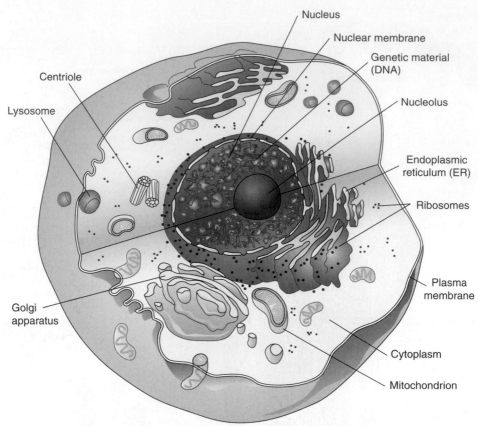

Nucleus
Nuclear membrane
Genetic material (DNA)
Nucleolus
Centriole
Lysosome
Endoplasmic reticulum (ER)
Ribosomes
Plasma membrane
Golgi apparatus
Cytoplasm
Mitochondrion

FIGURE 3-2 Basic structure of a cell. The basic structure of a cell includes the cell membrane, the nucleus, and the cytoplasm. Modified from Cohen BJ, Wood DL. Memmler's The Human Body in Health and Disease, 9th Ed. Philadelphia: Lippincott Williams & Wilkins, 2000.

TISSUE LEVEL

The next level of organization in the body is the tissue level. Tissues are composed of similar cells that work together to perform common tasks. For example, muscle cells group together to form muscles, which contract to produce movement. The four types of body tissues are muscle, connective, nervous, and epithelial.

- Muscle tissue: There are both voluntary and involuntary muscles. Voluntary muscle tissue is found in areas of your body that you have control over, such as your arms and legs. Involuntary muscle tissue is found in those parts over which you lack direct control, such as your intestines.
- Connective tissue: This type of tissue supports the internal structures of the body. An example is cartilage, which is found primarily in the joints.
- Nervous tissue: This type of tissue is made up of nerve cells or neurons. Neurons transmit electrical impulses that control body activity.
- Epithelial tissue: This type of tissue covers the body outside and also lines the cavities on the inside of the body. It helps to support and protect the body while allowing for excretion of fluids.

ORGAN LEVEL

Tissues with common functions come together to form the organs in the body. Organs are structures that perform specialized functions. Examples are the brain, stomach, and heart.

SYSTEM LEVEL

A group of organs forms a system in the body. Each system has a common purpose to perform specialized functions. The body systems and a brief description of the function of each are listed below:

- Integumentary system: Protects the body against invasion by bacteria; regulates body temperature and water content.
- Skeletal system: Provides support and gives shape to the body; stores minerals; manufactures some blood cells.
- Muscular system: Enables movement of the body; holds the body erect.
- Nervous system: Transmits messages throughout the body; coordinates the reception of stimuli.
- Endocrine system: Integrates all body functions; produces hormones.
- Circulatory system: Pumps nutrients and oxygen in the blood to all parts of the body; carries waste products to the kidneys and lungs.
- Immune system: Protects the body from harmful substances; returns excess fluids and cellular waste to the circulatory system.
- Respiratory system: Brings oxygen into the body for transportation to the cells; removes carbon dioxide.
- Digestive system: Breaks down ingested food so that it can be absorbed into the bloodstream; eliminates solid wastes.
- Urinary system: Maintains fluid and electrolyte balance in the body; filters blood to remove wastes and excretes liquid waste.
- Reproductive system: Permits the creation of new life.

Navigating the Body

Health care professionals need to be familiar with directional and positioning terms, which are frequently used during examinations, diagnostic procedures, and treatments of patients.

ANATOMICAL POSITION AND DIRECTIONAL AND POSITIONAL TERMS

Directional terms are always relative to the **anatomical position**. In the anatomical position, the body is erect and facing forward, and the arms are at the sides with the palms of the hands facing forward (Fig. 3-3). Left and right are from the subject's perspective, not the observer's. The directional terms help to describe a complaint, symptom, body part, or process as it relates to another. **Superior** refers to above or nearer to the head. You might use this term when describing an observation such as, "The bruise is superior to the eyebrow" (above the eyebrow). **Inferior** refers to below or toward the feet. **Anterior** and **ventral** are directional terms that relate to the front of the body. An example of anterior would be, "The rash covered the entire anterior portion of the thigh" (front of the thigh). **Posterior** and **dorsal** are terms that relate to the back side of the body or toward the back. **Medial** means toward the midline of the body, and **lateral** refers to away from the midline or toward the side. You may see the directional term lateral used for descriptive purposes as in, "The tumor is located on the lateral wall of the left lung." The last two directional terms are **proximal** and **distal**. Proximal refers to something nearer to the point of attachment or origin. An example of this would be, "The shoulder is proximal to the elbow." Distal, on the other hand, means further from the origin or point of attachment. See Figure 3-4 for an illustration of the directional terms.

Two terms used for positioning patients are supine and prone. **Supine** refers to a position in which the patient is horizontal and lying face up. Noticing that the word "up" is included in the

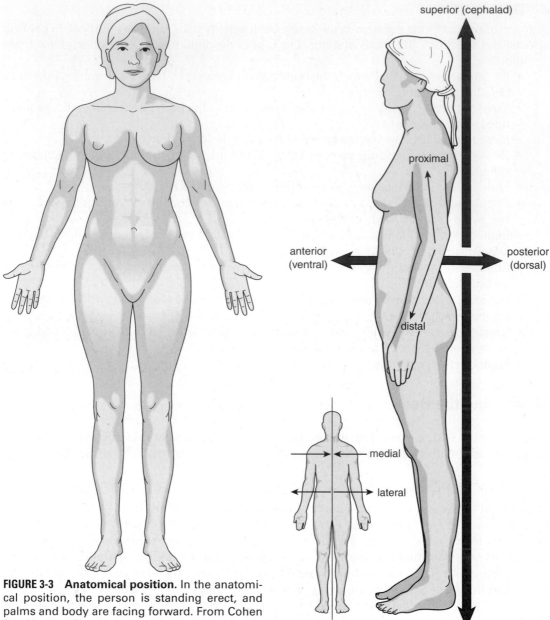

FIGURE 3-3 Anatomical position. In the anatomical position, the person is standing erect, and palms and body are facing forward. From Cohen BJ. Medical Terminology, 4th Ed. Philadelphia: Lippincott Williams & Wilkins, 2003.

FIGURE 3-4 Directional terms. Directional terms are frequently used to describe a symptom, a body part, or how one part is related to another. For example, the shoulder is proximal to the elbow. Modified from Cohen BJ, Wood DL. Memmler's The Human Body in Health and Disease, 9th Ed. Philadelphia: Lippincott Williams & Wilkins, 2000.

first syllable of the word "supine" will help you remember its meaning. **Prone** is the opposite of supine, with the patient lying face down. These two terms are frequently used in operating room and X-ray reports. For example, "The patient was placed in the supine position and the abdomen was prepped." This means that the patient was placed on the operating table on his or her back, lying face up. See Figure 3-4 and Table 3-1 for a listing of directional terms and additional examples of the terms.

Table 3 1   Body Position and Directional Terms

Term	Direction	Example
anterior or ventral	toward the front; away from the back of the body	The nose is on the anterior side of the face; the toes are anterior to the ankle.
posterior or dorsal	near the back; toward the back of the body	The spine is on the posterior side of the body.
superior or cephalad	above; toward the head	The neck is superior to the chest.
inferior or caudal	below; toward the soles of the feet	The knee is inferior to the hip; the stomach is inferior to the chest.
proximal	near the point of attachment to the trunk	The elbow is proximal to the wrist.
distal	farther from the point of attachment to the trunk	The fingers are distal to the wrist.
lateral	pertaining to the side; away from the middle	The eyes are lateral to the nose.
medial	toward the middle of the body	The nose is medial to the eyes.
prone	lying horizontal and face up	
supine	lying horizontal and face down	

BODY PLANES

Body planes are imaginary, flat surface areas of the body (Fig. 3-5). Always remember that the anatomical position of the body is the reference point. Three planes are frequently used to locate structural arrangements:

- Frontal: This plane separates the body into front and back portions, also called anterior and posterior portions.

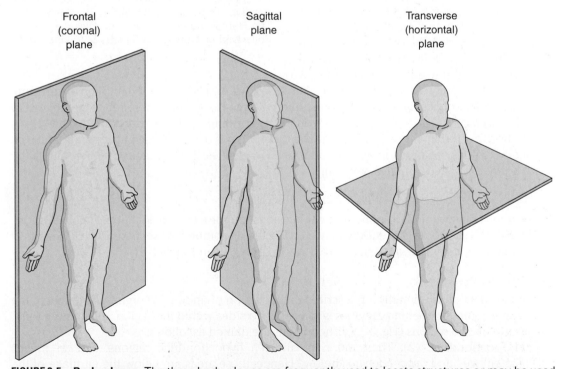

Frontal (coronal) plane   Sagittal plane   Transverse (horizontal) plane

FIGURE 3-5   Body planes. The three body planes are frequently used to locate structures or may be used for diagnostic testing. For example, planes are used to describe positioning or views in X-rays and other special radiographic tests. From Cohen BJ, Wood DL. Memmler's The Human Body in Health and Disease, 9th Ed. Philadelphia: Lippincott Williams & Wilkins, 2000.

- Sagittal: This vertical plane divides the body or organ into unequal left and right sides. The midsagittal plane divides the body or organ into equal left and right sides.
- Transverse or horizontal: This plane separates the body into upper and lower portions, also called superior and inferior portions. Think of the root *trans*, which means "across," as in transcontinental. This plane cuts "across" the body.

In a clinical setting, X-rays or radiographic studies use body planes to describe the images taken. Imaging tests can be taken along the vertical plane or along the transverse plane by a computed tomography (CT) scan.

The Body Cavities and Divisions

A body cavity is defined as a hollow space that contains body organs. The body has two major cavities, one in the front of the body and one in the back. The front body cavity is called the ventral cavity. The adjective ventral comes from the Latin word *venter*, meaning "belly." The cavity in the back of the body is called the dorsal cavity, from the Latin word *dorsum*, which means "back." The dorsal cavity is subdivided into the cranial and spinal cavities, which house the brain and spinal cord (Fig. 3-6).

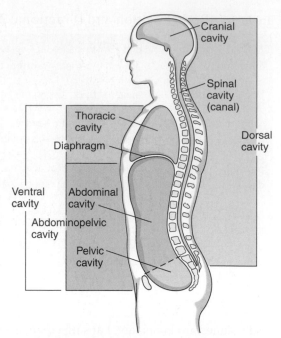

FIGURE 3-6 Body cavities. The body is divided into two major cavities—ventral and dorsal—five cavities within the ventral and dorsal cavities: The ventral cavity includes the thoracic, abdominal, and pelvic cavities, and the dorsal cavity includes the cranial and spinal cavities. *Reprinted with permission from:* Cohen BJ, Wood DL. Memmler's The Human Body in Health and Disease, 9th Ed. Philadelphia: Lippincott Williams & Wilkins, 2000.

The ventral cavity extends from the neck to the pelvis and is subdivided into the **abdominopelvic** and **thoracic** cavities. It contains the internal organs sometimes referred to as the *viscera* (singular *viscus*), both of which are Latin words. The abdominopelvic cavity contains the organs of digestion, excretion, and reproduction. The diaphragm is a muscle used in respiration; it also physically divides the thoracic and abdominopelvic cavities. The thoracic cavity contains the heart, aorta, esophagus, trachea, and lungs.

DIVISIONS OF THE ABDOMINOPELVIC CAVITY

An examiner may want to describe surgical incisions and procedures, location of pain, tumors, or organs. In order to do this effectively, we divide the abdomen into sections, which consist of either nine regions or four quadrants (Fig. 3-7A, B; Table 3-2; and Table 3-3).

Nine Regions

Region designation is primarily for describing the location of underlying organs. Note that in the following list, the number in parentheses refers to two sides within the region, a left and a right, and counts as two regions (Fig. 3-7A). The regions are named as follows:

- Hypochondriac (2): There are right and left hypochondriac regions. *Chondr-* means "cartilage," and *hypo-* refers to "below." Hence, these areas are below the cartilage of the ribs on the left and right sides.
- Epigastric: This area is just above the stomach. *Epi-* is a prefix that means "above." This area is above the stomach and is situated between the left and right hypochondriac regions.

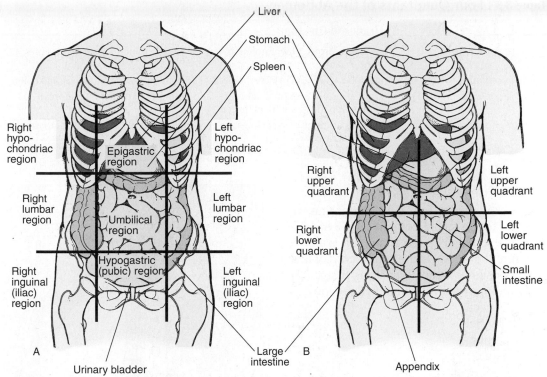

FIGURE 3-7   Abdominopelvic cavity. A. The nine regions of the abdomen. **B.** The four quadrants of the abdomen. From Stedman's Medical Dictionary, 27th Ed. Baltimore: Lippincott Williams & Wilkins, 2000.

- Lumbar (2): There are right and left lumbar regions. They are located at waist level on either side of the navel.
- Umbilical: If you look at the nine regions as a tic-tac-toe board, the umbilical region is the middle section. It contains the belly button or umbilicus.
- Hypogastric: This is the middle section right below the umbilical section.
- Inguinal (2): There are right and left inguinal sections. They lie on either side of the hypogastric section. Inguinal also refers to the "groin" area (Fig. 3-7A, Table 3-2).

Four Quadrants

Four quadrants identify the abdomen (Fig. 3-7B, Table 3-3). The center point is the navel, also known as the umbilicus or belly button. The quadrants are named as follows: right upper quadrant (RUQ), left upper quadrant (LUQ), right lower quadrant (RLQ), and left lower quadrant (LLQ).

Table 3-2   Nine Regions of the Abdomen

left hypochondriac region	left lateral region just below the ribs
left lumbar region	left lateral region in the middle row
left inguinal region	left lower region of the lower row by the groin
epigastric region	middle region in the upper row
umbilicus	middle region in the middle row
hypogastric region	middle section in the lower row
right hypochondriac region	right lateral region just below the ribs
right lumbar region	right lateral region in the middle row
right inguinal region	right lower region of the lower row by the groin

Table 3-3 Four Quadrants of the Abdomen

Term	Organs in Quadrant
left upper quadrant (LUQ)	left lobe of liver, spleen, stomach, portions of the pancreas, small intestines, and colon
right upper quadrant (RUQ)	right lobe of liver, gallbladder, portions of the pancreas, small intestines, and colon
right lower quadrant (RLQ)	contains portions of small intestines and colon, right ovary and fallopian tube, appendix, and right ureter
left lower quadrant (LLQ)	contains portions of small intestines and colon, left ovary and fallopian tube, and left ureter

DIVISIONS OF THE BACK

The back is divided into five sections that correspond to the spinal column (Fig. 3-8, Table 3-4). The spinal or vertebral column is a bony structure that protects the spinal cord, which is composed of delicate nervous tissue. The spinal column is divided into five sections:

1. Cervical
2. Thoracic
3. Lumbar
4. Sacral
5. Coccygeal

The spine is made up of 7 cervical, 12 thoracic, 5 lumbar, and 5 sacral vertebrae. There are also approximately 4 coccygeal vertebrae fused into 1 coccyx. Abbreviations are frequently used to denote the vertebrae:

- 7 **cervical** in the neck region: C1 to C7.
- 12 **thoracic** in the chest region: T1 to T12.
- 5 **lumbar** in the lower back region: L1 to L5.
- 5 **sacral** in just above the tail region: S1 to S5 (5 fused pieces).
- 1 **coccyx** in the tail region (3-4 fused pieces).

The human body has a unique design all of its own. It is composed of differing cells, tissues, and organs that all go together to make up the different body systems that work synergistically to sustain life. It is important for the student to learn the terms associated with the body components as well as the descriptive anatomical and position terminology. Some of these terms get to be quite lengthy; thus, health care professionals frequently use abbreviations. Abbreviations are used in all disciplines of medicine. It is important to note that some abbreviations have more than one meaning. For example, CRF may mean chronic renal failure or case report form. Abbreviations respective to the chapter topic will be presented in each subsequent chapter.

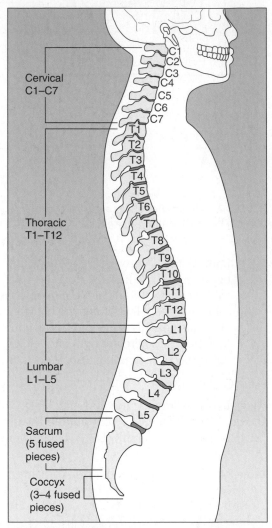

FIGURE 3-8 **Divisions of the back.** The five main divisions of the back include the cervical vertebra, the thoracic vertebra, the lumbar vertebra, the sacrum, and the coccyx. The sections are frequently named by the capital letter of the section (e.g., the second cervical vertebra is C2). From Willis MC, CMA-AC. Medical Terminology: A Programmed Learning Approach to the Language of Health Care. Baltimore: Lippincott Williams & Wilkins, 2002.

Table 3-4 Divisions of the Back

Term	Area of the Back	Number of Bones	Abbreviation
cervical	neck	7	C1-C7
thoracic	chest	12	T1-T12
lumbar	lower back below waist	5	L1-L5
sacral	lower back	5 fused bones	S1-S5
coccyx	tailbone	3-4 fused bones	—

Abbreviation Table • Body Organization

ABBREVIATION	MEANING
LUQ	left upper quadrant
RUQ	right upper quadrant
LLQ	left lower quadrant
RLQ	right lower quadrant

Study Table • Body Organization

TERM	PRONUNCIATION	MEANING
abdominopelvic	ab-DOM-ih-no-PELV-ihk	adjective meaning abdomen and pelvis; used to describe one of the body subcavities contained in the ventral cavity
anatomical position	an-ah-TOM-ih-kal	standing erect with palms facing forward
anterior	an-TEER-ee-uhr	toward the front of the body; can be a noun or an adjective
cervical	SUR-vih-kuhl	pertaining to the neck
chromosome	KROH-muh-sohm	component of the cell nucleus that contains the genes
coccyx	KOK-six	tailbone
diaphragm	DY-ah-fram	muscle that separates the thoracic and abdominopelvic cavities
distal	DISS-tahl	away from the attachment point to the body; can be a noun or an adjective
dorsal	DOR-sahl	adjective meaning the back
epigastric	epp-ih-GAS-trik	above the stomach

TERM	PRONUNCIATION	MEANING
hypochondriac	hy-poh-KON-dree-ak	below the ribs; also used as a noun to refer to a person who has imaginary illnesses
hypogastric	hy-poh-GAS-tric	below the stomach
inferior	ihn-FEER-ee-ohr	below or in the direction away from the cranium; can be a noun or an adjective
inguinal	IN-gwin-uhl	groin
lateral	LAT-eh-rahl	adjective meaning away from the middle of and toward the side of the body
medial	MEE-dee-ahl	toward the midline of the body
myalgia	my-AL-jee-ah	muscle pain
posterior	poss-TEE-ree-ohr	toward the back of the body
proximal	PROX-ih-mahl	toward the point of fixation to the body
sacrum	SAY-krum	5 fused bones of the lower back
superior	soo-PEER-ee-ohr	above; toward the cranium
thoracic	tho-RASS-ik	adjective for chest area
thorax	THOR-ax	chest
umbilicus	um-BILL-ih-kuhs	navel, belly button
ventral	VEHN-trahl	adjective meaning toward the front of the body and away from the back of the body
viscera	vih-SER-ah	internal organs

EXERCISES

 EXERCISE 3-1   Matching

Insert the letter from the right-hand column that matches each numbered item in the left-hand column.

A. PLANES OF THE BODY

1. _____ frontal plane

2. _____ sagittal plane

3. _____ transverse plane

A. divides the body into upper and lower

B. divides the body into left and right

C. divides the body into anterior and posterior

B. DIRECTIONAL TERMS

1. _____ superior

2. _____ lateral

3. _____ posterior

4. _____ medial

5. _____ distal

6. _____ prone

7. _____ supine

8. _____ inferior

9. _____ anterior

10. _____ proximal

A. lying horizontal and face up

B. near the point of attachment to the trunk

C. toward the front; away from the back of the body

D. below; toward the soles of the feet

E. lying horizontal and face down

F. above; toward the head

G. pertaining to the side; away from the middle

H. near the back; toward the back of the body

I. farther from the point of attachment to the trunk

J. toward the middle of the body

EXERCISE 3-2   Fill in the Blank

Select the correct word from the following list and complete the sentence.

anterior	dorsal	lateral	posterior	superior
distal	inferior	medial	proximal	ventral

1. The wrist is _____ to the elbow.

2. The _____ end of the lower leg communicates with the ankle.

3. The sternum is _____ to the spinal cord.

4. The knee cap is on the _____ side of the body.

5. The head is _____ to the neck.

6. The ears are located on the _____ of the head.

7. The shoulder blades are on the _____ side of the body.

8. The chin is _____ to the forehead.

EXERCISE 3-3   Word Building

Add the correct prefix or suffix to the word root to make a new term. Select from the following word elements: *-itis, -ic, -al, hypo-, hyper-, epi-, and trans-*. The first exercise is an example.

WORD ROOT OR COMBINING FORM	ADD PREFIX OR SUFFIX	MEANING	TERM
1. gastr/o	*hypo-* *-ic*	below the stomach	*hypogastric*
2. dors/o	_____	pertaining to the back	_____
3. chondr/o	_____	inflammation of the cartilage	_____
4. thorac/o	_____	across the chest or thorax	_____
5. neur/o	_____	inflammation of a nerve	_____
6. cardi/o	_____	pertaining to the region above or upon the heart	_____

EXERCISE 3-4   Body Organization

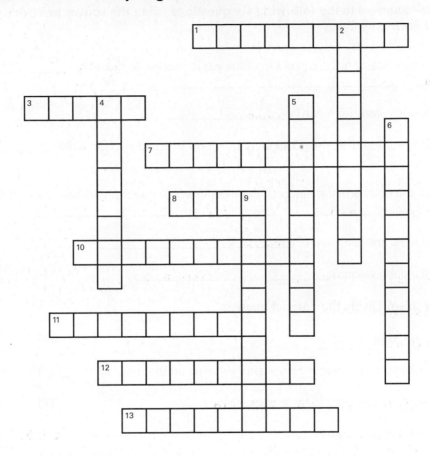

ACROSS
1. Belly button
3. Groups of these make a body system
7. Lungs are part of this system
8. Number of body cavities
10. Type of supportive tissue
11. Stomach is in this system
12. Towards the back
13. Watery fluid in the cells

DOWN
2. Contains the genetic code
4. Towards the front
5. Separates the body into upper and lower parts
6. Region below the umbilicus
9. Type of tissue that lines the body cavities

CHAPTER 3 QUIZ

Write the answers to the following six questions using the spaces provided to the right of each question.

1. What word describes the position of the ear in relation to the nose? _____
   lateral

2. What does posterior mean? _towards the back_

3. What word describes the position of the elbow in relation to the wrist? _____
   proximal

4. When the body is in the anatomical position, which direction are the palms of the hands facing? _anterior / forward_

5. What does myalgia refer to? _muscle pain_

6. What are the viscera? _guts, internal organs_

True or false? Circle the correct answer.

7. Prone is lying face up.	TRUE	~~FALSE~~
8. The left hypochondriac region is above the left lumbar region.	TRUE	FALSE
9. The little toe is medial to the big toe. (lateral)	TRUE	~~FALSE~~
10. The diaphragm is a muscle.	~~TRUE~~	FALSE
11. There are five divisions to the back.	~~TRUE~~	FALSE
12. The sacrum is also called the tailbone. (coccyx)	TRUE	~~FALSE~~
13. The sagittal plane divides the body into right and left portions.	~~TRUE~~	FALSE

CHAPTER 4

The Integumentary System

LEARNING OBJECTIVES

Upon completion of this chapter, you should be able to:

- Name the two layers of the skin.
- Name the accessory structures of the integumentary system.
- Build and pronounce medical terms of the integumentary system.
- Name the disorders and treatments relating to the integumentary system.
- Name the major classifications of pharmacologic agents used to treat skin disorders.
- Analyze and define the new terms introduced in this chapter.
- Interpret abbreviations associated with the integumentary system.

Introduction

The largest organ of the body is the skin. The skin covers the entire body—more than 20 square feet on average—and weighs about 24 pounds. It is part of the integumentary system, which also includes the accessory structures: hair, nails, and **sebaceous** (oil) and **sudoriferous** (sweat) glands. *Integumentum* is Latin for "covering" or "shelter." The physician who specializes in the diagnosis and treatment of skin disorders is called a **dermatologist** (dermat/o being one of the combining forms for skin). Coupling the root dermat/o with the previously learned suffix -logy gives us the term **dermatology**, which is the term for the specialty practice that deals with the skin.

Word Elements

The major word elements that relate to the integumentary system consist of various anatomical components, accessory structures, colors of the skin, and abnormal conditions. The Word Elements table lists many of the roots, their meanings, and examples associated with the integumentary system.

Word Elements • *Integumentary System*

WORD ELEMENT	MEANING	EXAMPLE
albin/o	white	albinism
cirrh/o, jaund/o, xanth/o	yellow	cirrhosis, jaundice, xanthoderma
cutane/o	skin	cutaneous
cyan/o	blue	cyanosis
-cyte, cyt/o	cell	melanocyte
derm/o, dermat/o	skin	dermatitis
epi-	upon	epidermal
erythr/o	red	erythema
ichthy/o	dry, scaly (fish-like)	ichthyosis
kerat/o	horn-like	keratosis
leuk/o	white	leukoderma
melan/o	black	melanoma
myc/o	fungus	dermatomycosis
onych/o	nail	onychophagia
pil/o	hair	pilonidal
scler/o	hardening	scleroderma
seb/o	sebum	seborrhea
sub-	below	subcutaneous
sudor/i	sweat	sudoriferous
xer/o	dry	xeroderma

Structure and Function

The skin consists of two layers, the **epidermis** (epi- is a prefix meaning "on" or "over") and **dermis**. Beneath the skin (epidermis and dermis) is a layer of connective tissue called the **subcutaneous** layer. (Sub- is a prefix meaning "beneath" or "under"; cutane/o is another root for skin; and -ous is an adjective suffix meaning "pertaining to.") This layer is composed of **adipose** or fatty tissue. The subcutaneous layer is important because it connects the dermis to the muscles and organs beneath it (Fig. 4-1).

The epidermis is composed of several thin sublayers of **epithelial** (adjective form of **epithelium**) tissues. There are no blood vessels or nerves in epithelial tissues. The epidermis provides a protective covering for the entire body. The deepest layer of the epidermis contains special cells called **melanocytes** (melan/o is a root word meaning "pigment," and -cyte is a suffix meaning "cell"). These cells produce a pigment called **melanin**, which gives the skin its color and also protects against sunlight.

The dermis or **corium** (another term for dermis) is the thick layer of tissue just below the epidermis. It contains blood vessels, nerves, and a few of the accessory structures: hair follicles and sebaceous and sudoriferous glands. The blood vessels in the dermis provide nourishment to the skin and help maintain temperature control. The nerves in this layer receive sensory impulses that enable the body to recognize pain, touch, heat, cold, and pressure.

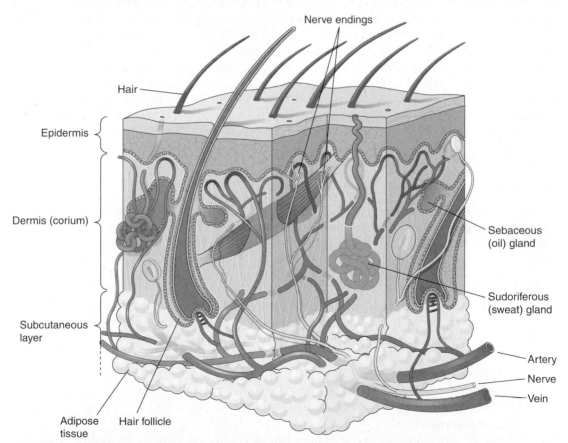

FIGURE 4-1   Cross-section of the skin. The three layers of the skin: epidermis (epi- is a prefix meaning "upon" or "on top"; dermis is a root for skin), dermis or corium, and the subcutaneous layer (sub- is a prefix meaning "under"; cutane is a root meaning "skin"). Modified from Cohen BJ, Taylor J. Memmler's Structure and Function of the Human Body, 8th Ed. Baltimore: Lippincott Williams & Wilkins, 2005.

The hair follicles produce hair that is distributed over much of the body. The fibers of the hair are composed of a hard protein called **keratin** (kerat/o means "keratin" or "hard, horn-like"). Like skin, hair color is determined by the pigment melanin, which was described earlier as being produced from special cells called melanocytes. These melanocytes surround the hair shaft, and when a small quantity of melanin is produced, the hair color is lightly colored or blonde. Production of larger quantities contributes to darker hair. Gray hair, the result of diminished or no production of melanin, frequently occurs as people age.

The sebaceous or oil glands are closely associated with the hair follicles. These glands secrete **sebum**, an oily fluid, into the hair shaft. The sebum moves along the shaft toward the surface of the epidermis and provides lubrication to the skin and hair.

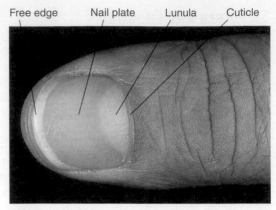

Free edge   Nail plate   Lunula   Cuticle

FIGURE 4-2 Superior view of a nail. The cuticle is the thin band of tissue that seals the nail plate to the skin. From Cohen BJ, Taylor J. Memmler's Structure and Function of the Human Body, 8th Ed. Baltimore: Lippincott Williams & Wilkins, 2005.

The sudoriferous glands are found over most of the body but are most numerous in the palms of the hands, soles of the feet, forehead, and armpits. These glands secrete a watery fluid that evaporates and helps cool the body. The nails, also accessory structures of the integumentary system, are composed of the protein keratin. A nail is a hard plate that covers the dorsal surface of the last bone of each toe and finger and offers protection from injury. Besides providing protection, the fingernails aid the fingertips in picking up small objects. The free edge of the nail is the part that extends beyond the tip of the finger or toe. The nail plate rests on the finger; the **lunula** (which means "half moon") is the pale half-moon–shaped region at the proximal end of the nail; and the **cuticle** (*cutis* is the Latin word for skin) is the thin band of tissue that seals the nail plate to the skin (Fig. 4-2).

Disorders and Treatments

DISORDERS

The skin is the only system that can be observed in its entirety for abnormalities and disease. It can provide clues to underlying disease in the body and reflect the state of its own health. Such clues consist of changes in skin color, **turgor** (the distension and displacement of fluid in the skin), **lesions**, and eruptions.

Skin Lesions

A lesion is a wound or other injury to the skin. It can be caused by systemic diseases; underlying infections; exposure to bacteria, fungi, viruses, and parasites; or an allergic reaction to food or drugs. Lesions can be categorized as flat, elevated, or depressed. There are numerous types of lesions, each having its own medical term, as shown in the following list:

Flat lesions:
- **Macule:** Flat, colored spot less than 1 cm in diameter (e.g., freckle).
- **Plaque:** Flat or lightly raised lesion more than 1 cm in diameter.

Elevated lesions:
- **Bulla:** Raised, fluid-filled lesion or blister greater than 1 cm (e.g., severe poison oak).
- **Nodule:** Solid, raised lesion larger than a papule, 0.6 to 2 cm in diameter (e.g., small tumor).
- **Papule:** Small, circular, solid elevation of the skin less than 1 cm in diameter (e.g., wart, pimple).

- **Pustule:** Small, circular, pus-filled elevation of the skin, usually less than 1 cm in diameter (e.g., pustular psoriasis or scabies).
- **Vesicle:** Small, circular, fluid-filled elevation of the skin less than 1 cm (e.g., poison ivy, chickenpox).
- **Wheal:** Smooth, rounded, slightly raised area often associated with itching (e.g., hives, insect bites).

Depressed lesions:
- **Fissure:** Crack or break in the skin; a slit of any size.
- **Ulcer:** An open sore or crater that extends to the dermis resulting from destruction of the skin; usually heals with scarring (e.g., pressure or bed sore).

These common types of lesions are illustrated in Figure 4-3.

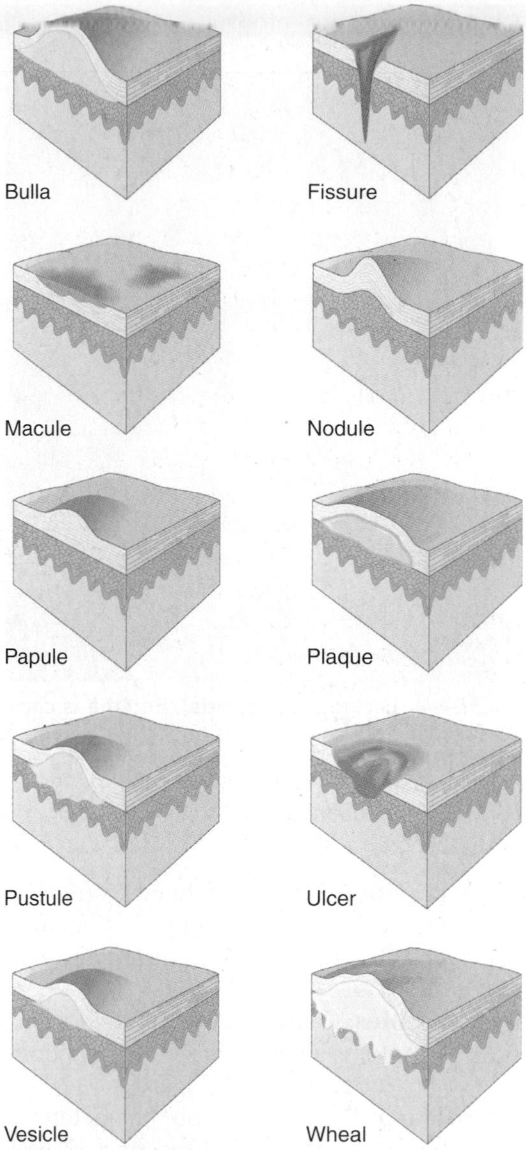

Inflammatory Disorders

There are numerous types of skin disorders that are characterized by the inflammatory process. Contact **dermatitis** (dermat/o means "skin"; -itis means "inflammation") can be caused by exposure to an allergen or by direct contact with a chemical or plant. Poison ivy, for example, may be the diagnosis when the skin becomes **erythematous** (erythemat/o means "redness"; -ous means "pertaining to"), is covered with tiny vesicles, and is often itchy or **pruritic** (prurit/o means "to itch"; -ic is the adjective suffix that means "pertaining to"; the noun is **pruritus**; the suffix -us means "condition").

Eczema is a type of chronic dermatitis that may begin in childhood and progress through adulthood (Fig. 4-4). This disorder is characterized by red, vesicular lesions that are crusted and pruritic. Another common chronic inflammatory condition is **psoriasis** (*psor* is French meaning "to itch"; -iasis means "a condition or process") (Fig. 4-5). Patches of crusty papules with erythematous or red circular borders and silvery scales are evidence of this disorder.

Scleroderma (scler/o means "hard"; derma means "skin") may occur as a skin disorder or sometimes suggests a systemic disease. The skin becomes taut, thick, and leather-like, causing the joints to become immovable.

Bulla — Fissure — Macule — Nodule — Papule — Plaque — Pustule — Ulcer — Vesicle — Wheal

FIGURE 4-3 Skin lesions. Illustrations of some of the more common skin lesions. From Cohen BJ. Medical Terminology: An Illustrated Guide, 5th Ed. Philadelphia: Lippincott Williams & Wilkins, 2007.

Skin Infections

Skin is our protective barrier, and when it breaks down, bacteria, viruses, fungi, and parasites have an opportunity to invade our body. Many infections, however, can be more annoying than they are serious. Symptoms of an infection may be **edema** (swelling), redness of the skin, and drainage from lesions. Terms naming some of the more common skin infections are provided in the following list.

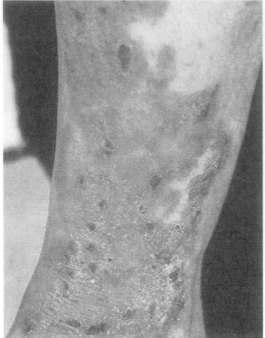

FIGURE 4-4 Eczema (dermatitis). Eczema is characterized by red, vesicular lesions that are crusted and pruritic. From Cohen BJ. Memmler's The Human Body in Health and Disease, 10th Ed. Philadelphia: Lippincott Williams & Wilkins, 2005.

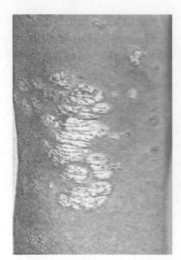

FIGURE 4-5 Psoriasis. Psoriasis is characterized by patches of crusty papules with erythematous or red circular borders and silvery scales. From Cohen BJ. Memmler's The Human Body in Health and Disease, 10th Ed. Philadelphia: Lippincott Williams & Wilkins, 2005.

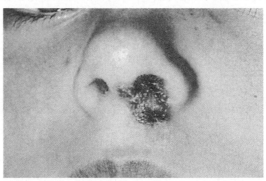

FIGURE 4-6 Impetigo. Impetigo is characterized by pustules that may become crusted and rupture. From Cohen BJ. Medical Terminology: An Illustrated Guide, 5th Ed. Philadelphia: Lippincott Williams & Wilkins, 2007.

- **Impetigo:** Caused by bacteria (*Staphylococcus aureus*); symptoms include pustules that become crusted and rupture (Fig. 4-6).
- **Scabies:** Caused by an egg-laying mite; symptoms include vesicular eruptions with intense itching (Fig. 4-7).
- **Tinea:** Fungal infection; characterized by irregularly shaped red rings of vesicles or papules; itchy (Fig. 4-8).
  - **Tinea barbae** (barbae refers to barber or beard): Fungal infection of the beard.
  - **Tinea capitis** (capitis refers to head or scalp): Fungal infection of the scalp.
  - **Tinea pedis** (pedis refers to foot): Fungal infection of the foot (athlete's foot).
  - **Tinea cruris** (cruris refers to upper leg or groin): Fungal infection of the groin or genital region (jock itch).
- **Shingles** (**herpes zoster**): Caused by a virus; symptoms include pain and a vesicular rash that develops along the path of a nerve.

Burns

A burn is an injury to the skin caused by heat (flames, heat, sun), chemicals (alkalis or acids), or electricity. The severity of the burn is categorized by the depth of the layers of skin involved. See Table 4-1 for the classification of burns. Superficial burns, such as those caused by sunburn, damage the epidermis and usually heal in about 2 to 7 days. Partial-thickness burns are more painful because they involve the epidermis and part of the dermis. Full-thickness burns affect all of the skin layers and may not always be as painful since the nerve endings may be destroyed.

Skin Cancer

Sun exposure is the biggest cause of skin cancer. **Melanoma** is a common type of skin cancer. It is also one of the more dangerous types because it has a tendency to spread, or **metastasize** (the verb form of **metastasis**; meta- means "beyond" and -stasis means "place").

Other Skin Disorders

Some skin and nail disorders that do not fit into the previously mentioned categories include pressure or **decubitus** (from a Latin word that means "to lie down") **ulcers**, better known as bedsores; **acne**, a disease of the sebaceous glands common in teens and young adults; **vitiligo**, which is depigmented blotches or macules that appear on the skin (Fig. 4-9); and **paronychia** (para- means "next to"; onych means "nail"; -ia is a suffix that means "a condition of"), which is an infection of the skin around the nails (Fig. 4-10).

    Alopecia, or baldness, can be caused by stress, medicine (chemotherapy in which the hair follicles are affected), systemic diseases, or male pattern baldness. (Alopecia comes from a Greek word that means to "eat away" as a parasite eats away at the host.) Alopecia can also be a symptom of a disease. Other skin conditions that may be disease symptoms are **erythema** (erythro means "red"), **ichthyosis** (ichthy means "dry, fish-like"; -osis means "an abnormal condition"), and **edema** (swelling). Some of these disorders may be a mere irritation, whereas others may become serious and require surgical and/or other medical treatment.

FIGURE 4-7 Scabies. Scabies is caused by an egg-laying mite and has symptoms that include vesicular eruptions with intense itching. From Fleisher GR, MD, Ludwig S, MD, Baskin MN, MD. Atlas of Pediatric Emerg Medicine, Philadelphia: Lippincott Williams & Wilkins, 2004.

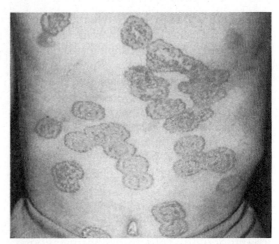

FIGURE 4-8 Tinea (ringworm). Tinea is a fungal infection that is characterized by irregularly shaped red rings of vesicles or papules. From Cohen BJ. Memmler's The Human Body in Health and Disease, 10th Ed. Philadelphia: Lippincott Williams & Wilkins, 2005.

TREATMENTS

Surgical procedures are frequently performed on the integumentary system to diagnose or treat abnormal conditions. A **biopsy** is the surgical removal of a small piece of skin or tissue for the purpose of diagnosis. **Cryogenic surgery**, also called **cryosurgery** or **cryotherapy** (*cryo* is

Table 4-1 Classification of Burns

Type of Burn	Layers of Skin Involved
superficial burn, sunburn	erythema (redness); superficial damage to epidermis; no blisters
partial-thickness burn	blisters; erythema
full-thickness burn	damage to the epidermis, dermis, and subcutaneous layers, muscle, and bone; may require skin grafts

from the Greek word *kruos* meaning "frost"; thus, the root cry/o means "to freeze"), is a technique used to destroy abnormal tissues such as warts, moles, and tumors by exposure to extreme cold. Cryogenic surgery often involves the use of liquid nitrogen.

Burned skin frequently becomes charred and necrotic (necr/o is a root that means "dead"; -ic is an adjective suffix that means "pertaining to"). For new healthy tissue to grow, the damaged skin must be removed or **debrided**, which is a verb form for the process known as **debridement** (French *débridement*, from *débrider*, which means "to remove adhesions" or, literally, "to unbridle").

Many types of plastic surgery are performed on specific areas of the skin for either cosmetic or treatment purposes. These surgeries are discussed in the respective body system chapters. Other types of treatments involving the integumentary system include medications, which may be administered by various means. One method of administration is called **transdermal** (trans- is a prefix meaning "across"; derm/o is a root for skin; -al is an adjective suffix meaning "pertaining to") in which the medication is absorbed continuously through the skin to produce a systemic effect. These medications may come in patches, ointments, or creams.

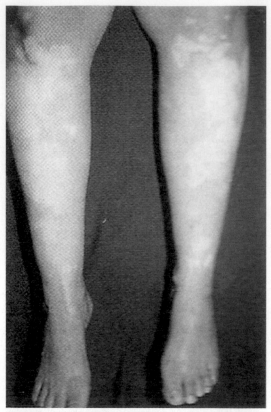

FIGURE 4-9   Vitiligo. Vitiligo is a condition with depigmented blotches or macules that appear on the skin. From Cohen BJ. Medical Terminology: An Illustrated Guide, 5th Ed. Philadelphia: Lippincott Williams & Wilkins, 2007.

Pharmacology

Pharmacology (pharm/o, pharmacy/o means "drug"; -logy means "the study of") is defined as the study of drugs and how they affect living organisms. Thousands of drugs are on the market, and learning about all of them is impractical. One way to begin learning about drugs, though, is to understand the drug classification system. Drugs that affect the body similarly are classified according to that particular therapeutic effect. Some drugs have more than one therapeutic effect and fit into multiple classifications. For example, aspirin can reduce inflammation (anti-inflammatory), reduce fever (**antipyretic**: anti- is a prefix meaning "against"; pyret is the root for "fever"; -ic is an adjective suffix that means "pertaining to"), and relieve pain (**analgesic**; an- is a prefix meaning "without"; alges is a root for "pain"; -ic is an adjective suffix that means "pertaining to").

Skin disorders frequently cause discomfort ranging from minor annoyances to major

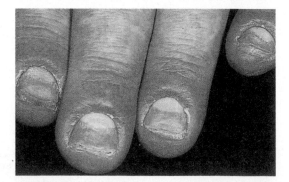

FIGURE 4-10   Paronychia. Paronychia is an infection of the skin around the nails. From Cohen BJ. Medical Terminology: An Illustrated Guide, 5th Ed. Philadelphia: Lippincott Williams & Wilkins, 2007.

ailments such as burns. Treatment is usually topical and local (a cream, lotion, or ointment applied to the affected area). It may also be oral or by injection. Classifications of topical medications are listed below.

- **Antipruritics** (anti- means "against"; pruritic refers to itching): Used to relieve discomfort and itching caused by rashes or dermatitis:
  - Local anesthetics: Used to relieve pain (the "-caines" such as lidocaine, benzocaine)
  - **Anti-inflammatory** agents: Used to reduce inflammation (corticosteroids such as Cortaid, Topicort)
  - Drying agents: Used to prevent itching from rash or irritation (Benadryl, Caladryl)
- **Antifungals** (anti- means "against"; fungal is the adjective form of fungus): Used to treat infections such as thrush, diaper rash, vaginitis, athlete's foot, and jock itch. Examples include Mycostatin, Tinactin, Desenex, and Lamisil.
- **Antiseptics** (anti- means "against"; septic refers to "decay or breaking down of bacteria"): Drugs that inhibit the growth of bacteria (**bacteriostatic**; bacteri/o means "bacteria"; static means "stationary" or, in this case, "not growing") on the skin. Examples include Hibiclens and Betadine.
- **Antivirals** (anti- means "against"; viral refers to a virus): Cold sores, chickenpox, and genital herpes are viral skin conditions that are treated with antiviral medications. An example of a drug in this classification is acyclovir.
- **Scabicides** (scabo means "to scratch" and scabies causes intense itching; -cide means "to kill") and **pediculicides** (pedicul means "lice"): Scabies is caused by a mite that burrows under the skin. An infestation of lice causes **pediculosis**. Both conditions are treated topically by applying agents such as Lindane and Kwell, respectively.
- Acne medication: Topical drugs such as sulfur, salicylic acid, and benzoyl peroxide are used to treat the common skin condition called acne.
- Burn medications: Infection is the major complication of burns, and topical agents are used to prevent infection. Examples in this classification include Silvadene and Sulfamylon. Sometimes oral or intravenous **antibiotics** (anti- means "against"; bio means "life") are necessary to eradicate the infection.

Many skin conditions manifest themselves as a break in the continuity of the skin, eruptions, or infections. The medications prescribed are usually applied directly to the lesions as mentioned earlier. At times, **sedatives** (comes from the Latin *sedatio*, which means "to calm") are necessary to help patients relax so they don't irritate the lesions or scratch the skin. Patient compliance with the medication regimen is a major factor for improvement and healing.

Abbreviation Table • The Integumentary System

ABBREVIATION	MEANING
BSA	body surface area (used in describing skin damage assessment caused by burns)
LE	lupus erythematosus
SLE	systemic lupus erythematosus
SPF	sun protection factor
STSG	split-thickness skin graft
UV	ultraviolet

Study Table • *Integumentary System*

TERM AND PRONUNCIATION	ANALYSIS	MEANING
adipose (AD-ih-pohs)	from the Latin word *adeps* (fat)	fatty tissue
corium (KO-ree-uhm)	from the Latin word *cutis* (skin)	synonym for dermis
cutaneous (cue-TAYN-ee-uhs)	from the Latin word *cutis* (skin)	adjective referring to the skin
cuticle (CUE-tih-kuhl)	from the Latin word *cutis* (skin)	the thin band of tissue that seals the nail plate to the skin
dermatologist (dur-muh-TAHL-uh-jist)	*dermat/o* (skin); *-logist* (practitioner)	a specialist who diagnoses and treats skin diseases
dermatology (dur-muh-TAHL-uh-jee)	*dermat/o* (skin); *-logy* (study)	study of the integumentary system
dermis (DUR-mis)	from the Greek word *derma* (skin)	inner layer of skin
epidermis (epp-ih-DUR-mis)	*epi-* (upon); *dermis* (skin)	outer layer of the skin
follicle (FAWL-ik-uhl)	from the Latin word *folliculus* (a small sac)	small sac in the skin from which a hair grows
keratin (KERR-uhtin)	from the Greek word *kera* (horn)	protein that forms hair, nails, and the tough outer layer of skin
lunula (LOO-new-luh)	from the Latin word *luna* (moon)	white, crescent-shaped area of a nail
melanin (MELL-uh-nihn)	from the Greek word *melas* (black)	dark pigment present in skin and other parts of the body
melanocyte (MEL-uh-no-site)	from the Greek word *melas* (black); *-cyte* (cell)	cell that produces melanin
sebaceous (se-BAY-shus)	from the Latin word *sebum* (tallow and by extension, grease, oil, fat)	oil-producing gland
subcutaneous (sub-ku-TAY-nee-us)	*sub-* (beneath); *cutane* (skin); *-ous* (adjective suffix)	beneath the skin
sudoriferous (soo-doe-RIFF-uh-russ)	from two Latin words: *sudor* (sweat) and *fero* (to carry)	sweat-producing glands

Disorders and Symptoms

abscess (AB-sehs)	from the Latin word *abscessus* (a going away)	localized collection of pus in any body part, frequently associated with swelling and inflammation

TERM AND PRONUNCIATION	ANALYSIS	MEANING
acne (ak-nee)	a common English word	inflammatory papular and pustular eruption of the skin
albinism (al-BY-nih-zm)	from a Latin word *albus* (white) and *-ism* (condition)	partial or total absence of pigment of the skin, hair, eyes
alopecia (al-oh-PEE-shee-uh)	from a Greek word *alopekia* (fox mange)	partial or complete loss of hair; baldness
comedo (KOM-eh-do)	a Latin word (glutton)	blackhead; dilated hair follicle filled with bacteria; primary lesion in acne
cyanosis (SY-uh-no-siss)	*cyan/o* (blue); *-osis* (abnormal condition)	abnormal condition signaled by bluish discoloration of tissue
cyst (sih-st)	from the Greek word *kystis* (bladder)	closed sac or pouch in or under the skin that contains fluid or solid material
dermatitis (dur-muh-TY-tiss)	*dermat/o* (skin); *-itis* (inflammation)	inflammation of the skin
dermatomycosis (DUR-matt-oh-MI-ko-sis)	*dermat/o* (skin); *myc/o* (fungus); *-osis* (abnormal condition)	fungal infection of the skin
diaphoresis (dy-ah-for-EE-sis)	a Greek word (perspiration)	synonym for perspiration
ecchymosis (ek-ee-MOH-sis)	*ec-* (out); from *chymos* (Greek word for juice); *-osis* (abnormal condition)	a purple patch more than 3 mm in diameter caused by blood under the skin; see also petechiae
eczema (EK-zee-ma)	from the Greek word *eczeo* (boil over)	inflammatory condition of the skin characterized by erythema, vesicles, and crusting with scales
epidermitis (epp-ih-dur-MY-tiss)	*epi-* (upon); *-dermis* (skin); *-itis* (inflammation)	inflammation of the epidermis
erythema (ehr-ih-THEE-ma)	Greek word (flush)	abnormal redness of the skin
excoriation (ex-COR-ee-at-shun)	from the Latin verb *excorio* (to skin)	scratch mark; linear break (caused most often from scratching) in the skin surface
hemangioma (hee-man-jee-OH-ma)	*hem/o* (blood); *angi/o* (vessel); *-oma* (tumor)	benign tumor of blood vessels; birthmark
hyperhidrosis (hyper-HY-droh-sis)	*hyper-* (above normal); *hidr* (sweat); *-osis* (condition)	profuse sweating; increased or excessive perspiration; may be caused by heat, menopause, or infection

(continued)

TERM AND PRONUNCIATION	ANALYSIS	MEANING
ichthyosis (ik-thee-OH-sis)	*ichthy/o* (fish-like); *-osis* (abnormal condition)	abnormally dry skin; scaly; resembling fish skin
impetigo (im-peh-TYE-goh)	from the Latin verb *impeto* (attack)	inflammatory skin disease with pustules that rupture and become crusted
keloid (KEE-loid)	from the Greek word *kelis* (tumor); and *-oid* (like)	overgrowth of scar tissue
lesion (LEE-shun)	from the Latin verb *laedo* (to injure)	wound, injury, or pathological change in body tissue
macule (MAK-yul)	from the Latin word *macula* (spot)	flat, discolored area that is flush with the skin; birthmark or freckle
melanoma (mel-uh-NO-muh)	*melan/o* (black); *-oma* (tumor)	tumor of the melanocytes; skin cancer characterized by dark pigmented, irregular-shaped lesion
nevus (NEE-vuhs)	Latin word for birthmark	mole; pigmented skin blemish that is usually benign but may become cancerous
nodule (NOD-yul)	from the Latin word *nodus* (knot)	a small node or circumscribed swelling
onychomalacia (ON-ih-ko-muh-LAY-shee-uh)	*onych/o* (nail); *-malacia* (softening)	softening of the nails
onychopathy (on-ih-KOP-uh-thee)	*onych/o* (nail); *-pathy* (disease)	any disease of the nails
papule (pap-yul)	from the Latin word *papula* (pimple)	small, circumscribed solid elevation of the skin
paronychia (pahr-oh-NIK-ee-ah)	*para-* (adjacent); *onych/o* (nail); *-ia* (condition)	infection around a nail
petechia (peh-TEEK-ia); petechiae (plural)	from the Italian word *peticchie* (small hemorrhagic spots)	tiny hemorrhagic spot(s) on the skin less than 3 mm in diameter; see also ecchymosis
polyp (PAHL-ip)	from the Latin word *polypus* (a growth on a stem)	a mass of tissue that bulges outward from the skin's surface on a stem or stalk of mucous membrane
pruritus (pru-RY-tis)	from the Latin verb prurio (to itch)	itching

TERM AND PRONUNCIATION	ANALYSIS	MEANING
psoriasis (soh-RY-ih-sis)	Greek word for itch	chronic skin disease characterized by itchy, red, silvery-scaled patches
pustule (PUHST-yul)	from the Latin word *pustula* (pimple)	small (up to 1 cm in diameter) circumscribed elevation of the skin containing pus
scabies (SKAY-bees)	from the Latin verb *scabo* (to scratch)	contagious infection caused by a mite
scleroderma (sklehr-oh-DER-ma)	*scler/o* (hardness); *-derma* (skin)	chronic disease characterized by thickening and hardening of the skin
shingles; herpes zoster (HER-peez ZAHS-tuhr)	from the Greek word *herpo* (to creep)	viral infection producing the eruption of highly painful vesicles that may follow a nerve path
tinea (TIN-ee-uh)	Latin word for worm	any fungal infection of the skin (tinea barbae = beard; tinea capitis = head; tinea pedis = athlete's foot)
ulcer (UL-ser)	from the Latin word *ulcus* (a sore)	an open sore or lesion of the skin; a lesion through the skin or a mucous membrane resulting from loss of tissue
urticaria (ur-tih-KAR-ee-uh)	from the Latin word *uro* (to burn)	hives; allergic reaction of the skin characterized by eruption of pale red elevated patches
verruca (ve-ROO-kah)	Latin word for wart	wart; caused by a virus
vesicle (VES-ih-kal)	from the Latin word *vesicula* (blister)	small, fluid-filled, raised lesion; a blister
vitiligo (vit-il-IH-go)	from the Latin word *vitium* (blemish)	localized loss of skin pigmentation characterized by milk-white patches

Diagnoses, Procedures, and Treatments

analgesic (an-uhl-GEE-sik)	*ana-* (without); *gesic* (pain)	agent that relieves pain
antibiotic (an-ty-BYE-ah-tik)	*anti-* (against); *biotic* (organism)	agent that kills bacteria
antifungal (an-ty-FUNG-ul)	*anti-* (against); *fungal* (fungus)	agent that kills fungus

(continued)

TERM AND PRONUNCIATION	ANALYSIS	MEANING
anti-inflammatory (an-ty-ihn-FLAM-ah-tor-ee)	*anti-* (against); *inflammatory* (inflammation)	agent to reduce inflammation
antipruritic (an-ty-pryu-RIH-tik)	*anti-* (against); *pruritic* (itching)	agent that reduces itching
antipyretic (an-ty-PEYE-reh-tik)	*anti-* (against); *pyretic* (burning)	agent that reduces fever
antiseptic (an-tih-sehp-tik)	*anti-* (against); *septic* (poison)	agent that inhibits the growth of infectious agents
antiviral (an-ty-VY-rahl)	*anti-* (against); *viral* (virus)	agent that destroys viruses
debridement (deh-BREED-ment)	*de-* (removal); *bridement* (from the word *bridle*, the part of the riding harness by which a rider controls the horse)	removal of necrotic or dead tissue from a wound or burn
dermatoplasty (dur-MAT-oh-plass-tee)	*dermat/o* (skin); *-plasty* (surgical repair)	plastic surgery repair performed on the skin
incision and drainage (I&D)	common English words	cutting open of a wound or lesion, such as an abscess, and letting out or draining the contents, such as pus
onychectomy (ON-ihk-EHK-toh-mee)	*onych/o* (nail); *-ectomy* (excision)	surgical removal of a nail
onychotomy (on-ih-KOT-oh-mee)	*onych/o* (nail); *-tomy* (incision)	incision into a nail
scabicide (SKA-bih-seyed)	*scabies* (see above); *-cide* (destruction)	agent lethal to mites
transdermal (trans-DUR-mahl)	*trans-* (across); *derm/o* (skin); *-al* (adjective suffix)	a method of administering medication through the unbroken skin via patch or ointment

EXERCISES

 EXERCISE 4-1   Case Study

Read the following case study out loud to a friend. Define the underlined medical terms in the space provided below.

CHIEF COMPLAINT: Rash on the face

PRESENT ILLNESS: 29 y/o white female states that last week she started having some itching on her forehead. She went to the doctor who prescribed erythromycin, an (1) <u>antibiotic</u>, and (2) <u>Benadryl</u>. Two days later, the rash covered her entire face. The patient was diagnosed with (3) <u>impetigo</u> and was admitted to the hospital for treatment.

CONSULTATION: Dr. Smith, a (4) <u>dermatologist</u>, saw the patient. The chart was reviewed, and the patient was examined. She is married and has no children and no pets. She developed (5) <u>dermatitis</u> on her forehead 2 weeks ago that has spread to her entire face. The rash has become more (6) <u>erythematous</u>, and she now has (7) <u>pustules</u> on her forehead, nose, and cheeks. Facial (8) <u>edema</u> persists, and she is almost unable to open her eyes. She has been given additional antibiotics and an (9) <u>antipruritic medication</u>.

She developed (10) <u>pruritus</u> on her feet, which was thought to be a reaction to the antibiotic, so the medication was changed to Cleocin.

IMPRESSION: Impetigo; allergic response to erythromycin. Patient responding to Cleocin. Continue with current antibiotic regimen and continue to monitor patient. Thank you for allowing me to participate in this interesting case. I will follow patient and provide additional suggestions if warranted.

Dr. Smith

TERM   **DEFINITION**

1. _____   _____

2. _____   _____

3. _____   _____

4. _____   _____

5. _____   _____

6. _____   _____

7. _____   _____

8. _____   _____

9. _____   _____

10. _____   _____

EXERCISE 4-2 Labeling the Skin

adipose tissue	epidermis	nerve	subcutaneous layer
artery	hair	nerve endings	sudoriferous gland
dermis	hair follicle	sebaceous gland	vein

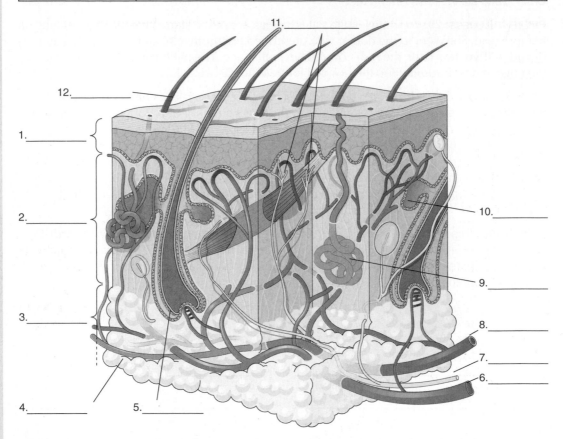

EXERCISE 4-3 Word Building

Add the correct prefix or suffix to the word root to make a new term. Select from the following word elements: *-pathy*, *-osis*, *-logy*, *-oma*, *-itis*, and *epi-* to make a new term.

WORD ROOT OR COMBINING FORM	ADD PREFIX OR SUFFIX	MEANING	TERM
1. dermat/o	_____	inflammation of the skin	_____
2. melan/o	_____	malignant black tumor	_____

3. dermis _____   outer layer of skin   _____

4. onych/o _____   disease of the nail   _____

5. dermat/o _____   study of the skin   _____

6. ichthy/o _____   dry, scaly, fish-like skin   _____

Use the following prefixes to write the term for the following definitions.

epi- on, upon, over   *per-* through   *intra-* within   *sub-* under

7. under the skin _____

8. through the cutaneous layer _____

9. within the skin _____

10. on the surface of the skin _____

EXERCISE 4-4   Matching

Match the terms in Column 1 with the best definitions in Column 2.

TERM

DEFINITION

1. _____ nevus   A. birthmark

2. _____ verruca   B. thickened scar

3. _____ macule   C. blackhead

4. _____ alopecia   D. mole

5. _____ keloid   E. wart

6. _____ comedo   F. baldness

7. _____ diaphoresis   G. profuse sweating; increased perspiration

8. _____ erythema   H. abrasion of upper skin layers

9. _____ excoriation   I. flat, colored spot

10. _____ hemangioma   J. redness of the skin

EXERCISE 4-5   Pronunciation

In the online student resources, go to the Audio Glossary and select Chapter 4, The Integumentary System. Select a term that you are unfamiliar with and "listen" to the pronunciation. Write the term and definition of the term below. Repeat for a total of 20 terms. Be prepared to pronounce these terms in class.

AUDIO PRONUNCIATION GLOSSARY: THE INTEGUMENTARY SYSTEM

TERM	DEFINITION
1.	
2.	
3.	
4.	
5.	
6.	
7.	
8.	
9.	
10.	
11.	
12.	
13.	
14.	
15.	
16.	
17.	
18.	
19.	
20.	

EXERCISE 4-6   Integumentary System Crossword Puzzle

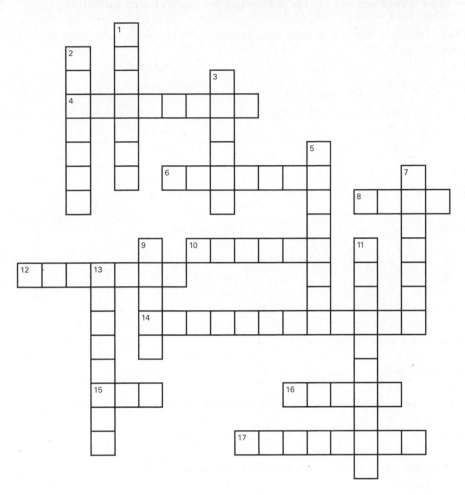

ACROSS

4. vesicular rash that develops along the path of a nerve
6. fatty tissue
8. root word that means "dead"
10. wound or injury
12. pigment that determines hair and skin color
14. term for "redness"
15. root word for "freezing"
16. root word for "nail"
17. depigmented blotches that appear on the skin

DOWN

1. thin band of tissue that seals the nail plate to the skin
2. small, circular, pus-filled elevation of the skin
3. thick layer of tissue just below the epidermis
5. a very common type of skin cancer with irregular borders and a variance in color that progresses to a dark or almost black shade
7. infection caused by an egg-laying mite
9. fungal infection
11. an infection of the skin around the nails
13. baldness

CHAPTER 4 QUIZ

Choose the correct answer for the following multiple choice questions.

1. If **myc** is the root word for fungus, what is the term that means "condition of the nail caused by fungus"?
   a. mycosis
   b. onychomycosis
   c. trichomycosis
   d. onychomalacia

2. If **ichthy** is the root word for dry, fish-like, what is the term for a condition of being extremely dry?
   a. ichthyioma
   b. ichthyosis
   c. ichthyema
   d. ichthiitis

3. The term to describe a lesion of the skin containing pus is:
   a. verruca
   b. pustule
   c. bulla
   d. macule

4. A large blister filled with fluid is called:
   a. hemangioma
   b. furuncle
   c. cutis
   d. bulla

5. **Tinea** means a fungal infection. Which term best describes a fungal infection of the skin and/or accessory structures?
   a. tinea pedis
   b. tinea cruris
   c. tinea capitis
   d. all of the above

6. The term for natural or abnormal baldness that may be total or partial is:
   a. amastia
   b. alopecia
   c. urticaria
   d. desquamation

7. The term used for a condition of profuse sweating is:
   a. diaphoresis
   b. sebaceous
   c. halitosis
   d. peristalsis

8. The term that best describes the thin band of tissue that seals the nail plate to the skin is:
   a. corium
   b. follicle
   c. cuticle
   d. epidermis

9. The term that best describes the cell that produces the pigment that provides color to the skin and hair is:
   a. keratocyte
   b. melanocyte
   c. erythrocyte
   d. leukocyte

10. Which term describes a fungal infection of the skin?
    a. dehiscence
    b. dermatomycosis
    c. dermatitis
    d. evisceration

Match the diagnoses listed here with the definitions that follow.

albinism	cyanosis	keloid	scleroderma
alopecia	ecchymosis	petechia	urticaria
biopsy	fissure	polyp	vitiligo

11. A firm scar that forms in the healing of a sore or wound is a _____.

12. _____ is a small slit or crack-like lesion.

13. _____ is a condition with a bluish discoloration of tissue.

14. A chronic disease characterized by thickening and hardening of the skin is called _____.

15. Absence or loss of hair is a condition called _____.

16. Partial or complete absence of pigment of the skin, hair, and eyes is termed _____.

17. A loss of skin pigmentation with milk-white skin patches is a condition known as _____.

18. _____, or hives, is an allergic reaction of the skin characterized by pale red eruptions.

19. The removal of a small piece of living tissue for examination under a microscope is called a(n) _____.

20. A(n) _____ is a mass of tissue that bulges outward and grows on a stem or stalk.

CHAPTER 5

The Skeletal System

LEARNING OBJECTIVES

Upon completion of this chapter, you should be able to:

- Name the major structures and functions of the skeletal system.
- Name the medical specialists and health care professionals who treat disorders of the skeletal system.
- Build skeletal medical terms from word parts.
- Differentiate between the axial and appendicular skeletons.
- Give the medical terms used for the three types of joints.
- Name the major drug classifications used to treat skeletal disorders.
- Interpret abbreviations associated with the skeletal system.
- Analyze and define the new terms introduced in this chapter.

Word Elements • Skeletal System

ROOT	REFERS TO
ankyl/o	stiff, fused, closed
arthr/o	joint
brachi/o	arm
calcane/o	calcaneus, heel bone
carp/o	wrist
cheir/o	hand
chondr/o	cartilage
cost/o	rib
crani/o	cranium
dactyl/o	finger, toe
electr/o	electricity
femur/o	femur, thigh bone
humer/o	humerus, upper arm bone
kinesi/o	movement
kyph/o	hump
lord/o	swayback, curve
lumb/o	lower back
my/o, muscul/o	muscle
myel/o	bone marrow
orth/o	correct, straight
oste/o	bone
ped/o	foot, child
pelv/o	pelvis
phalang/o	bones of fingers and toes
spondyl/o, vertebr/o	vertebrae
thorac/o	thorax, chest
SUFFIX	**REFERS TO**
-algia	pain
-desis	stabilize or fuse
-ectomy	removal of, excision of

(continued)

SUFFIX	REFERS TO
-gram	written record of
-itis	inflammation
-kinesia	movement
-logy	study of
-malacia	softening
-oma	tumor
-physis	to grow
-plasty	surgical repair
-porosis	porous
-scopy	to visually examine

An Overview of the Skeletal System

The human skeleton begins to form about 6 weeks after fertilization and continues to grow and develop until the person is 25 years old. The human skeleton, which includes approximately 206 bones, performs many duties. It serves as a rigid but articulating (which means "allowing for movement") framework for all our muscles and other tissues. It also protects our vital organs by forming a shield to ward off blows. Its less obvious jobs are to produce and store essential minerals and to make blood cells.

In this chapter, you will learn that the skeleton may be divided into two parts: the **axial** and **appendicular** skeletons (Fig. 5-1). The axial skeleton consists of the skull and the chest bones, along with those of the spinal column, and the appendicular skeleton includes all the bones that are attached to the trunk of the body.

The appendicular skeleton comprises the arms and legs, along with the shoulder and pelvic girdles. The adjective "appendicular" indicates that the "appendages" (smaller parts that project from the main part) attach to the trunk (central core of the body). You may see a more common word, "appendix," in the term "appendicular." While the appendicular skeleton has nothing to do with the body's "appendix," the two do have a common classical word origin. *Appendix* is a Latin word referring

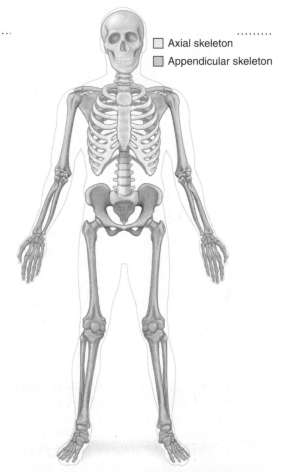

☐ Axial skeleton
☐ Appendicular skeleton

FIGURE 5-1   Axial and appendicular skeletons. The axial and appendicular skeletons differentiated. The axial skeleton is shown in yellow; the appendicular (consisting of the arms and legs) is in gray.

to something that is attached to something else. Thus, the appendicular skeleton is attached to the axial skeleton, the main hub of the body.

In addition to bones, the skeletal system includes ligaments, tendons, and joints. Movement is possible because bones provide points of attachment for ligaments and tendons, along with muscles, which are discussed in Chapter 6.

Structure and Function

Bone formation begins early in fetal development when the skeleton is composed mostly of cartilage. **Ossification** (ossify means "to form bone") occurs during the second and third month of fetal development as the cartilage hardens and turns into bone. Bone, made up of **osseous** (osse/o means "bone" or "bony") tissue, comprises special mature bone cells called osteocytes (oste/o also means "bone"; -cyte means "cell"). The bones of the skeleton are of different shapes and sizes. They may be flat, like those found in the cranium and ribs, or short, such as those in the wrist and ankles. One of the more familiar shapes is the long bone, which is found in the arms, legs, hands, and feet.

The general structure of the long bone consists of the **diaphysis** (dia- means "through"; -physis means "growth") or shaft and the **distal** and **proximal epiphysis** (epi- means "upon"; -physis means "growth"), its two ends. Bone marrow is found in the middle of the shaft or the **medullary** (marrow) **cavity**. The bone marrow is where blood cell formation occurs. Most bones are covered with a membrane called the **periosteum** (peri- is a prefix that means "around"; oste means "bone"). The periosteum provides for bone repair and general bone nutrition. An inner layer membrane, the **endosteum** (endo- is a prefix meaning "within") lines the medullary cavity. This inner lining also contributes to growth and repair of bone tissue (Fig. 5-2).

DIVISIONS OF THE SKELETON

There are two divisions of the skeleton: the axial skeleton and the appendicular skeleton.

The Axial Skeleton

The bones of the axial skeleton are the cranial, facial, and thoracic bones, along with the *spinal column*. The six main **cranial** (crani/o means "skull") bones are the **frontal bone**; two **parietal bones** (pariet/o means "a wall of the body"; -al is a suffix that means "pertaining to"), one on each side; two **temporal bones** (temper/o means "temple," which is the area on the side of the head back by the ears); and the **occipital** bone (occiput means "the back of the head"). The cranial bones are joined by **sutures**, which are fibrous membranes that occur between them (Fig. 5-3). Cranial bones enclose and protect the brain and hearing organs.

The main facial bones are the **nasal bone**, **zygomatic** (zygo means "yoke" or "to join," and this bone joins with four other bones)

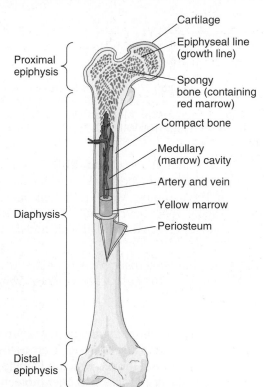

Cartilage
Epiphyseal line (growth line)
Proximal epiphysis
Spongy bone (containing red marrow)
Compact bone
Medullary (marrow) cavity
Artery and vein
Yellow marrow
Diaphysis
Periosteum
Distal epiphysis

FIGURE 5-2 Structure of a long bone. The epiphyses, or ends of the bones, are shown in relation to the diaphysis or shaft of the bone. The periosteum covers the bone's outer surface. The medullary is the middle of the bones and houses the blood vessels and marrow. From Cohen BJ. Medical Terminology: An Illustrated Guide, 5th Ed. Philadelphia: Lippincott Williams & Wilkins, 2007.

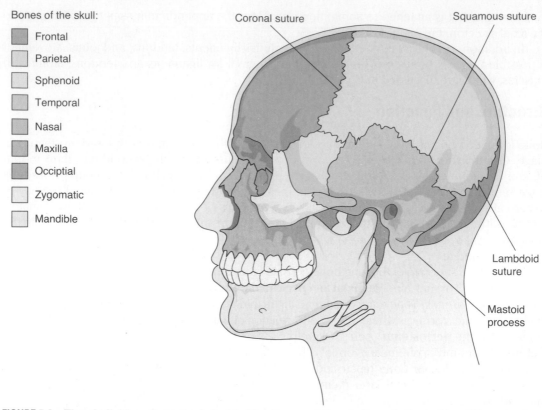

Bones of the skull:
- Frontal
- Parietal
- Sphenoid
- Temporal
- Nasal
- Maxilla
- Occiptial
- Zygomatic
- Mandible

Coronal suture

Squamous suture

Lambdoid suture

Mastoid process

FIGURE 5-3   The skull. View from the left side. The bones of the skull are indicated by different colors. The sutures, also known as suture joints, are the lines of junction between the two bones. These joints are usually immovable. Modified from Cohen BJ. Medical Terminology: An Illustrated Guide, 5th Ed. Philadelphia: Lippincott Williams & Wilkins, 2007.

bones (two), **maxilla**, and **mandible**. The nasal bone forms the bridge of the nose, and the two zygomatic bones form the cheeks. The maxilla is the upper jawbone, and the mandible is the lower jawbone. The mandible, which is the only facial bone that moves, allows for speaking and chewing. The facial bones have several functions, including providing structure for the face, placement of the teeth, openings for food and air, and cavities for the sense organs of taste, sight, and smell.

> *Although the mandible is regarded as "the jawbone,"* maxilla *is the Latin word for jawbone. The Latin verb* mandere, *from which "mandible" is derived, means "to chew or devour."*

The **thoracic** (thorac/o means "chest") bones, which include the sternum, the ribs, and associated cartilage, are known collectively as the thoracic cage (Fig. 5-4). The adjective thoracic is formed from the word thorax, which is Latin for "breastplate" (chest armor); thus, thoracic refers to the chest area. Its purpose is to offer protection of the internal organs from injury. The two major organs inside the thoracic cage are the heart and lungs.

At the back (posterior), each rib pair is attached to its correspondingly numbered **vertebra** (vertebr/o means "vertebra" or "backbone"). The anterior (front) rib attachments are to the **sternum** (stern/o means "chest"), but the last two rib pairs "float," which means that they do not attach to the sternum, but only to the vertebrae. The lower end of the sternum is a bony dagger-like projection called the **xiphoid process**. This term comes from the Greek word, *xiphos*, which means "sword."

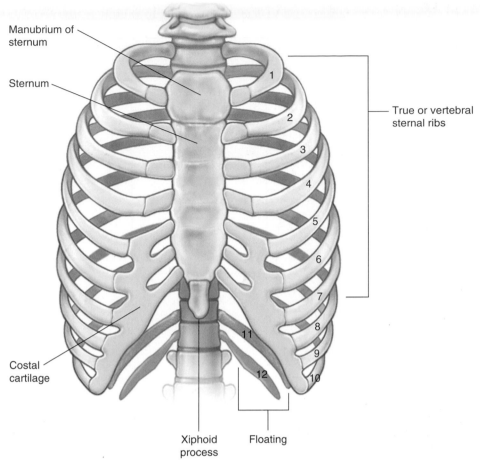

Manubrium of
sternum

Sternum

True or vertebral
sternal ribs

1
2
3
4
5
6
7
8
9
10
11
12

Costal
cartilage

Xiphoid
process

Floating

FIGURE 5-4   Thoracic cage. The thorax comprises the sternum, manubrium of the sternum, ribs, and costal cartilage. The first seven ribs articulate or join the sternum or breastbone by means of the costal cartilage. The last five ribs are not directly joined to the sternum, and the last two ribs are attached posteriorly to the thoracic vertebrae.

> The medical phrase for floating ribs is **costae fluctuantes**. *Since rib pairs 8, 9, and 10, together with the "floating ribs" 11 and 12, are sometimes collectively called **false ribs** or **costae spuriae**, it follows that the first seven pairs of ribs are **costae verae** ("true ribs"). If you know the English words* fluctuate, spurious, *and* verify, *you can associate them with the three terms above as a help in remembering them. If you are unfamiliar with those English words, you might want to look them up in a good dictionary and make them part of your general vocabulary.*

The spinal column includes five sections of vertebrae (singular: vertebra). The naming of a vertebra consists of a prefix letter (C for cervical; T for thoracic; and L for lumbar), followed by a number indicating the placement on the column. A couple of examples would be C1 for the first cervical vertebra (*cervix* is Latin for "neck") and L5 for the fifth lumbar vertebra in the lower back region. *Lumbus* is Latin for "loin," and thus, the lumbar region is part of the lower back. The distribution of the vertebrae of the cervical, thoracic, and lumbar regions is shown in Figure 5-5. The illustration shows the **sacrum** and **coccyx** at the base of the spine. These are formed by the fusion of rudimentary bones.

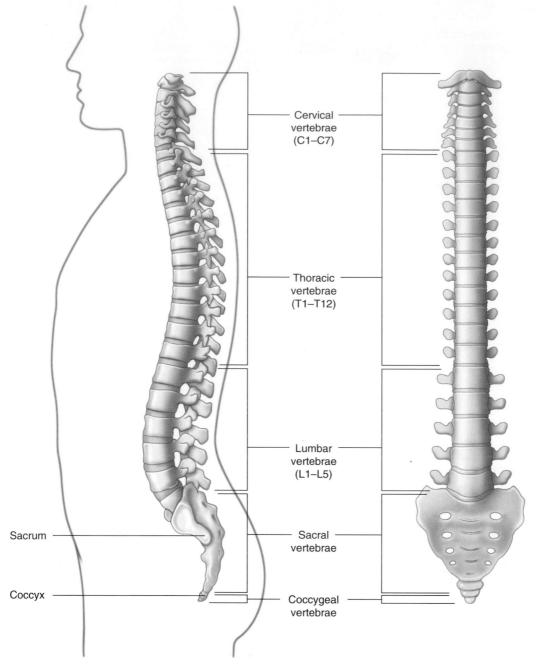

FIGURE 5-5   Vertebral column. The vertebral, or spinal, column is composed of bones called vertebrae. It is divided into five regions: cervical, thoracic, lumbar, sacral, and coccygeal. These are often abbreviated by their first letter. For example, C7 is the seventh cervical vertebra.

 The words cervix *and* cervical *also refer to the "neck" of the uterus, part of the female reproductive system (see Chapter 14).*

The sacrum is joined to the hip bones and, therefore, is part of the pelvic girdle, which is in turn part of the appendicular skeleton. Although the sacrum is not part of the axial skeleton, it is mentioned here because it is associated with the spinal column.

The Appendicular Skeleton

As mentioned earlier, the appendicular skeleton consists of the body's "appendages" (arms and legs) and the areas to which these appendages are attached: shoulder and pelvic girdles. Shoulder bones, although associated with the chest, are part of the appendicular skeleton. The main bones of the shoulder girdle are the **clavicle** (collarbone) and the **scapula** (shoulder blade) (Fig. 5-6).

The long bone extending from the shoulder and ending at the elbow is called the **humerus**, not because it is the "funny bone" but because *humerus* is the Latin word for "shoulder." However, there is a connection with the word "humorous." The phrase "funny bone" was most probably coined as a joke because the ulnar nerve, which causes the pins-and-needles sensation when it is struck, is located where the humerus joins the elbow.

The forearm consists of the **ulna** and **radius**, which extend from the elbow down to the wrist (Fig. 5-7). The wrist includes eight bones called **carpals**, from the Greek word *karpos*, meaning "wrist." As we learned in Chapter 2, meta- is a prefix meaning "beyond," and therefore, the **metacarpals** lie "beyond" the carpals, connecting the wrist to the fingers. The **phalanges** make up the fingers. The term

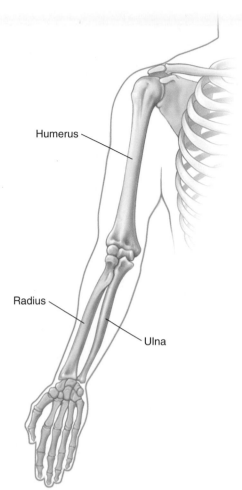

FIGURE 5-7 **The bones of the arm.** The bones of the arm include the humerus, radius, and ulna. The humerus, or upper arm bone, articulates with the scapula at the shoulder and the radius and ulna at the elbow. The radius and ulna, or lower arm bones, articulate with the humerus at the elbow and the carpals at the wrist.

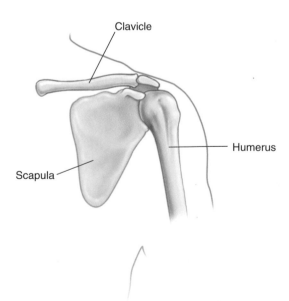

FIGURE 5-6 **The bones of the shoulder.** The bones of the shoulder include the clavicle, humerus, and scapula.

phalanges is the plural form of *phalanx*, which is Greek for "line of soldiers." The bones of the wrist and hand are shown in Figure 5-8.

The pelvic girdle, so named because it surrounds and protects the pelvic organs, consists of the two hip bones, right and left, along with the sacrum, noted earlier in connection with the spinal column. The hip bone, also called the **os coxae**, is a fusion of three bones: the **ilium**, the **ischium**, and the **pubis**.

The **femur**, Latin for "thigh," is a long bone that extends from the hip to the knee, and the **tibia** and **fibula** are long bones that extend from the knee to the ankle (Fig. 5-9).

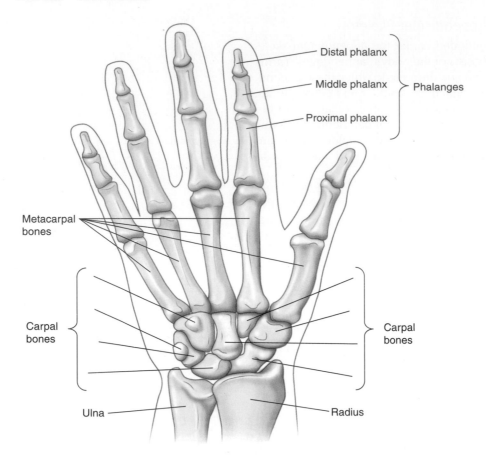

FIGURE 5-8 **Hand and wrist bones.** The wrist is made up of eight carpal bones. They join the metacarpals, which extend out to the phalanges or fingers. Meta- means "beyond," so the metacarpals, or bones of the palm of the hand, are beyond the wrist bones.

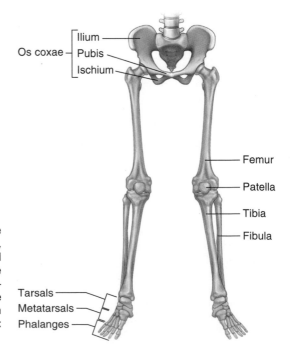

FIGURE 5-9 **Bones of the pelvic girdle and legs.** The pelvis is formed from three fused bones, the ilium, ischium, and pubis, which are collectively termed the os coxae. The femur is the longest bone in the body and is located in the thigh. The tibia and fibula are the lower leg bones. The tarsals or ankle bones join the metatarsal bones in the foot, which are connected to the phalanges or toes. (Note: Phalanges are both finger and toe bones.)

The tibia, Latin for "shin," is the shin bone or heavy bone of the lower leg; the fibula, from the Latin word *figibula*, meaning "fastener," does not bear the body's weight, but together with the tibia, it is connected to the **talus** (ankle bone). The **patella** (kneecap) is a "floating" bone that is imbedded in the tendon of the thigh muscle. It offers protection to the knee joint.

Tarsus (from the Greek *tarsos*, meaning "a flat surface") is sometimes used as a technical name for the ankle. The **tarsals** and **metatarsals** (meta- means "beyond," and tarsal refers to the ankle bones, so these are the bones in the foot) of the ankle and foot correspond with the carpal and metacarpal bones of the wrist and hand. The bones making up the fingers and toes are both called **phalanges** (phalang/o and dactyl/o are roots for fingers and toes). The bony protrusions at the distal end of the fibula are called the **medial** and **lateral malleolus**. These

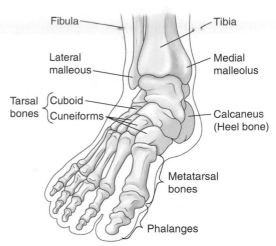

FIGURE 5-10 The bones of the ankle and foot. The medial and lateral malleolus are protrusions from the lower leg bones that we know as "ankle" bones. The tarsals are the ankle bones, and the metatarsals (meta- means "beyond") are the bones just beyond the tarsals.

may be referred to as the "ankle bones," but they are really part of the tibia and fibula. The heel bone, or **calcaneus**, is one of the larger bones in the foot. Figure 5-10 shows the bones of the ankle and foot.

JOINTS

A **joint** (from the Latin *junctio*, meaning "junction") is simply a "meeting place" between bones. Some joints, such as the knee and elbow joints, are highly movable (articulating), and some are capable of little or no movement. A joint with no movement is called a **synarthrosis** (syn- is a prefix meaning "together, joined"; arthr/o is a root meaning "joint"; -osis is a suffix meaning "condition of"). A joint with little movement is called an **amphiarthrosis** (amphi- is a prefix meaning "on both sides"). Any of the suture joints in the cranium would be a good example of a synarthrosis, and the vertebral bodies within the spinal column are examples of amphiarthroses.

A joint that has free movement is called a **diarthrosis** or a **synovial joint**. The spaces within each synovial joint are filled with a viscous (thick) liquid called **synovial fluid**. Although the spaces in even a large joint are so tiny that less than 1/100th of an ounce of synovial fluid is needed to fill each one, the fluid is needed to lubricate the joint as it moves and to cushion it against shock. The synovial joints permit a variety of movements. The knee and elbow joints, for example, are synovial joints and are called "hinge joints." They provide **flexion** and **extension**. The ball and socket joint of the shoulder, also a synovial joint, provides a range of motions including rotation. Figure 5-11 shows the various movements of the synovial joints, and Table 5-1 describes their various movements.

Cartilage, a precursor to bone tissue, is classified as connective tissue, but the term is included here because cartilage enables movement (articulation) in the synovial joints.

Bursae (singular: **bursa**) are found wherever tendons or ligaments impinge on other tissues and consist of spaces within connective tissue that are filled with synovial fluid. **Bursitis** has become a common English word that means "inflammation of a bursa," which may be, but is not always, connected to a joint cavity.

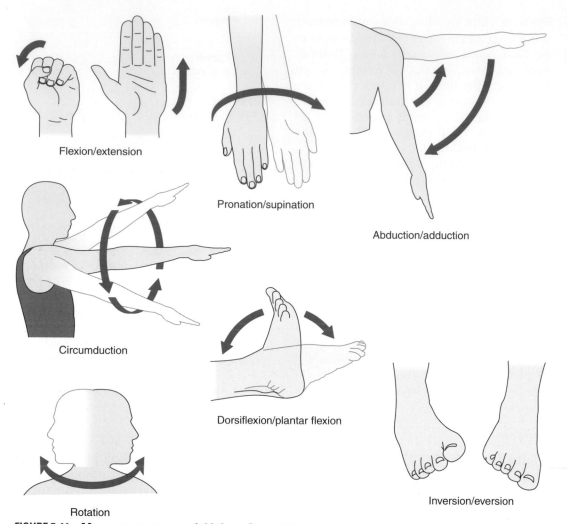

Flexion/extension

Pronation/supination

Abduction/adduction

Circumduction

Dorsiflexion/plantar flexion

Inversion/eversion

Rotation

FIGURE 5-11   Movements at synovial joints. Synovial joints are more freely moving joints. From Cohen BJ, Taylor J. Memmler's Structure and Function of the Human Body, 8th Ed. Baltimore: Lippincott Williams & Wilkins, 2005.

Table 5-1   Movements of Synovial Joints

Movement	Description
abduction	movement away from the midline of the body
adduction	movement toward the midline of the body
circumduction	movement in a circular direction from a central point
dorsiflexion	backward bending as of the hand or foot
eversion	turning outward
extension	movement that brings the limb into a straight position
flexion	bending or being bent
inversion	turning inward
plantar flexion	bending the sole of the foot or pointing the toes downward
pronation	to turn downward or backward as with the hand or foot
rotation	moving around a central axis
supination	turning the palm or foot upward

Practice and Practitioners

There are a number of specialists who work in the branch of **orthopedic** medicine (orth/o means "straight" or "correct"; ped comes from the Greek word *pais*, meaning "child"). These specialists diagnose and treat patients with musculoskeletal disorders. Orthopedic physicians employ medical, physical, and surgical methods to ensure the correct functioning of the skeletal system. They may coordinate patient care with physical and occupational therapists or specialists in sports medicine.

Another medical specialist who works in this field is a **rheumatologist** (rheum/o, rheumat/o means "to flow"), which is a physician who specialize in the treatment of joint disorders such as arthritic conditions. This specialist works with patients who have rheumatoid arthritis or other systemic (involves the entire body) connective tissue disorders.

Disorders and Treatments

Disorders of the skeletal system can be attributed to several causes including trauma, disease, neoplasms, joint disorders, and disorders of the spine. Assessments can be made by a variety of diagnostic tests such as X-rays, bone scans, certain hematologic laboratory studies, and noninvasive or surgical procedures. We will discuss these procedures as they relate to each class of disorder.

Trauma to the skeletal system frequently produces a **sprain** (tear in a ligament or the fibrous tissues that connects two bones) or **fracture** (break in the bone). A sprain is usually quite painful and results in swelling, tenderness, and sometimes discoloration over the affected area. X-rays of the injured bone can detect a break. In some cases, an **MRI** (magnetic resonance imaging), which is a noninvasive radiologic procedure, is needed for a detailed view of the injury. Sometimes **arthroscopy** (arthr/o means "joint"; -scopy means "examination with an instrument") is required. This procedure involves insertion of a scope into the joint for direct visual examination (Fig. 5-12).

A fracture or broken bone can include a deformity, pain, and tenderness. Complications may set in depending on the nature of the break. If the fracture is a simple or **closed fracture**, then there is no wound or open skin. If the broken bone protrudes through the skin, then it is called an open or **compound** fracture. A compound fracture is more severe and can lead to infection. **Osteomyelitis** (oste/o means "bone"; myel/o means "marrow"; -itis is a suffix meaning "inflammation") is an inflammation or infection of the bone caused by bacteria entering through a wound or carried by the blood into the bone. Intense antibiotic treatment is usually required to eradicate an infection.

Treatment of the fracture consists of **reduction** or realignment of the broken bones. This may be accomplished through the use of **traction** (using elastics or pulley and weights to maintain alignment) or may include the use of surgically placed rods, plates, and/or screws. Immobilization of the bone during the healing process is achieved with a cast or splint. Table 5-2 lists the most common types of fractures.

Osteoporosis (-porosis is a condition of being porous) is a bone disorder that is

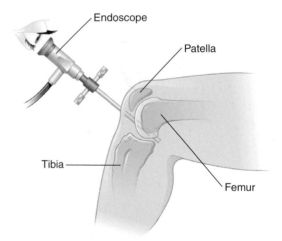

FIGURE 5-12 Arthroscopic examination of the knee. An endoscope or arthroscope (arthr/o means "joint"; -scopy is a suffix meaning "to examine with a viewing instrument") is inserted between projections at the end of the femur to view the interior of the knee. From Cohen BJ. Medical Terminology: An Illustrated Guide, 5th Ed. Philadelphia: Lippincott Williams & Wilkins, 2007.

Table 5-2   Common Fractures

Fracture	Description	Example
closed	simple fracture with no open wound	
Colles	break in the distal end of the radius (wrist)	
comminuted	break in which the bone is crushed or splintered	
compression	fracture or break caused by a squeezing or opposing force; loss of height in a vertebra due to disease or trauma	
greenstick	incomplete break; one side of the bone is broken and the other is bent	

Table 5-2 Common Fractures *(continued)*

Fracture	Description	Example
impacted	break where one bone fragment is pushed or driven into another	
oblique	break is at an angle to the bone	
open	skin is broken through the fracture; bone protrudes through the skin	
Pott	fracture of the distal end of the fibula	
spiral	break is S-shaped, usually caused by twisting injury	

(continues)

TABLE 5-2   Common Fractures *(continued)*

Fracture	Description	Example
transverse	break is straight across the bone, at a right angle to the long axis of the bone	

exhibited by a decrease in bone density and mass. This disease is frequently seen in older individuals, more commonly in postmenopausal women with estrogen deficiency. Compression fractures of the vertebrae resulting in **kyphosis** (humpback) and loss of height are characteristic. Treatment may include estrogen supplements, weight-bearing exercises, and dietary supplements.

Two other bone disorders are **rickets** and **osteomalacia** (oste/o means "bone"; -malacia is a suffix that means "softening"). These two conditions occur from a deficit of vitamin D and the resultant lack of calcium absorption. Rickets (skeletal deformities, particularly bowed legs) is seen in children who have soft bones caused by poor calcification, the result of a vitamin D deficit. Osteomalacia is seen in adults who have poor vitamin D absorption as well, resulting in compression fractures of the vertebrae.

Neoplasms or tumors of the bone may be primary or secondary (from other sites in the body). **Osteosarcoma** (oste/o means "bone"; sarc/o means "flesh") is a highly malignant (spreads easily) tumor of the bone. It is more commonly seen in children, and treatment may require amputation of the limb. **Chondrosarcoma** (chondr/o means "cartilage"; sarc/o means "flesh"; -oma means "tumor") is a tumor that arises from the cartilage and is more often seen in adults.

Joint disorders include various types of **arthritis** (arthr/o means "joint"; -itis means "inflammation"), which can impair joint function and cause disability at all ages. Arthritis is a general term that is widely used to denote joint inflammation. General wear and tear on joints causes a gradual degeneration of the cartilage and may involve the weight-bearing joints such as the hips, knees, and fingers. This type of arthritis is called **osteoarthritis** (oste/o means "bone"; arthr/o means "joint"; -itis means "inflammation"), or **OA**. Symptoms include pain and swelling in the joints. Treatment may include medication for pain and inflammation and/or physical therapy. If fluid accumulates in the joint, an **arthrocentesis** (arthr/o means "joint"; -centesis is a suffix meaning "to puncture") may be necessary to drain the fluid and relieve the pressure in the joint.

Rheumatoid arthritis (rheumat/o means "to flow"; -oid means "resemblance of"; arthr/o means "joint"; -itis means "inflammation"), or **RA**, is a systemic inflammatory joint disorder

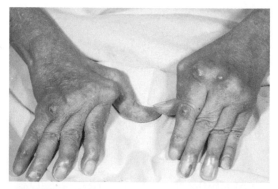

FIGURE 5-13   Advanced rheumatoid arthritis. The hands show swelling of the joints and deviation of the fingers. From Cohen BJ. Medical Terminology: An Illustrated Guide, 5th Ed. Philadelphia: Lippincott Williams & Wilkins, 2007.

commonly seen in women (Fig. 5-13). It is thought to be based on an immunologic abnormality that causes an inflammatory response with subsequent tissue destruction. It usually begins in small joints such as the fingers and progresses to weight-bearing joints. Chronic inflammation and fluid accumulation in the joint causes swelling and pain. Deformities of the joints occur in advanced stages. Treatments consist of medication to reduce pain and inflammation, rest, and physical therapy.

Anyone who has ever had low back pain knows how debilitating and limiting it can be to normal activity. Disorders of the spine can cause severe pain and limit mobility. A disc that protrudes into the spinal canal and puts pressure on the spinal nerve is called a **herniated disc**. It can be diagnosed with a **CT scan** (noninvasive test using computed tomography), **MRI** (magnetic resonance imaging), or a **myelogram** (myel/o means "marrow" or "spinal cord"; -gram means "a record of"). Medications are used to reduce the inflammation and decrease pain and muscle spasms. Rest is often encouraged along with strengthening exercises, depending on the extent of the herniation.

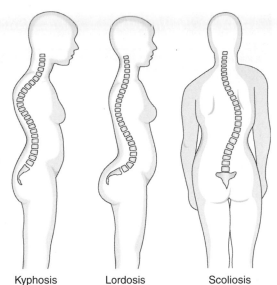

Kyphosis   Lordosis   Scoliosis

FIGURE 5-14   Curvatures of the spine. Kyphosis is an exaggerated thoracic curve; lordosis is an exaggerated lumbar curve; scoliosis is a sideways curve in any region. From Cohen BJ. Medical Terminology: An Illustrated Guide, 5th Ed. Philadelphia: Lippincott Williams & Wilkins, 2007.

Other spinal disorders may involve curvature of the spine. Causes include paralysis, disc degeneration, diseases, osteoporosis, or a congenital transmission. As mentioned earlier, kyphosis, which can occur as a result of osteoporosis, causes a humpback. **Lordosis** (comes from the Greek word *lordos*, which means "to bend backward") is sometimes known as "swayback" and involves the lumbar region. **Scoliosis** (scoli/o means "crooked"; -osis means "abnormal condition") is a sideways curvature of the spine that may occur in any region of the spine (Fig. 5-14).

Many skeletal disorders require surgical intervention and physical therapy with pharmacologic agents. The following drug classifications are some of the more common ones used to attain therapeutic responses in bone disorders.

Pharmacology

Most people who have bone pain find it very debilitating. They often take **analgesics** (an- is a prefix meaning "without"; algesia is a root meaning "without sensation") or other medication to relieve the pain. Examples of over-the-counter analgesics include aspirin (Bayer), acetaminophen (Tylenol), and ibuprofen (Motrin, Advil). Strong pain medications, or **narcotics** (narc/o means "to sleep"), are derived from the opium plant or are made synthetically. They relieve severe pain but can be addicting. Examples of narcotics include morphine and Demerol.

Anti-inflammatory agents, another drug classification, are also useful in treating skeletal system disorders. These are frequently taken with joint disorders, such as arthritis, or an injury, such as a sprain, to reduce swelling. **NSAIDs (nonsteroidal anti-inflammatory drugs)** are used to treat the inflammatory response. Naproxen (Aleve) and ibuprofen (Motrin, Advil) are examples of drugs found in this classification.

Abbreviation Table • The Skeletal System

ABBREVIATION	MEANING
ACL	anterior cruciate ligament
C (C1, C2, etc.)	cervical
CT	computed tomography
CTS	carpal tunnel syndrome
Fx	fracture
L (L1, L2, etc.)	lumbar
LE	lower extremity
RA	rheumatoid arthritis
ROM	range of motion
S	sacral
T	thoracic
THR	total hip replacement
TKA	total knee arthroplasty
TKR	total knee replacement
Tx	traction

Study Table • The Skeletal System

TERM AND PRONUNCIATION	ANALYSIS	MEANING
Structure and Function		
amphiarthrosis (AM-fee-ar-THRO-sihs)	*amphi-* (both sides); *arthr/o* (joint); *-osis* (abnormal condition)	joint with little movement
appendicular (APP-ehn-DIHK-yu-lahr)	adjective referring to something that is added or attached	having to do with something attached
axial (AX-ee-uhl)	adjective form of axis, a common English word	straight line through a physical body
brachial (BRAY-kee-uhl)	*brachi/o* (arm); *-al* (adjective suffix)	having to do with an arm
bursa (BUR-sah)	a Latin word meaning "purse"	sac-like connective structure found in some joints; protects moving parts from friction

TERM AND PRONUNCIATION	ANALYSIS	MEANING
calcaneus (kal-KAY-nee-uhs)	Latin word for heel	the heel bone
carpal (KAR-pahl)	adjective form of carpus (wrist)	a wrist bone
cartilage (CAR-tih-lij)	from the Latin word *cartilagin* (gristle)	dense, flexible connective tissue
cervical (SUR-vih-kuhl)	*cervic/o* (neck); *-al* (adjective suffix)	adjective describing the vertebrae (C1–C7) in the neck region; also used in connection with the uterus, which is part of the female reproductive system
cervix (SUR-vix); the adjective is cervical	Latin word for neck	neck (also the neck of the uterus)
chondrogenesis (konn-droh-JENN-uh-sihs)	*chondr/o* (cartilage); *-genesis* (origin)	formation of cartilage
chondroid (KONN-droyd)	*chondr/o* (cartilage); *-oid* (similar to)	resembling cartilage
clavicle (KLAV-ih-cuhl); the adjective is clavicular (kla-VIK-yu-luhr)	from the Latin word *clavicula* (a small key)	the collarbone
coccyx (KOK-six); the adjective is coccygeal (kok-SIH-jee-uhl)	from the Greek word *kokkyx* (cuckoo)	the tailbone, made up of the four fused vertebrae at the base of the spinal column
cranial bones (KRAY-nee-uhl)	*crani/o* from the Greek word *kranion* (skull); *-al* (adjective form)	collectively, and along with other minor bones, the frontal bone, two parietal bones, two temporal bones, and the occipital bone
diaphysis (dye-AFF-ih-sihs)	a Greek word (growing between)	shaft of the long bone
diarthrosis (dy-ar-THRO-sihs)	a Greek word (articulation)	synonym for synovial joint
endosteum (ehn-DOST-ee-um)	*endo-* (inside); *oste/o* (Greek word for bone)	inner membrane layer of the bone
epiphysis (eh-PIFF-ih-sihs)	*epi-* (upon); *-physis* (growth)	end of the long bone (distal, proximal)
extension (ehx-TEN-shun)	a common English word	to straighten a joint
femur (FEE-muhr)	a Latin word (thigh)	thighbone
fibula (FIHB-yu-lah)	a Latin word (clasp)	the lateral leg bone
flexion (FLEHX-shun)	from the Latin verb *flecto* (bend)	bending a joint
frontal bone (FRUN-tuhl)	frontal (adjective form of English noun: front)	one of the six main cranial bones

(continued)

TERM AND PRONUNCIATION	ANALYSIS	MEANING
humerus (HUE-muh-ruhs)	a Latin word (shoulder)	the long bone extending from the shoulder to the elbow
ilium (IL-ee-uhm)	a Latin word (flank)	one of the three bones fused together to form the hip bone
ischium (IS-kee-uhm)	a Latin word (hip)	one of the three bones fused together to form the hip bone
lumbar (LUM-bar)	from *lumbus* (Latin for loin); *-ar* (adjective suffix)	adjective describing the vertebrae (L1–L5) in the lower spinal column
malleolus (mahl-ee-OHL-us)	from the Latin word *malleus* (hammer)	bony protrusion on either side of the ankle (medial and lateral)
mandible (MAN-dih-buhl); the adjective is mandibular (man-DIB-yu-luhr)	a Latin word (jaw)	the lower jawbone
maxilla (MAX-ih-luh); the adjective is maxillary (MAX-ih-lahr-ee)	a Latin word (jawbone)	the bone above the upper teeth
medullary cavity (MED-yul-her-ee)	an adjective form of *medulla* (Latin for marrow)	bone marrow cavity
metacarpal (MEHT-uh-KAR-puhl)	*meta-* (beyond); carp from *carpus* (wrist); *-al* (adjective suffix)	short for metacarpal bone; one of the five bones extending from the wrist to the first knuckle in each hand
metatarsals (MEH-tah-TAHR-sahlz)	*meta-* (beyond); tarsal from *tarsos* (flat surface); *-al* (adjective suffix)	short for metatarsal bones; the bones between the tarsals and the phalanges (toes) of the foot
nasal bone (NAY-zuhl)	*nas/o* (nose); *-al* (adjective suffix)	a facial bone (nose)
occipital bone (ox-SIP-it-uhl)	*occiput* (Latin for back of the head); *-al* (adjective suffix)	one of the six main cranial bones
os coxae (OSS COX-ay)	*os* (Latin for bone); *coxae* (Latin: genitive case for hip)	hip bone
osseous (OSS-ee-us)	from the Latin word *osseus* (bony); *-ous* (adjective suffix)	bone tissue
ossification (OSS-ihf-ih-KAY-shun)	*oss* (bone); *facio* (Latin verb for make)	bone formation
osteocytes (OSS-tee-oh-syt)	*oste/o* (bone); *-cyte* (cell)	mature bone cells

TERM AND PRONUNCIATION	ANALYSIS	MEANING
osteogenesis (oss-tee-oh-JENN-uh-suhs)	*oste/o* (bone); *-genesis* (origin)	formation of bone
parietal bones (puh-RY-uh-tuhl)	from a Latin word *paries* (wall) and *-al* (adjective suffix)	two of the six main cranial bones
patella (pah-TELL-ah)	a Latin word (small plate)	kneecap
pectoral girdle (pek-TOR-uhl)	from *pectus*, a Latin word (chest); *-al* (adjective suffix)	the shoulder girdle
periosteum (pair-ee-OST-ee-um)	*peri-* (around); *oste/o* (bone)	membrane that surrounds the outside of the bone
phalanges (FAY-lanj-es)	plural of the Greek word *phalanx* (a column of soldiers)	fingers (singular form is phalanx)
pubis (PYU-bihs)	short for "os pubis"; from the Latin word *pubertas* (grown up)	one of the three bones fused together to form the hip bone
radius (RAY-dee-uhs); the adjective is radial (RAY-dee-uhl)	a Latin word (a rod or a spoke of a wheel)	one of the two bones (the other is the ulna) extending from the elbow to the wrist
sacrum (SAK-rum); the adjective is sacral (SAK-ruhl)	short for "os sacrum," a Latin word meaning sacred	bone formed from five vertebrae fused together near the base of the spinal column
scapula (SKAP-yu-luh); plural is scapulae (SKAP-yu-lay); the adjectival form is scapular (SKAP-yu-luhr)	a Latin word for shoulder blade	the shoulder blade
sternum (STUR-nuhm)	from a Greek word *sternon* (chest)	the breastbone
suture (SOO-chur)	from the Latin word *sutura* (seam)	in the skeletal system, a fibrous membrane joining bones, especially the cranial bones
synarthrosis (syn-AR-thr-oh-sihs)	*syn-* (together); *arthr/o* (joint); *-osis* (condition)	joint with no movement
synovial (sy-NOH-vee-ahl)	*syn-* (together); Latin *ovum* (egg); *-al* (adjective suffix)	adjective form of synovia, a synonym for synovial fluid
talus (TAY-luhs)	a Latin word (ankle)	the bone in the ankle that articulates with the tibia and fibula
tarsals (TAR-sahlz)	from Greek *tarsos* (a flat surface, sole of the foot)	the bones of the sole of the foot

(continued)

TERM AND PRONUNCIATION	ANALYSIS	MEANING
tarsus (TAR-suhs)	from Greek *tarsos* (a flat surface)	instep or sole of the foot; collectively, the seven bones making up the bottom of the foot
temporal bones (TEMP-uh-ruhl)	from the Latin *tempus* (time, temple)	two of the six main cranial bones; located on the side of the head near the ears
thoracic (tho-RASS-ik)	from the Greek *thorax* (breastplate, the chest)	adjective form of thorax
thorax (THOR-ax)	from Greek *thorax* (breastplate, the chest)	chest
tibia (TIH-bee-ah); the adjective form is tibial (TIH-bee-al)	a Latin word (flute)	shin bone
ulna (ULL-nah); the adjective is ulnar (ULL-nahr)	a Latin word (elbow; forearm)	one of the two bones (the other is the radius) extending from the elbow to the wrist
vertebra (VUR-tuh-bruh); plural is vertebrae (VUR-tuh-bray)	From the Latin *verto* (to turn)	one of the 33 segments making up the spinal column
xiphoid process (ZEYE-foyd)	from the Greek *xipho* (sword), *-oid* (resemblance to)	bony, dagger-like structure at the lower end of the sternum
zygomatic bones (ZI-go-MAT-ik)	from Greek *zygoma* (bolt or bar); *-tic* (adjective suffix)	a facial bone (cheek, one of two)

Common Disorders

arthralgia (ar-THRAL-jee-uh)	*arthr/o* (joint); *-algia* (pain)	pain in a joint
arthritis (ar-THRY-tuhs)	*arthr/o* (joint); *-itis* (inflammation)	inflammation of a joint
arthrocele (ARTH-roh-seel)	*arthr/o* (joint); *-cele* (hernia)	swelling of a joint
arthrochondritis (ARTH-roh-konn-DRY-tihs)	*arthr/o* (joint); *chondr/o* (cartilage); *-itis* (inflammation)	inflammation of cartilage in a joint
arthrodynia (arth-roh-DINN-ee-uh)	*arthr/o* (joint); *-dynia* (pain)	pain in a joint
arthropathy (ar-THROP-ah- thee)	*arthr/o* (joint); *-pathy* (disease or disorder)	any disorder of a joint
arthrosis (ar-THROW-sihs)	*arthr/o* (joint); *-osis* (abnormal condition of)	disintegration of a joint
brachialgia (BRAY-kee-AL-jee-uh)	*brachi/o* (arm); *-algia* (pain)	pain in the arm

TERM AND PRONUNCIATION	ANALYSIS	MEANING
bursitis (burr-SY-tihs)	*burs/o* (bursa); *-itis* (inflammation)	inflammation of a bursa
carpal tunnel syndrome (KAR-puhl TUN-uhl SINN-druhm)	*carp/o* (wrist); *-al* (adjective suffix); *syn-* (together); from the Greek *dromos* (a running)	condition characterized by wrist pain, often occurring during sleep
chondrodynia (konn-droh-DINN-ee-uh)	*chondr/o* (cartilage); *-dynia* (pain)	pain originating in cartilage
chondromalacia (konn-droh-muh-LAY-she-uh)	*chondr/o* (cartilage); *-malacia* (softening)	softening of cartilage
chondropathy (kon-DROP-ah-thee)	*chondr/o* (cartilage); *-pathy* (disease or disorder)	disease of cartilage
chondrosarcoma (KONN-droh-sar-KOH-ma)	*chondr/o* (cartilage); *sarc/o* (flesh); *-oma* (tumor)	malignant tumor arising from the cartilage
compound fracture (KOM-pound FRAK-chur)	from the Latin *fractura* (a break)	break in the bone where the bone comes through the skin; open fracture
costalgia (koss-TAL-jee-uh)	*cost/o* (rib); *-algia* (pain)	pain in a rib(s)
costochondritis (KOSS-toh-kon-DRY-tihs)	*cost/o* (rib); *chondr/o* (cartilage); *-itis* (inflammation)	inflammation of rib cartilage
dactylalgia (DAKK-tihl-AL-jee-uh)	*dactyl/o* (finger, toe); *-algia* (pain)	pain in a finger (or toe)
dactylodynia (DAKK-tihl-oh-DINN-ee-uh)	*dactyl/o* (finger, toe); *-dynia* (pain)	pain in a finger (or toe)
dactylomegaly (DAKK-tih-lo-MEG-uh-lee); more often called megadactyly (meg-uh-DAKK-tuh-lee), probably because "mega" has so many common uses as an English prefix	*dactyl/o* (finger, toe); *-megaly* (enlargement)	enlargement of one or more fingers or toes
fracture (FRAK-chur)	from Latin word *fractura* (break)	break in a bone
herniated disc (HER-nee-ay-ted disk)	from Latin word *hernia* (rupture); *disc/o* (disk)	protrusion of a fragmented intervertebral disc in the intervertebral foramen with potential compression of a nerve
kyphosis (ky-FOH-sihs)	*kyph/o* (humped); *-sis* (condition)	humpback; anteriorly concave curvature of the thoracic and sacral region of the spine

(continued)

TERM AND PRONUNCIATION	ANALYSIS	MEANING
lordosis (lohr-DOH-sihs)	from the Greek word *lordosis* (a bending backwards)	swayback; abnormal anteriorly convex curvature of the lumbar part of the spine
ostealgia (oss-tee-AL-jee-uh)	*oste/o* (bone); *-algia* (pain)	pain in a bone
osteitis (oss-tee-EYE-tihs)	*oste/o* (bone); *-itis* (inflammation)	inflammation of bone
osteochondritis (OSS-tee-oh-konn-DRY-tihs)	*oste/o* (bone); *chondr/o* (cartilage); *-itis* (inflammation)	inflammation of bone and associated cartilage
osteodynia (oss-tee-oh-DINN-ee-uh)	*oste/o* (bone); *-dynia* (pain)	pain in a bone
osteomalacia (OSS-tee-oh-muh-LAY-she-uh)	*oste/o* (bone); *-malacia* (softening)	softening of bone
osteomyelitis (OSS-tee-oh-my-eh-LY-tihs)	*oste/o* (bone); *myel/o* (marrow); *-itis* (inflammation)	inflammation of bone marrow
osteopenia (oss-tee-oh-PEEN-ee-uh)	*oste/o* (bone); *-penia* (deficiency)	abnormally low bone density
osteoporosis (OSS-tee-oh-puh-RO-sihs)	*oste/o* (bone); *por/o* (porous); *-sis* (condition)	atrophy and thinning of bone tissue
osteosarcoma (OSS-tee-oh-sar-KOH-ma)	*oste/o* (bone); *sarc/o* (flesh-like); *-oma* (tumor)	highly malignant tumor of the bone
rheumatoid arthritis (ROO-mah-toid ar-THRY-tuhs)	from the Greek word *rheuma* (flux); *-oid* (resemblance of)	systemic disease occurring more often in women that affects the connective tissue; involves many joints, especially those of the hands and feet
rickets (RIH-kehts)	common English word	disease due to vitamin D deficiency characterized by deficient calcification and soft bones associated with skeletal deformities
scoliosis (skohl-ee-OH-sihs)	*scoli/o* (twisted); *-sis* (condition)	lateral curvature of the spine; S-shaped curvature
sprain (SPRAYN)	common English word	injury to a ligament
syndrome (SIN-drum)	*syn-* (together); from the Greek *dromos* (running)	collection of signs and symptoms occurring together and characterizing a medical condition

TERM AND PRONUNCIATION	ANALYSIS	MEANING
Practice and Practitioners		
orthopedics (or-thoh-PEE-diks)	*orth/o* (straight or correct); *ped-* (child); *-ic* (adjective suffix)	the medical specialty concerned with the development, preservation, restoration, and function of the musculoskeletal system
orthopedic surgeon (or-thoh-PEE-dik)	*orth/o* (straight or correct); *ped-* (child); *-ic* (adjective suffix)	a physician in the field of orthopedics (can be M.D. or D.O.)
rheumatologist (ROO-mah-tah-lo-gist)	*rheumat/o* (flux); *-logist* (one who studies a certain field)	physician who treats joint and connective tissue disorders such as arthritis
rheumatology (ROO-mah-tah-lo-gee)	*rheumat/o* (flux); *-logy* (the study of)	field of specialty that deals with joints and connective tissue disorders
Diagnosis and Treatment		
analgesics (an-al-GEE-ziks)	*an-* (absence); from the Greek word *gesis* (sensation)	medication used to relieve pain
anti-inflammatory (AN-ty-in-FLAMM-ah-tohr-ee)	*anti-* (against); inflammatory (common English word)	medication used to reduce inflammation (example: used to reduce joint inflammation in arthritis)
arthrocentesis (arth-roh-senn-TEE-sihs)	*arthr/o* (joint); *-centesis* (surgical puncture for aspiration)	removing fluid from a joint
arthrogram (ARTH-roh-gram)	*arthr/o* (joint); *-gram* (record or picture)	radiograph of a joint
arthrometry (arth-ROM-uh-tree)	*arthr/o* (joint); *-metry* (process of measuring)	measurement of the amount of movement in a joint
arthroscope (ARTH-roh-skope)	*arthr/o* (joint); *-scope* (instrument for viewing)	device used in arthroscopy
arthroscopy (ahr-THRAW-skoh-pee)	*arthr/o* (joint); *-scopy* (use of instrument for viewing)	examination of the interior of a joint
CT scan	abbreviation for computed tomography	noninvasive imaging test; imaging anatomic information from a cross-sectional plane of the body
MRI	abbreviation for magnetic resonance imaging	a diagnostic radiograph in which the magnetic nuclei of a patient are aligned in a magnetic field; these signals are converted into tomographic images

(continued)

TERM AND PRONUNCIATION	ANALYSIS	MEANING
myelogram (MY-el-loh-gram)	*myel/o* (bone marrow); *-gram* (record or picture)	X-ray of the spinal column using contrast medium
narcotic (nahr-KAH-tik)	*narc/o* (sleep)	drug derived from opium with potent analgesic effects; potential effects of dependency through prolonged use
NSAIDs	abbreviation for nonsteroidal anti-inflammatory drugs	medication that exerts analgesic and anti-inflammatory actions
reduction (ree-DUK-shun)	common English word	correcting a fracture by realigning the bone pieces
traction (TRAK-shun)	common English word	using elastics or pulley and weights to maintain alignment; a pulling or dragging force exerted on a limb in a distal direction

Surgical Procedures

arthrectomy (ar-THREK-tuh-mee)	*arthr/o* (joint); *-ectomy* (surgical removal)	excision of a joint
arthroplasty (ARTH-roh-plass-tee)	*arthr/o* (joint); *-plasty* (surgical repair)	surgical repair of a joint
arthrotomy (ar-THRAWT-uh-mee)	*arthr/o* (joint); *-tomy* (cutting operation)	surgical incision into a joint
carpectomy (kar-PEK-tuh-me)	*carp/o* (wrist); *-ectomy* (surgical removal)	excision of part of the wrist
chondroplasty (KONN-droh-plass-tee)	*chondr/o* (cartilage); *-plasty* (surgical repair)	surgical repair of cartilage
costectomy (koss-TEK-tuh-mee)	*cost/o* (rib); *-ectomy* (surgical removal)	excision of a rib
ostectomy (oss-TECK-tuh-mee)	*oste/o* (bone); *-ectomy* (surgical removal)	surgical removal of bone
osteoplasty (OSS-tee-oh-plass-tee)	*oste/o* (bone); *-plasty* (surgical repair)	surgical repair of bone
osteorrhaphy (OSS-tee-oh-raff-ee)	*oste/o* (bone); *-rrhaphy* (surgical suturing)	suturing together the parts of a broken bone
osteotomy (oss-tee-AW-tuh-mee)	*oste/o* (bone); *-tomy* (cutting operation)	surgical cutting of bone
vertebrectomy (ver-tuh-BREKK-tuh-mee)	from the Latin word *verto* (to turn); *-ectomy* (surgical removal)	excision (resectioning) of a vertebra

EXERCISES

EXERCISE 5-1   Figure Labeling: Skeleton

Write the name of each numbered part in the corresponding line below.

calcaneus	facial bones	mandible	pelvis	sternum
carpals	femur	metacarpals	radius	tarsals
clavicle	fibula	metatarsals	ribs	tibia
costal cartilage	humerus	patella	sacrum	ulna
cranium	ilium	phalanges	scapula	vertebral column

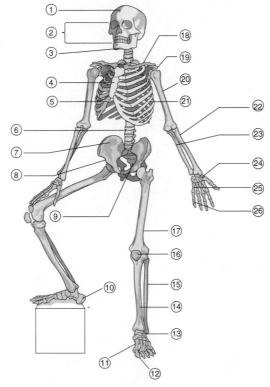

1. _____   10. _____   19. _____

2. _____   11. _____   20. _____

3. _____   12. _____   21. _____

4. _____   13. _____   22 _____

5. _____   14. _____   23. _____

6. _____   15. _____   24. _____

7. _____   16. _____   25. _____

8. _____   17. _____   26. _____

9. _____   18. _____

EXERCISE 5-2   Figure Labeling: Long Bone

Write the name of each numbered part in the corresponding line below.

cartilage	diaphysis	epiphyseal line	periosteum	spongy bone
compact bone	distal epiphysis	medullary canal	proximal epiphysis	yellow marrow

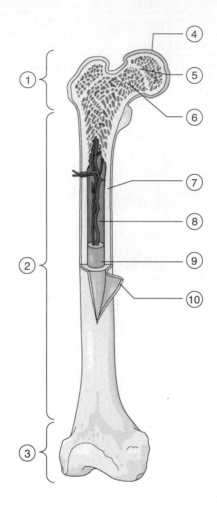

1. _____   6. _____

2. _____   7. _____

3. _____   8. _____

4. _____   9. _____

5. _____   10. _____

EXERCISE 5-3   Word Building

Use the word elements listed to build the terms defined below.

-algia = pain	-ectomy = removal	-logy = study	-plasty = plastic repair
arthr/o = joint	electr/o = electricity	-malacia = softening	-porosis = porous
cardi/o = heart	-gram = record	my/o = muscle	sarc/o = flesh
chondr/o = cartilage	inter- = between	myel/o = marrow/spine	-scopy = visual exam
cost/o = rib	-itis = inflammation	-oma = tumor	
-desis = fusion/fixation	kinesi/o = movement	oste/o = bone	

_____ means inflammation of the bone and bone marrow.

_____ means visual examination of a joint.

_____ means abnormal softening of cartilage.

_____ means a radiograph of a joint.

_____ means the fusion or fixation of a joint.

_____ means the study of movement of body parts.

_____ means surgical repair of cartilage.

_____ means pertaining to the area between the ribs.

_____ means inflammation of the bone.

_____ means a highly malignant tumor of the bone.

_____ means surgical repair of a joint.

_____ means X-ray of the spine.

_____ means inflammation of the cartilage.

_____ mean bones with diminished density; porous.

_____ means pain in the ribs.

EXERCISE 5-4   Matching: Terms of Joint Movement

Match the terms in Column 1 with the best definitions in Column 2.

TERM

DEFINITION

1. _____ abduction

A. backward bending of hand or foot

2. _____ rotation

B. bending the foot toward the ground

3. _____ plantar flexion

C. straightening or stretching

4. _____ extension

D. motion around a central axis

5. _____ dorsiflexion

E. motion away from the body

6. _____ flexion

F. bending motion

7. _____ adduction

G. motion toward the body

EXERCISE 5-5   Matching: Types of Fractures

Match the terms in Column 1 with the best definitions in Column 2.

TERM

DEFINITION

1. _____ comminuted

A. break at an angle

2. _____ greenstick

B. S-shaped break

3. _____ compound

C. bone splintered or crushed

4. _____ simple

D. bone pressed into itself

5. _____ impacted

E. broken straight across bone

6. _____ transverse

F. skin has been broken along with the bone

7. _____ oblique

G. no open wound, broken bone

8. _____ spiral

H. bone only partially broken

EXERCISE 5-6 Fill in the Blank

Use the following terms in the questions that follow.

arthroplasty   osteoporosis   rheumatoid arthritis
arthrocentesis   osteosarcoma   rickets
laminectomy   polydactylism   scoliosis

1. Mrs. Thomas, age 82, is being treated for a broken hip. Her physician will be running tests for what potential degenerative bone ailment? _____

2. Bobbie, age 6 months, is being given orange juice and vitamin supplements to avoid what condition? _____

3. Baby Smith was born with an extra digit at the side of her left hand. The doctor assures her mother that this can easily be removed. What is this condition called? _____

4. Mr. Johnson's physician has discovered a tumor on his femur. He has been admitted to the hospital for a biopsy to rule out what type of bone cancer? _____

5. The school nurse has asked Janelle to bend over so that she may examine her back. What is the nurse looking for? _____

6. Susan Smith is 26 years old and has been experiencing chronic joint pain in her fingers. X-rays show a degeneration of the cartilage and joint deformities. What condition may Susan have? _____

7. Bob Williams, a former professional football player, has had numerous knee injuries over the years. His physician says he has to have his knee replaced. This type of surgery is called a(n) _____.

EXERCISE 5-7 Case Study

The underlined definitions refer to a medical term. Read the case study and replace the underlined definitions with an appropriate medical term. Write this term in the space provided below.

COMPLAINT: Mrs. Smith, an 82-year-old female, was out walking her dog on a snowy day. She slipped on a patch of ice, fell, and incurred a wrist and hip injury.

ASSESSMENT: In the emergency room, a (1) <u>physician who treats and diagnoses skeletal conditions</u> examined her. He ordered X-rays of her right wrist and left hip. The X-rays revealed (2) <u>a wrist bone that was broken in many pieces</u>. She (3) <u>could not flex or move her wrist much</u>. The hip bone was (4) <u>broken and pressed into another part of the bone</u>. The surgeon performed a (5) <u>realignment of the wrist bones</u>. He ordered that Mrs. Smith be placed into (6) <u>a treatment using elastics or pulley and weights to maintain alignment of her hip</u>. He ordered a (7) <u>very strong pain medication</u> to relieve her pain and also (8) <u>a drug to decrease the swelling</u> at the site of her fractures.

CASE STUDY QUESTIONS

1. _____ surgeon

2. _____ fracture

3. _____ (*Hint*: The acronym for this term is ROM.)

4. _____

5. _____

6. _____

7. _____

8. _____

EXERCISE 5-8 Crossword Puzzle: The Skeletal System

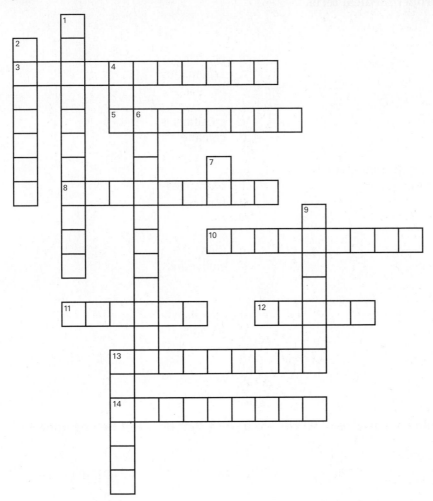

ACROSS

3. instrument used to view inside a joint
5. lower jaw bone
8. inflammation of a joint
10. fingers and toes
11. root for cartilage
12. root for cranium
13. heel bone
14. pain in a rib

DOWN

1. surgical repair of a bone
2. upper jaw bone
4. abbreviation for range of motion
6. joint pain
7. abbreviation for computed tomography
9. wrist bones
13. tailbone

CHAPTER 5 QUIZ

Identify the proper medical term.

1. Collar bone
   a. ischium
   b. ulna
   c. clavicle
   d. zygomatic

2. Bones of the hands
   a. tarsals
   b. metacarpals
   c. metatarsals
   d. calcaneus

3. Bones of the fingers and toes
   a. metatarsals
   b. carpals
   c. phalanges
   d. fibulas

4. Heel bone
   a. ilium
   b. zygomatic
   c. ulna
   d. calcaneus

5. Back bone/spine
   a. vertebrae
   b. temporals
   c. maxilla
   d. scapula

6. Shoulder blade
   a. scapula
   b. sternum
   c. maxilla
   d. scoliosis

Each of the following groups of words has a word that does not belong. Identify this term.

7. a. scoliosis	b. rickets	c. RA	d. diaphysis
8. a. humerus	b. fibula	c. radius	d. ulna
9. a. tibia	b. fibula	c. femur	d. ulna
10. a. deltoid	b. patella	c. sternum	d. carpal
11. a. sclerosis	b. kyphosis	c. scoliosis	d. lordosis
12. a. cervical	b. parietal	c. thoracic	d. lumbar
13. a. patella	b. sternum	c. phalanges	d. diaphragm
14. a. comminuted	b. insertion	c. compound	d. greenstick

Fill in the blank with the correct term.

15. An incision into the chest is termed _____.

16. The word that means "inflammation of a joint" is _____.

17. Aspiration of fluid from a joint by a needle puncture is a(n) _____.

18. The study and treatment of disorders of the musculoskeletal system is _____.

19. To "reduce" a fracture is to _____.

20. The specialist who treats disorders of the skeletal system is called a(n) _____.

CHAPTER 6

The Muscular System

LEARNING OBJECTIVES

Upon completion of this chapter, you should be able to:

- Identify the word elements of the muscular system.
- Give the terms for the three types of muscular tissue.
- Give the medical terms used to describe the function of muscles.
- Give the medical terms used for the main types of muscle movement.
- Build, spell, and pronounce medical terms that relate to the muscular system.
- Identify the terms related to disorders, treatments, and surgical procedures of the muscular system.
- Give the names of the major drug classifications used to treat muscular disorders.
- Identify and interpret selected abbreviations relating to the muscular system.
- Analyze and define the new terms introduced in this chapter.

Word Elements • Muscular System

WORD ELEMENT	REFERS TO
fasci/o	fibrous membrane
fibr/o	fiber
hemi-	half
kine-; kinesi/o	movement
ligament/o	ligament
muscul/o	muscle
my/o	muscle
para-	beside, beyond, near
-paresis	partial or incomplete paralysis
-plegia	paralysis
quadri-	four
sthen/o	strength
tend/o; tendin/o	tendon
ton/o	tone

An Overview of the Muscular System

The muscular system includes all of the muscles in our bodies: **skeletal**, such as the biceps and hamstrings muscles; **cardiac**, muscles of the heart; and **smooth**, such as the muscles in the stomach and bladder. Its main functions are to help maintain posture, produce heat, and help us move. There are three times as many muscles as there are bones in the human body. In fact, muscles make up about half of the average person's total body weight.

Structure and Function

Muscles are made up of fibers that are enclosed in a fibrous sheath of **fascia** (comes from the Latin word *fasces*, which means "a bundle"; therefore, this term means a bundle or band of tissue) and are attached to bones by **tendons** (tend/o means "tendon" or "to stretch"), which are made up of connective tissue (Fig. 6-1). **Ligaments**, from the Latin noun *ligament*, meaning "string," connect bones to bones and offer support to muscles.

Muscles have the ability to contract (shorten in length) and to relax. These two actions hold the body erect and make all movement possible, including all obvious activities, such as lifting objects, running, throwing a ball, and swinging a bat. However, muscles are also needed for seeing, talking, eating, digesting, breathing, smiling, frowning, blinking, and so on. Each muscle fiber receives its own nerve impulse and has its own supply of glycogen for energy.

TYPES OF MUSCLE TISSUE

As mentioned earlier, there are three types of muscles: skeletal, smooth, and cardiac (Fig. 6-2). Each type is discussed briefly in the following sections. Muscles can be characterized by their location, control action (voluntary or involuntary), and cell appearance (striated or nonstriated) (Fig. 6-3).

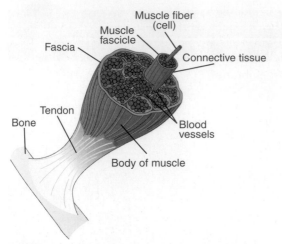

FIGURE 6-1   Structure of a skeletal muscle. Muscle cells are referred to as fibers that are held in bundles by connective tissue. A sheet of fascia covers the muscle. From Cohen BJ. Medical Terminology: An Illustrated Guide, 5th Ed. Philadelphia: Lippincott Williams & Wilkins, 2007.

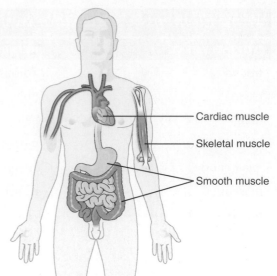

FIGURE 6-2   Types of muscles: skeletal, cardiac, and smooth. Smooth muscle makes up the wall of ducts and hollow organs, such as the stomach and intestine; cardiac muscle makes up the wall of the heart; skeletal muscle is attached to bones. From Cohen BJ. Medical Terminology: An Illustrated Guide, 5th Ed. Philadelphia: Lippincott Williams & Wilkins, 2007.

Comparison of the different types of muscle			
	Smooth	Cardiac	Skeletal
Location	Wall of hollow organs, vessels, respiratory passageways	Wall of heart	Attached to bones
Cell characteristics	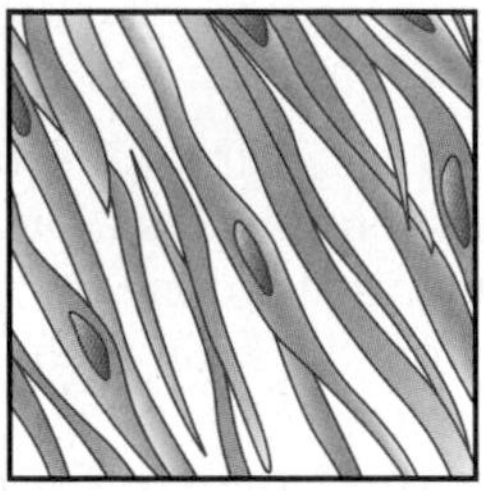 Tapered at each end, single nucleus, non-striated	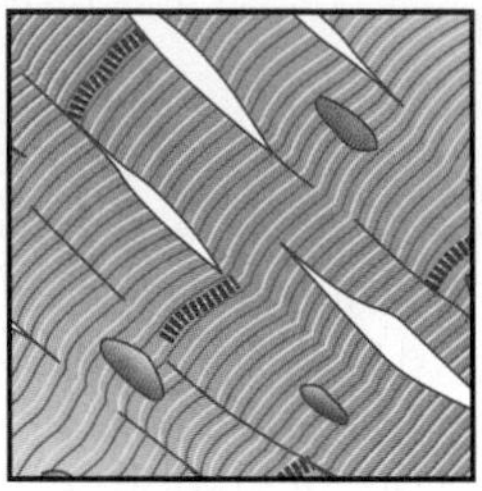 Branching networks, single nucleus, lightly striated	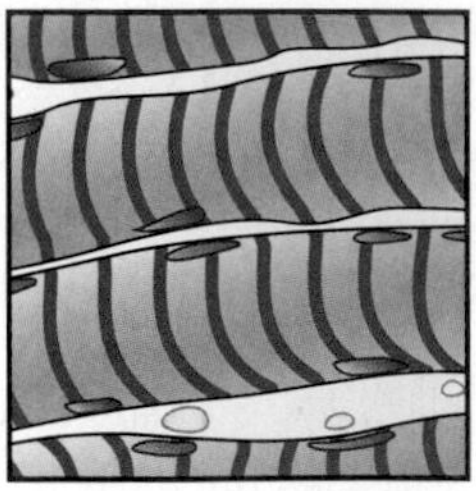 Long and cylindrical, multi-nucleated, heavily striated
Control	Involuntary	Involuntary	Voluntary

FIGURE 6-3   Comparison of muscle types. A comparison of the types of muscles, their location, cell characteristics, and type of control. From Cohen BJ, Wood DL. Memmler's The Human Body in Health and Disease, 9th Ed. Philadelphia: Lippincott Williams & Wilkins, 2000.

Skeletal Muscle

Of the three types of muscles, skeletal muscles form the largest group. There are more than 600 skeletal muscles responsible for movements in the body. These muscles are attached to bones and, during contraction, change the position or angles of the bones to which they attach, thus creating movement.

Skeletal muscle is also known as striated muscle because of the dark and light bands in the muscle fibers that create a "striped" or striated appearance. Skeletal muscle is responsible for voluntary movement, the generation of heat (accomplished through rapid small contractions known as shivering), and maintenance of posture.

Smooth Muscle

Smooth muscle is a nonstriated muscle and acts involuntarily. It is found in the blood vessels, respiratory passageways, and digestive tract, as well as in the walls of hollow internal organs. The functions of smooth muscle are to control and move substances through their passageways with wave-like motions, as well as to regulate the diameter of the openings of the vessels and hollow organs. The contents of the hollow organs may be expelled when the walls of the organs contract, as occurs in the uterus and urinary bladder during birth, urination, or elimination.

Cardiac Muscle

Cardiac muscle, also known as the **myocardial muscle** (my/o means "muscle"; cardi/o means "heart"), forms the muscular wall of the heart. It acts involuntarily and has a lightly striated appearance. The contraction and relaxation of the cardiac muscle is responsible for the heartbeat and pumping action of the heart. This subject will be discussed in greater detail in Chapter 9.

MUSCLE MOVEMENT

The skeletal muscles are stimulated by the nervous system and perform in groups or antagonistic pairs to accomplish movement. For example, the muscles in the posterior of the thigh flex the leg, while the muscles in the anterior of the thigh straighten the leg. Each skeletal muscle can be classified in terms of the following:

- **Prime mover:** contracts and produces movement.
- **Antagonist:** works in opposition to produce opposite movement (comes from the Greek word *antagonistes* meaning "competitor, opponent, rival"; anti- is a prefix meaning "against").

Table 6-1 describes the types of muscle movements.

Table 6-1   Types of Muscle Movements

Movement	Definition	Example
abduction	movement away from midline	moving the arms outward from the body
adduction	movement toward midline	return of the lifted arms to sides
eversion	turning outward	turning the sole of the foot outward
inversion	turning inward	turning the sole of the foot inward
extension	opening the angle of a joint	straightening of the knee
flexion	closing the angle of a joint	bending the knee
pronation	turning downward	turning the palm of the hand downward
supination	turning upward	turning the palm of the hand upward
dorsiflexion	bending backward	pointing the toes backward toward your nose
plantar flexion	bending the sole of the foot	pointing the toes downward
rotation	turning a body part on its own axis	turning the head

Practice and Practitioners

The medical specialists who treat disorders of the muscular system include **neurologists** (neur/o means "nerve"; -logist means "a practitioner of a medical specialty") and orthopedic surgeons, who also treat skeletal disorders, as noted in Chapter 5. A neurologist is a physician who specializes in the diagnosis and treatment of both the muscular system and the nervous system, and the area of study is called **neurology**. Many conditions involve joints as well as muscles, and orthopedic physicians diagnose and treat patients with these disorders. Other health care professionals who work with patients with muscular system disorders include occupational therapists (OT) and physical therapists (PT). Both of these professions require advanced academic degrees. An OT provides therapy based on engagement in meaningful activities of daily life; aids in motor learning, compensation, and adaptation; directs fabrication of splints; and assists patients to regain function to perform everyday activities. The PT provides services that help restore function, improve mobility, relieve pain, and prevent or limit permanent physical disabilities of patients suffering from injuries or disease. They restore, maintain, and promote overall fitness and health.

Disorders and Treatments

There are numerous disorders of the muscular system, some involving multiple systems and others affecting only the muscular system. The discussion that follows is specific to the muscular system only.

MUSCULAR SYSTEM DISORDERS

Abnormal muscle conditions are diagnosed by using techniques such as X-ray, magnetic resonance imaging **(MRI)**, or electromyography **(EMG)**. Various laboratory tests are used to evaluate levels of blood components that may be elevated or decreased in disease states. Treatments vary according to the condition and may involve medications, exercise regimens, and occupational and physical therapy.

Muscle disorders can be caused by physical trauma, such as sports injuries and accidents. They can also result from genetic disorders. Sometimes muscular abnormalities are related to autoimmune conditions and nervous system disorders. The following sections discuss common abnormal conditions of the muscles and some of their treatment procedures.

Muscular Dystrophy

Muscular dystrophy (dys- is a prefix meaning "bad, ill, difficult"; -trophy is a suffix meaning "nutrition" or "growth") is a group of inherited muscle disorders that cause muscle weakness without affecting the nervous system. The most common form, which affects only males, is Duchenne muscular dystrophy (DMD). It usually appears around ages 3 to 5 years, and by age 12 or so, the patient has limited mobility and may be confined to a wheelchair. Frequently, death results from respiratory failure and infection. There is no known cure, and treatment consists of using measures aimed at maintaining optimal motor functions through moderate exercise programs and the use of supportive appliances. Treatment plans usually involve a multidisciplinary approach with nutritional support, occupational and physical therapy, and sometimes drugs when secondary conditions such as infections result.

Myasthenia Gravis

Myasthenia gravis (my- means "muscle"; -asthen means "weakness"; -ia means "condition of"; *gravis* has a Latin origin and means "weighty, serious, heavy") is an immunologic disorder characterized by fluctuating weakness, especially of the facial and external eye muscles, that usually increases with activity. The muscles of the limbs, neck, and breathing can also be affected, in which case assisted ventilation may be needed. Other symptoms can include **dysphagia** (dys- is a prefix meaning "difficult"; phag- is a word element meaning "to swallow"; -ia is a suffix meaning "condition of"); **ptosis** (ptosis is a word element meaning "drooping") of one or both eyes; and

paralysis (para- is a prefix meaning "next to"; -lysis can mean "to destroy" or "to loosen," as when muscles lose their shape or become flaccid). Treatment usually consists of supportive measures, such as dietary interventions when difficulty with swallowing occurs, pharmacologic agents to alleviate respiratory difficulty, and occupational and physical therapy.

Fibromyalgia

Fibromyalgia (fibr/o is a root for "fiber"; my/o is a root for "muscle"; -algia is a suffix for "pain") is a chronic disorder characterized by widespread aching and stiffness of muscles and soft tissues, fatigue, tenderness, and sleep disorders. The cause of fibromyalgia is unknown; it may coexist with other chronic diseases. Treatment consists of a limited exercise program and medications such as pain relievers and muscle relaxants.

Amyotrophic Lateral Sclerosis (Lou Gehrig Disease)

Amyotrophic (a- is a prefix meaning "without"; my/o means "muscle"; troph- means "growth, food, nourishment"; -ic is an adjective suffix) **lateral sclerosis** (scler/o is a word element that means "hardening"; -sis is a suffix that means "condition of") **(ALS)**, named after Lou Gehrig, the professional baseball player who died from the disease, is a progressive degeneration of the nerve tracts of the spinal cord causing muscular **atrophy** (a- means "without"; troph- means "growth, food, nourishment"; -y is an adjective suffix) or **amyotrophy** (a- is a prefix meaning "without"; my/o means "muscle"; troph- means "growth, food, nourishment"; -y is an adjective suffix). General weakness, muscle cramping, and twitching occur early. The disease progresses to respiratory muscle paralysis that eventually leads to death. Treatment consists of physical and occupational therapy and speech therapy to help maintain the ability to talk.

CUMULATIVE TRAUMA DISORDERS

Cumulative trauma disorders (CTD) are often caused by repetitive, work-related motions that damage muscles, tendons, joints, or nerves. A few of the more common ones are described in the following sections.

Carpal Tunnel Syndrome

Carpal tunnel syndrome is a skeletal disorder because it involves the carpal bones, but it is also considered a CTD of the muscular system because it involves the tendons of the wrist. The carpal tunnel is a narrow bony passageway in the wrist. The median nerve and tendons pass through this tunnel. When the wrist is overused, the tendons going through the tunnel become chronically swollen and inflamed. The swelling causes compression of the median nerve, resulting in pain and numbness in the fingers (Fig. 6-4). Treatment consists of surgery to release pressure on the nerve. A temporary measure may include the use of wrist braces to maintain proper positioning of the wrist and relieve pressure on the nerve.

Rotator Cuff Injury

A **rotator cuff injury** is an injury of the shoulder and is seen in people who perform repeated activities such as swimming or throwing a baseball. The rotator cuff is formed by four muscles that may become inflamed and swollen when overused. Treatment initially consists of a short period of rest followed by gentle strengthening exercises to the affected area. Surgical repair may be necessary to restore functional mobility. Treatment consists of surgery followed by physical therapy.

Epicondylitis

Epicondylitis (epi- is a prefix meaning "upon, above"; condyl- means "rounded end surface of a bone"; -itis means "inflammation"), also known as golfer's and tennis elbow, is an inflammation of the medial and lateral epicondyles. The epicondyles are bony projections of the distal portion of the humerus and are attachment points for the tendons that connect the muscles to the bone. These

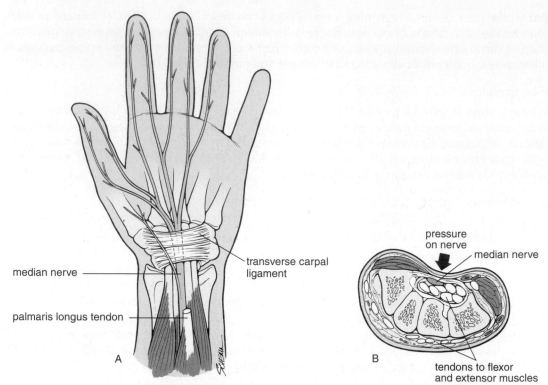

median nerve

palmaris longus tendon

transverse carpal
ligament

A

pressure
on nerve

median nerve

B

tendons to flexor
and extensor muscles

FIGURE 6-4   Carpal tunnel syndrome. (A) Pressure on the median nerve as it passes through the carpal (wrist) bone causes numbness and weakness in the areas of the hand supplied by the nerve. (B) Cross-section of the wrist showing compression of the median nerve. From Cohen BJ. Medical Terminology: An Illustrated Guide, 5th Ed. Philadelphia: Lippincott Williams & Wilkins, 2007.

muscles flex and extend the wrist and fingers. Repetitive arm motions, such as those common in golf and tennis, can cause inflammation of the tendons where they attach to the epicondyles (Fig. 6-5). The main symptom is pain at the elbow and in the forearm when lifting, squeezing, or carrying objects. A brace worn below the elbow to distribute the stress, along with anti-inflammatory medications and rest of the affected extremity, may provide temporary relief.

Plantar Fasciitis

Plantar fasciitis is an inflammation of the plantar fascia (connective tissue in the arch of the foot) that can cause intense pain when walking or running. It may be caused by long periods of weight bearing or sudden changes in activity. Obesity, jobs that require considerable walking on hard surfaces, shoes with little or no arch support, and inactivity are also associated with the condition. Stretching the plantar fascia, arch supports, shoes with good support and heels, weight loss, and anti-inflammatory medications are among some of the common noninvasive treatments.

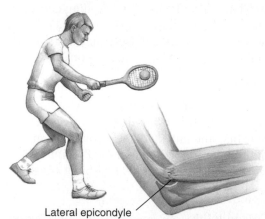

Lateral epicondyle

FIGURE 6-5   Tennis and golfer's elbow. Repetitive motions can cause an inflammation of the medial and lateral epicondyles, causing pain. Asset provided by Anatomical Chart Co.

SPORTS INJURIES

Participation in athletic competition frequently involves overuse of certain muscles, tendons, and joints. Injuries may occur as the athlete strives to achieve perfection. Even when the body is properly conditioned, injuries can occur. Two examples are the hamstring injury and shin splints.

Hamstring Injury

A **hamstring injury** is a strain or tear in one of the hamstring muscles (group of four posterior thigh muscles). Pain occurs suddenly during running or acceleration. This injury is common among sprinters, track hurdlers, and baseball or football players. Treatment consists of rest, ice, compression (bandaging), and elevation (RICE).

Shin Splints

A **shin splint** is pain caused by a number of conditions including overuse of the muscles in the lower leg, stress fractures (small sliver or crack in the bone usually caused by repeated use) of the tibia, or possibly an inflammation of the periosteum (as discussed in Chapter 5, which is the outer covering of the bone; peri- is a prefix meaning "around"; oste/o is the root for "bone"; -um is a singular noun ending) called **periostitis** (peri- is a prefix meaning "around"; oste/o is the root for "bone"; -itis means "inflammation"). Shin splint is more of a collective term describing the pain rather than a diagnosis. Pain occurs with walking, running, jumping, or other basic activity. Treatment may involve RICE or rest and ice initially and a compression bandage on the lower leg when activity resumes. Anti-inflammatory medications are frequently prescribed.

PARALYSIS

Paralysis (para- is a prefix meaning "alongside"; -lysis can mean "to destroy" or "to loosen," as when muscles lose their shape or become flaccid) is the loss of sensation and voluntary muscle movements caused by an injury or disease. The following terms name kinds of paralysis:
- **Hemiparesis:** slight paralysis of one side of the body (hemi- means "half"; -paresis means "partial" or "incomplete").
- **Myoparesis:** weakness or partial paralysis of a muscle (my/o means "muscle"; -paresis means "partial" or "incomplete").
- **Paraplegia:** paralysis of both legs and the lower part of the body (para- is a prefix meaning "alongside"; plegia means "paralysis").
- **Quadriplegia:** paralysis of all four extremities (quadri- means "four").
- **Hemiplegia:** total paralysis of one side of the body (hemi- means "half").

Any type of weakness or paralysis can be extremely incapacitating. A combination of occupational therapy, physical therapy, and drugs is used to restore muscles to an optimum level of movement and functional ability and to improve quality of life by relaxing muscles and decreasing discomfort.

Pharmacology

The major symptoms of skeletal muscle disorders are pain and muscle spasms. The pain is frequently caused by inflammation, and anti-inflammatory agents are often prescribed. These nonsteroidal anti-inflammatory drugs (NSAIDs) may include ibuprofen (Motrin, Advil) or naproxen (Aleve). A variety of analgesics, including aspirin, acetaminophen, and narcotics such as morphine, may be prescribed to relieve pain.

Skeletal muscle relaxants can also help reduce muscle spasms and/or tension. They sometimes are used to relieve pain with musculoskeletal disorders. Flexeril and Dantrium are examples of this drug classification.

Abbreviation Table • The Muscular System

ABBREVIATION	MEANING
CTD	cumulative trauma disorder
DMD	Duchenne muscular dystrophy
DTR	deep tendon reflexes
EMG	electromyography
IM	intramuscular
MG	myasthenia gravis
RICE	rest, ice, compression, elevation
ROM	range of motion

Study Table • The Muscular System

TERM AND PRONUNCIATION	ANALYSIS	MEANING
Structure and Function		
antagonist (an-TAG-oh-nihst)	a common English word	something (or in common use, someone) opposing or resisting the action of another
fascia (FASH-ee-ah)	the Latin word for band	fibrous sheath of connective tissue that covers a muscle
ligament (LIG-ah-ment)	from the Latin noun *ligamen* (string)	a type of muscle tissue connecting bones, cartilage, or other tissue structures
myocardial muscle (my-oh-CARD-ee-al)	*my/o* (muscle); *cardi/o* (heart); *-al* (adjective)	heart muscle
prime mover	two common English words	muscle that has the principal responsibility for a given movement
striated (STRY-ayted)	from the Latin verb *striare* (to groove)	adjective describing skeletal muscles
tendon (TEN-dun)	from the Latin verb *tendo* (stretch)	a type of muscle structure, such as the Achilles tendon, associated with appendicular muscles
tone, tonicity	from the Greek word *tonos*	tension present in resting muscles
Common Disorders		
amyotrophic lateral sclerosis (ALS) (ay-my-oh-TROH-fik) or Lou Gehrig disease	*a-* (deficient); *my/o* (muscle); lateral (side); *scler/o* (hard); *-osis* (abnormal condition)	a progressive degeneration of the nerve tracts of the spinal cord, causing muscular atrophy

TERM AND PRONUNCIATION	ANALYSIS	MEANING
asthenia (as-THEEN-ee-ah)	*a-* (deficient); *sthenos* (Greek word for strength)	weakness
atonia (AY-toh-nee-ah)	*a-* (deficient); *tonia* (tone)	flaccidity; lack of muscle tone; relaxation of muscle
atrophy (a-TROH-fee)	*a-* (deficient); *-trophy* (from the Greek word *trophé* meaning "nourishment")	wasting of the muscles
carpal tunnel syndrome	carpal (a wrist bone); tunnel (common English word); syndrome (a Greek word meaning "running together")	the tendons going through the carpal tunnel in the wrist be come chronically swollen and inflamed
epicondylitis (EP-ih-KON-dih-LYE-tis)	*epi-* (around); *condyl* (rounded end surface of a bone); *-itis* (inflammation)	inflammation of the tissues around the elbow; golfer or tennis elbow
fibromyalgia (FY-broh-MY-al-jee-ah)	*fibr/o* (fiber); *my/o* (muscle); *-algia* (pain)	a chronic disorder characterized by widespread aching and stiffness of muscles and soft tissues and fatigue
hamstring injury	hamstring muscle	strain or tear of the hamstring muscle group (posterior femoral muscle group)
hemiparesis (hem-ee-PAH-ree-sis)	*hemi-* (half); *-paresis* (paralysis)	slight paralysis of one side of the body
hemiplegia (hem-ee-PLEE-jee-ah)	*hemi-* (half); *-plegia* (paralysis)	total paralysis of one side of the body
kinesialgia (kin-ee-SAL-jee-uh); kinesialgia (kih-nee-see-AL-jee-uh)	kines (from the Greek word *kinesis* meaning "motion"); *-algia* (pain)	pain resulting from movement
muscular dystrophy (DIS-tro-fee)	muscular (common English word); *dys-* (difficult); *-trophy* (from the Greek word *trophé* meaning "nourishment")	group of inherited muscle disorders that cause muscle weakness without affecting the nervous system
myasthenia gravis (MY-ahs-THEE-nee-ah GRA-viss)	*my/o* (muscle); asthenia (from the Greek word *astheneia* meaning "weakness")	MG; an immunologic disorder characterized by fluctuating weakness, especially of the facial and external eye muscle
myocele (MY-oh-seel)	*my/o* (muscle); *-cele* (hernia)	hernia of a muscle
myodynia (my-oh-DINN-ee-yuh); myalgia (my-AL-jee-a)	*my/o* (muscle); *-dynia* (pain); *-algia* (pain)	pain in a muscle
myoma (my-OH-muh)	*my/o* (muscle); *-oma* (tumor)	benign neoplasm of muscle tissue

(continued)

TERM AND PRONUNCIATION	ANALYSIS	MEANING
myoparesis (MY-oh-pah-REE-sis)	*my/o* (muscle); *-paresis* (paralysis)	weakness or partial paralysis of a muscle
myositis (my-oh-SY-tihs)	*my/o* (s) (muscle); *-itis* (inflammation)	inflammation of muscle
myospasm (MY-oh-spaz-uhm)	*my/o* (muscle); *-spasm* (involuntary motion)	involuntary contraction of a muscle
paralysis (pah-RAL-ih-sis)	*para-* (not normal); *-lysis* (loosening)	loss of sensation and voluntary muscle movements caused by an injury or disease
paraplegia (PAR-ah-PLEE-jee-ah)	*para-* (not normal); *-plegia* (paralysis)	paralysis of both legs and the lower part of the body
periostitis (PEHR-ee-os-TY-tihs)	*peri-* (around); *oste/o* (bone); *-itis* (inflammation)	inflammation of the periosteum or the covering that surrounds the bone
plantar fasciitis (FASH-ee-eye-tis)	plantar (sole of the foot); fasci- (from *fascia*, Latin for band); *-itis* (inflammation)	inflammation of the plantar fascia causing heel pain
quadriplegia (kwah-drah-PLEE-jee-ah)	*quadri* (four); *-plegia* (paralysis)	paralysis of all four extremities
rotator cuff injury	rotator cuff (four muscles in the shoulder); injury (common English word)	inflammation of the rotator cuff in the shoulder caused by overuse
shin splint	two common English words used in an uncommon expression	term given to describe pain in the anterior portion of the lower leg during running, walking, and other similar activities
tenalgia (tehn-AL-jee-uh), tenodynia (ten-oh-DINN-ee-uh)	*ten/o* (tendon); *-algia* (pain); *-dynia* (pain)	pain in a tendon
tendonitis (ten-doe-NY-tiss); also sometimes spelled tendinitis (TEN-dih-NY-tiss)	*tendon/o* (tendon); *-itis* (inflammation)	inflammation of a tendon

Practice and Practitioners

kinesiology (kih-nee-see-AWL-uh-jee)	*kinesi/o* (movement); *-logy* (study of)	study of muscle motion
kinesiologist (kih-nee-see-AWL-uh-jist)	*kinesi/o* (movement); *-logist* (one who studies)	a specialist in kinesiology
myology (my-AWL-uh-jee)	*my/o* (muscle); *-logy* (study of)	study of muscles

TERM AND PRONUNCIATION	ANALYSIS	MEANING
orthopedic (or-thoh-PEE-dik)	*orth/o* (straight); *pedics* (child); note: the word was coined in the 18th century, originating with the study of skeletal disorders in children	pertaining to orthopedics or the study of the musculoskeletal system
orthopedic surgeon (or-thoh-PEE-dik)	*orth/o* (straight); *pedics* (child); surgeon (common English word)	a physician in the field of orthopedics (can be M.D. or D.O.)
neurologist (new-ROL-oh-gist)	*neur/o* (nerve); *-logist* (one who studies)	a physician who diagnoses and treats disorders of the nervous system

Diagnosis and Treatment

electromyography (ee-LEK-troh-my-OG-rafee)	*electr/o* (electricity); *my/o* (muscle); *-graphy* (process of writing)	abbreviation is EMG; records the strength of muscle contractions by means of electrical stimulation
myectomy (my-EKK-tuh-mee)	*my/o* (muscle); *-ectomy* (excision)	excision of part of a muscle
physical therapy (PT)	common English phrase	treatment to prevent disability and restore function through the use of heat, exercise, and massage to improve circulation, strength, flexibility, and muscle strength
RICE	acronym derived from <u>r</u>est, <u>i</u>ce, <u>c</u>ompression, and <u>e</u>levation	treatment used for common muscular disorders (hamstring injuries, sprains, strains, etc.)
skeletal muscle relaxants	*skelet/o* (skeleton); *-al* (adjective suffix); relaxant: that which relaxes	medications used to reduce muscle spasm
tenontoplasty (teh-NON-toe-plass-tee); tendinoplasty (TEN-dih-no-plass-tee); tendoplasty (TEN-doe-plass-tee); tenoplasty (TEN-oh-plass-tee)	*tenont/o, tendin/o, tend/o, ten/o* (tendon); *-plasty* (surgical repair)	surgical repair of a tendon
tenorrhaphy (TEN-oh-raff-ee)	*ten/o* (tendon); *-rrhaphy* (suturing)	suturing of a tendon
tenotomy (ten-AW-tuh-mee); also sometimes tendotomy (ten-DAW-tuh-mee)	*ten/o* (tendon); *-tomy* (incision)	incision into a tendon

EXERCISES

 EXERCISE 6-1   Case Study

PHYSICAL THERAPY PROGRESS NOTE

CHIEF COMPLAINT: Cervical neck pain with limited movement and right shoulder pain with limited ROM.

PROGRESS: The patient states that he is the same as he was the last time he was in for therapy.

AGGRAVATING FACTORS: Working.

PAIN/DISCOMFORT LEVEL: The patient states that the pain is 5/10.

TREATMENT: Treatment today consisted of moist heat and ultrasound of the cervical spine; therapeutic exercise to the neck and shoulder × 45 minutes.

PATIENT'S PROGRESS: The patient is doing well with his cervical spine exercises. His neck flexion, and neck extension and rotation are relatively improved. His radiating pain is reduced. His right shoulder is very painful. He has pain on flexion and abduction. He has pain on resisted abduction. He has a rotator cuff tendonitis, probable impingement.

The patient was put on a four-step treatment approach to decrease pain and increase neck and shoulder movement. He was advised to limit the use of his right arm as much as possible for 2 weeks, use ice and NSAIDs for pain, and keep his arm in a sling. He demonstrated improved ROM following his therapy. He is advised to use the exercise program on a regular basis.

QUESTIONS

1. What medical terms are associated with the patient's limited neck movements?

   _____

   _____

2. What does "tendonitis" (or "tendinitis") mean?

   _____

   _____

3. Explain what ROM is.

   _____

   _____

4. What are NSAIDs? Give an example of an NSAID.

   _____

   _____

5. What is the purpose of physical therapy?

   _____

EXERCISE 6-2   Word Building

Use the word elements listed to build the terms defined below.

-algia	hemi-	-logy	para-	tendin/o
-cele	-itis	muscul/o	-paresis	ten/o
fasci/o	kinesi/o	my/o	-pathy	-tomy
fibr/o	-logist	neur/o	-plegia	-trophy

1. Slight paralysis of one side of the body _____

2. Pain resulting from movement _____

3. Incision into a tendon _____

4. Inflammation of a muscle _____

5. Any disease of the muscle _____

6. A chronic disorder characterized by widespread aching _____

7. Hernia of a muscle _____

8. Physician who diagnoses and treats diseases of the nervous system _____

9. Paralysis of both legs and the lower part of the body _____

10. Inflammation of the fascia _____

EXERCISE 6-3   Fill in the Blank

Fill in the blank with the correct answer.

1. What are the three types of muscles?

    _____

2. Name two medical specialists who treat disorders of the muscular system?

    _____

3. What is the difference between a paraplegic and a hemiplegic?

    _____

4. Identify and define the word elements in the term "amyotrophic."

    _____

5. What is a prime mover? _____

    _____

6. What is the medical term for tennis elbow?

    _____

7. What does the abbreviation EMG stand for?

_____

_____

8. Define "muscular dystrophy."

_____

_____

9. What does each letter in RICE stand for?

_____

_____

10. Why would skeletal muscle relaxants be prescribed?

_____

_____

EXERCISE 6-4   True or False

Circle the correct answer.

1. Plantar fasciitis can cause heel pain.
   True   False

2. Duchenne disease is a type of arthritis.
   True   False

3. An antagonist is a muscle that opposes or resists the action of another muscle.
   True   False

4. Tennis elbow is another name for myositis.
   True   False

5. Shin splints may be caused by periostitis.
   True   False

6. Myoparesis is contraction of the muscle.
   True   False

7. Motrin is an example of an anti-inflammatory medication.
   True   False

8. Myocardium is the heart muscle.
   True   False

9. Tendons attach bone to bone.
   True   False

10. Kinesi/o is a root word for movement.
    True   False

EXERCISE 6-5 Crossword Puzzle: Muscular System

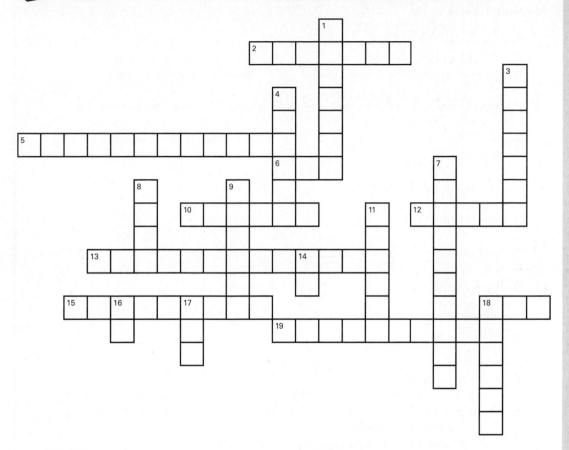

ACROSS

2. suffix for incomplete paralysis
5. widespread muscle aches, fatigue, unknown cause
6. abbreviation for Duchennes Muscular Dystrophy
10. suffix for paralysis
12. lack of muscle tone
13. tennis elbow
15. muscle group in the back of the thigh
18. abbreviation for straight leg raises
19. heart muscle

DOWN

1. triangular shoulder muscle
3. wasting of tissue
4. prefix meaning "four"
7. opposes a prime mover
8. prefix meaning "half"
9. fibrous band that connects muscle to bone
11. band of connective tissue that covers the muscle
14. abbreviation for intramuscular
16. root word for muscle
17. abbreviation for range of motion
18. hollow internal organ muscle type

CHAPTER 6 QUIZ

Multiple Choice

1. The three types of muscle tissue are:
   a. smooth, cardiac, deltoid
   b. cardiac, epicardium, skeletal
   c. cardiac, skeletal, smooth
   d. skeletal, trapezius, deltoid

2. Physicians in which of the following medical specialty(s) take care of muscular disorders?
   a. neurology
   b. orthopedic
   c. neurology and orthopedics
   d. chiropractic and orthopedics

3. Kinesiology is the study of:
   a. dance
   b. movement
   c. aerobics
   d. athletics

4. A quadriplegic is paralyzed in _____ limbs.
   a. one
   b. two
   c. three
   d. four

5. Carpal tunnel syndrome involves the _____.
   a. wrist
   b. knee
   c. elbow
   d. ankle

6. A muscle antagonist is a:
   a. muscle that resists the action of another
   b. muscle that has the principal responsibility for a given movement
   c. type of muscle that connects one muscle to another
   d. none of the above

7. The muscular disease in which a person is diagnosed usually by age 3 to 5 years and is confined to a wheelchair by age 12 and that is characterized by progressive muscle weakness is called:
   a. myasthenia gravis
   b. multiple sclerosis
   c. muscular dystrophy
   d. paraplegia

Fill in the Blank

8. Pointing the toes downward is called _____.

9. _____ is the term for weakness.

10. A hernia of a muscle is called _____.

11. _____ causes intense pain in the heel region upon walking.

12. A(n) _____ records the strength of muscle contractions.

13. The surgical repair of a tendon is called _____.

14. _____ is the study of muscles.

15. Muscle pain is called _____.

Define

16. antagonist _____

17. myoparesis _____

18. DTR _____

19. RICE _____

20. abduction _____

CHAPTER 7

The Nervous System

LEARNING OBJECTIVES

Upon completion of this chapter, you should be able to:

- Name the major parts of the nervous system and describe their functions.
- Identify the word elements that build terms related to the nervous system.
- Name the parts of a nerve.
- Identify the major divisions of the nervous system.
- Build, spell, and pronounce medical terms that relate to the nervous system.
- Identify the terms that relate to disorders and procedures of the nervous system.
- Describe the major drug classifications used to treat nervous system disorders.
- Identify and interpret selected abbreviations relating to the nervous system.
- Analyze and define the terms introduced in this chapter.

Word Elements • The Nervous System

WORD ELEMENT	REFERS TO
arachn/o	spider
cephal/o	head
cerebell/o	the cerebellum
cerebr/o	the cerebrum; also, the brain in general
cortic/o	outer layer or covering
encephal/o	brain
gangli/o; ganglion/o	ganglia (singular: ganglion)
gli/o	glue
hydr/o	water
iatr/o	physician; to treat
-mania	suffix meaning "morbid attraction to" or "impulse toward"
meningi/o	a membrane
ment/o	referring to the mind
-mnesia	memory
myel/o	in connection with the nervous system, refers to the spinal cord and medulla oblongata
neur/o	a nerve cell; nervous system
-oid	like
-paresis	weakness, loss of movement
-phasia	speech
-phobia	suffix meaning "morbid or unreasonable fear"
-plegia	paralyzed
schiz/o	to split
psych/o	referring to the mind
spin/o	referring to the spinal cord

An Overview of the Nervous System

The nervous system is one of the most complex systems in the body. It coordinates both the body's involuntary or unconscious functions, such as reflexes and thought processes, and the voluntary movements of walking, eating, talking, etc. The nervous system works in conjunction with the endocrine system to maintain homeostasis (home/o is the combining form for alike or the same; the term means "a state of equilibrium" or "staying the same") and is responsible for quick changes that are short lived to maintain this balance; the endocrine system initiates slow changes that are longer term. It also controls voluntary and involuntary movement, detects environmental changes, and registers sensory information (like pulling your hand away from a hot stove).

The nervous system has two main divisions: the **central nervous system (CNS)** and the **peripheral nervous system (PNS)** (Fig. 7-1). The CNS consists of the brain and spinal cord. The PNS, which may be divided into the **somatic** and **autonomic nervous subsystems**, controls skeletal muscles by means of the cranial and spinal nerves (Fig. 7-2).

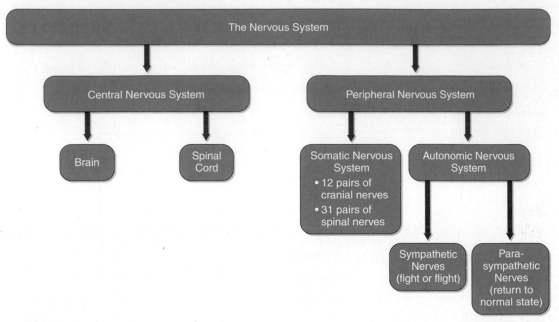

FIGURE 7-1   Divisions of the nervous system. The flow chart identifies the two main divisions of the nervous system: central and peripheral. Furthermore, it identifies how the peripheral nervous system is divided into the somatic and autonomic nervous systems and the main functions each performs.

Structure and Function

The structures that help the body perform the functions mentioned earlier are directed by **neurons** (neur/o means "nerve"), or nerve cells, and assisted by **neuroglia** (-glia means "glue"), the supporting tissues of the nervous system. The neurons carry electrical messages that coordinate the exchange of information between the body's internal and external environments (think of them as the "messengers"), whereas the neuroglia offer protection and support to the nerve tissue (think of them as "assistants").

The three principal parts of a neuron cell are the **cell body**, the **dendrites**, and the **axon** (Fig. 7-3). The cell body contains the nucleus and receives impulses from other cells through the dendrites. The dendrites, which project outward from the cell body, act as antennae that receive and transmit messages between the neuron and muscles, skin, or other neurons. The cell body passes these messages to the axon, which conducts electrical impulses away from the cell body. The connecting points for these message transfers are called **synapses. Synaptic** (adjective form of synapse) connections can occur between two nerve cells. The stimulus between the two cells is usually passed by means of a chemical called a **neurotransmitter** (neur/o means "nerve"; *transmitto* is Latin meaning "to send across"). For example, hormones are typical neurotransmitters.

When groups of neuron cell bodies occur within the PNS, each one is called a **ganglion** (plural: **ganglia**). Groupings of axons are called nerves wherever they occur in the body. Axons are covered by the **myelin sheath**, a white fatty material that provides protection and electrical insulation. Neurons are grouped together to carry out the highly complex sensing and processing actions required for everything we do. A stimulus from the environment creates a sensation we

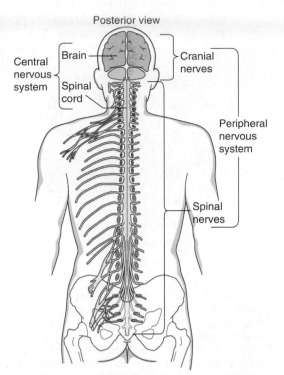

FIGURE 7-2 **Posterior view.** Divisions of the nervous system. The central nervous system is further divided into the brain and spinal cord. The cranial and spinal nerves are shown here as part of the peripheral nervous system. From Cohen BJ. Medical Terminology: An Illustrated Guide, 5th Ed. Philadelphia: Lippincott Williams & Wilkins, 2007.

experience and causes a reaction to the stimulus. This reaction requires complex interactions between the various body systems. For example, when a person senses trouble, the nervous system reacts by increasing the heart rate and blood pressure and dilating the blood vessels to the skeletal muscles. Dilation of the respiratory tubes occurs to permit a greater amount of oxygen into the lungs. All of this takes place so the person can react to the perceived problem by using muscles to "escape."

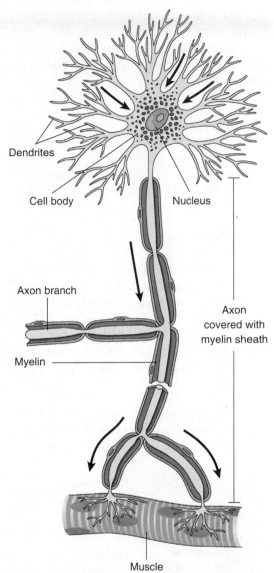

FIGURE 7-3 **Motor neuron.** The neuron is the basic functional unit of the nervous system. The arrows show the direction of the nerve impulse. Note the myelin sheath that covers the axon of the nerve. From Cohen BJ. Medical Terminology: An Illustrated Guide, 5th Ed. Philadelphia: Lippincott Williams & Wilkins, 2007.

CENTRAL NERVOUS SYSTEM

The CNS is the body's control center. All nerve messages originate and/or terminate in the brain or spinal cord. The brain and spinal cord interpret the messages and determine the body's responses.

The brain is one of the largest organs in the body and is responsible for most activities, including thought and memory processes. Sections of the brain control different body functions, such as breathing and temperature regulation. From the outside, the brain is separable into two hemispheres, each consisting of four lobes: the **frontal, parietal, occipital,** and **temporal** (Fig. 7-4). The names of the lobes relate to their location relative to the skull (i.e., frontal relates to the front part of the head; parietal refers to the sides or "walls" of the head; occipital relates to the back of the head; temporal relates to the temples or area posterior to the eyes on the side of the head).

The major parts of the brain include the following (Fig. 7-5):

- **Cerebrum:** The cerebrum, the largest part of the brain, is where memories and conscious thoughts are stored. It also directs some of our bodily movements. An outer layer of gray matter called the **cerebral cortex** protects the cerebrum, which is divided into two hemispheres: left and right. Please note that although groups of neuron cell bodies that exist within the PNS are called ganglia, a group of neuron cell bodies within the CNS is normally called a **nucleus** (plural: **nuclei**).

- **Cerebellum:** The cerebellum, like the larger cerebrum situated above it, also has two hemispheres. The cerebellum helps us perform learned body movements smoothly and helps maintain our equilibrium.

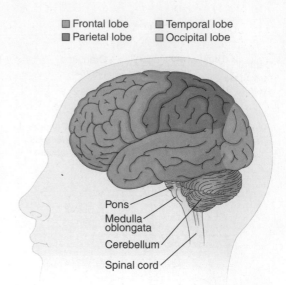

☐ Frontal lobe   ☐ Temporal lobe
☐ Parietal lobe   ☐ Occipital lobe

Pons
Medulla oblongata
Cerebellum
Spinal cord

FIGURE 7-4 Lateral view of the brain, external surface. The four main lobes (frontal, parietal, temporal, and occipital) are shown in this figure along with the major structures of the brain. Modified from Cohen BJ. Medical Terminology: An Illustrated Guide, 5th Ed. Philadelphia: Lippincott Williams & Wilkins, 2007.

- **Diencephalon:** The diencephalon contains both the **thalamus** and the **hypothalamus**. The thalamus processes sensory information, such as touch, taste, and sight, and directs the

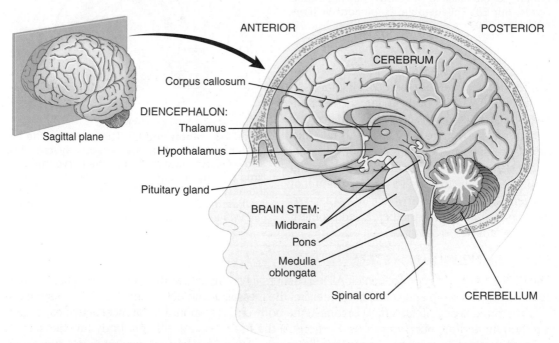

ANTERIOR   POSTERIOR

CEREBRUM

Corpus callosum

Sagittal plane

DIENCEPHALON:
   Thalamus
   Hypothalamus

Pituitary gland

BRAIN STEM:
   Midbrain
   Pons
   Medulla oblongata

Spinal cord   CEREBELLUM

FIGURE 7-5 Sagittal section of the brain. The major parts of the interior brain structures are shown. From Cohen BJ. Medical Terminology: An Illustrated Guide, 5th Ed. Philadelphia: Lippincott Williams & Wilkins, 2007.

impulses to certain parts of the brain. The hypothalamus, which is the hormone and emotion center of the brain, controls autonomic functions such as heart rate, dilation of blood vessels, and hormone secretion.

- **Brain stem:** The brain stem contains the **mesencephalon** (or **midbrain**), the **pons,** and the **medulla oblongata.** The mesencephalon processes visual and audible sensory information. Visual tracking, such as moving the eyes to read or following an object with your eyes, is an example of a midbrain function. It also transmits hearing impulses to the brain. The pons (Latin for "bridge") passes information to the cerebellum and the thalamus to control subconscious somatic activities such as regulating respiration. The medulla oblongata sends sensory information to the thalamus to direct the autonomic functions of the heart, lungs, and other organs of the body. The cavities between the brain stem and the cerebrum are called ventricles.

The spinal cord and the brain communicate continuously with one another. The messages exchanged produce all the actions and functions that make life pleasurable, painful, and even possible. In the average-sized adult, the spinal cord is about a foot and a half long and a half-inch wide. It is surrounded by membranes called spinal **meninges**, which absorb physical shocks that could damage the neural tissue (Fig. 7-6). The outer layer of the brain and spinal cord consists of **dura mater,** a dense collection of collagen fibers. The middle layer is termed the **arachnoid**

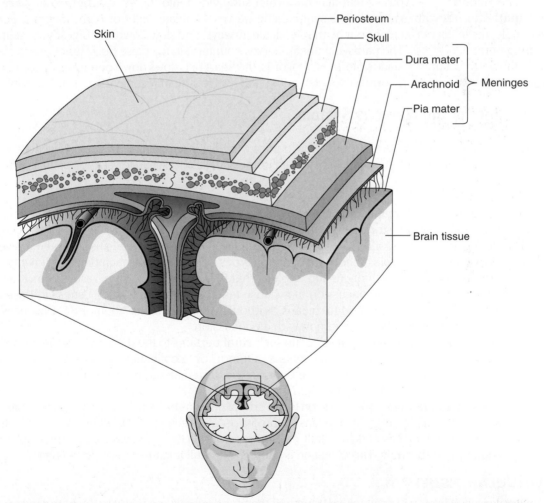

FIGURE 7-6   Meninges. The three protective layers of the meninges and adjacent tissues are shown. Modified from Cohen BJ. Medical Terminology: An Illustrated Guide, 5th Ed. Philadelphia: Lippincott Williams & Wilkins, 2007.

(arach means "spider"; -oid means "like") **layer** and is a thin delicate web-like layer. The inner layer, or **pia** (pia means "soft, tender") **mater,** is in direct contact with the brain tissue. The spinal cord is further protected by ligaments, tendons, and muscles.

PERIPHERAL NERVOUS SYSTEM

The PNS includes the 12 pairs of cranial nerves and 31 pairs of spinal nerves that run along the periphery of the body (see Fig. 7-2) (peri- means "around"; *pherein* is Greek meaning "to carry"). This term makes reference to something that is around or is connected to a major part. For example, a computer is a major object, and a printer that is connected to the computer is considered a "peripheral." The printer receives its direction from the computer or central object, much as the brain or CNS gives direction to an arm or leg in the periphery of the body. This system carries both sensory information from the body to the CNS and motor instructions from the CNS back to the body's muscles and glands.

The PNS is divided into two subsystems: the **somatic nervous system** and the **autonomic nervous system** (see Fig. 7-1). Conscious and habitual actions are called somatic, which comes from a Greek word meaning "body." Since some organs, such as the heart and lungs, work on their own, their performance is said to be autonomic. The noun autonomy is a common English word that means "self-sufficiency."

The autonomic nervous system may be further subdivided into the **sympathetic** and **parasympathetic nervous systems**. The sympathetic nerves stimulate "fight or flight" actions. For example, these nerves increase our heart rate, dilate airways, and slow down our digestive system during periods of stress. The parasympathetic nerves counterbalance these body functions to return the body to a homeostatic state. In other words, the heart rate slows down or returns to normal, the airways return to their normal diameter, and the digestive system resumes its normal activity.

Disorders of the Nervous System

Disorders of the nervous system can result from trauma, vascular insults, tumors, systemic degenerative diseases, and seizures, to name a few. Behavioral disorders make up a separate category of their own.

BRAIN TRAUMA

Head injuries can inflict trauma on the skull and brain. This may result in skull fractures, hemorrhage or bleeding, swelling, or direct injury to the brain itself. The injury may be mild, involving bruising to the brain tissues, or it can be severe, causing destruction of the brain tissue and massive swelling to the brain. A couple of the more common types of brain injuries include the following:
- **Concussion** (cerebral concussion: violent shaking of the brain) may result from a fall or blow to the head. A concussion may cause temporary loss of consciousness followed by a short period of *amnesia* (a- means "without"; -mnesia means "memory"). Dizziness, nausea, and headache are common with a concussion.
- **Subdural hematoma** (sub- means "under"; dural pertains to the dura layer of the meninges; hemat/o means "blood"; -oma means "a tumor" or "a collection of") is a collection of blood trapped in the subdural space beneath the dura mater and may result from a blow to the front or back of the head (Fig. 7-7).
- **Epidural hematoma** (epi- means "on top of"; dural pertains to the dura layer of the meninges; hemat/o means "blood"; -oma means "a tumor" or "a collection of") is when blood collects between the dura mater and the skull, causing pressure on the blood vessels and interrupting blood flow to the brain. This condition is caused by a skull fracture or blow to the head.

VASCULAR INSULTS

A vascular insult is an injury, attack, or trauma to the blood vessels. An injury to the blood vessels in the brain can result from an aneurysm (localized dilation of a vessel wall or chamber) that ruptures or an embolus or blood clot that blocks the blood flow to the brain tissues.

FIGURE 7-7 Cranial hematomas. Locations of epidural, subdural, and intracerebral hematomas are shown. **A.** Epidural hematoma occurs with a traumatic brain injury when blood accumulates between the dura and the skull. **B.** Subdural hematoma occurs within the dura layer. From Cohen BJ. Medical Terminology: An Illustrated Guide, 5th Ed. Philadelphia: Lippincott Williams & Wilkins, 2007.

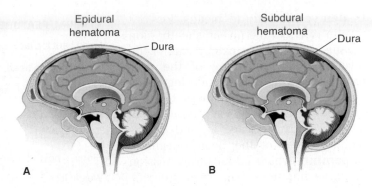

- **Cerebrovascular accident (CVA):** Also known as a stroke, a CVA results from oxygen deprivation caused by a blockage in or rupture of a blood vessel. Symptoms may include **hemiparesis** (hemi- means "half"; -paresis means "partial paralysis"), **hemiplegia** (hemi- means "half"; -plegia means "paralysis"), or **aphasia** (a- means "without"; -phasia means "speech").
- **Transient ischemic attack (TIA)**: A TIA is a temporary interruption in the blood supply to the brain. Dizziness and weakness are common symptoms with TIAs.
- **Aneurysm:** An aneurysm is a localized dilation of an artery, caused by weakness in the vessel wall or heart chamber (Fig. 7-8).

Most people think of an insult as a verbal assault, such as when someone calls someone else a name that causes hurt feelings. But the Latin verb insulto literally means "to physically jump on." So a vascular insult is a physical matter that has nothing to do with hurt feelings.

TUMORS

Tumors are lesions or neoplasms that may cause localized dysfunction, producing an increase in **intracranial pressure (ICP)**. Tumors may be benign or malignant. Two examples of tumors occurring in the nervous system include **astrocytomas** (*astr/o* means "star shaped"; *cyt/o* means "cell"; *-oma* means "tumor") and **meningiomas** (*mening/o* means "meninges"; *-oma* means "tumor"). Tumors may metastasize from other parts of the body such as the breast or lung.

SYSTEMIC DEGENERATIVE DISEASES

Degenerative diseases frequently develop slowly over time. There usually is a progressive deterioration that may start out affecting individual components of the body and end up involving one or more body systems. Examples of systemic degenerative diseases include **multiple sclerosis**, **Parkinson** and **Alzheimer disease.**

Multiple sclerosis (MS) is a progressive degenerative disease with symptoms caused

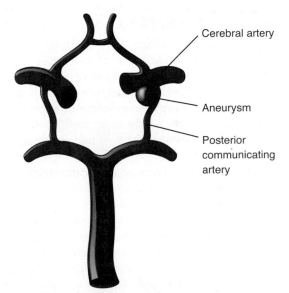

FIGURE 7-8 Cerebral aneurysm. The circle of arteries that supply blood to the brain is called the circle of Willis named after Thomas Willis, an English physician. (It is located near the center of the brain.) The aneurysm is a bulge or weakening of the artery. Reprinted with permission from Porth CM. Pathophysiology, 6th Ed. Philadelphia: Lippincott Williams & Wilkins, 2002:443.

by **demyelination** (de- means "loss of"; myelin refers to the myelin sheath; -tion means "state of") or patchy loss of the myelin sheath (covering of the neurons). The symptoms include leg weakness, double vision, numbness, tingling, and paralysis. Parkinson disease usually develops after age 60 and occurs with the loss of the neurotransmitter **dopamine**, which inhibits transmission of nerve impulses. Weakness, tremors, facial mask (no expression), and muscle rigidity are some of the symptoms (Fig. 7-9). As the disease progresses, dysphagia (dys- means "difficult"; phag/o means "swallowing"; -ia is a suffix meaning "condition of") and difficulty with mastication (chewing) may develop. Alzheimer disease, one of the most common types of **dementia** (de- is a prefix meaning "apart from"; ment refers to mind; -ia is a suffix meaning "condition of"), is a degenerative and eventually fatal condition involving atrophy of the cerebral cortex that produces a progressive loss of intellectual function.

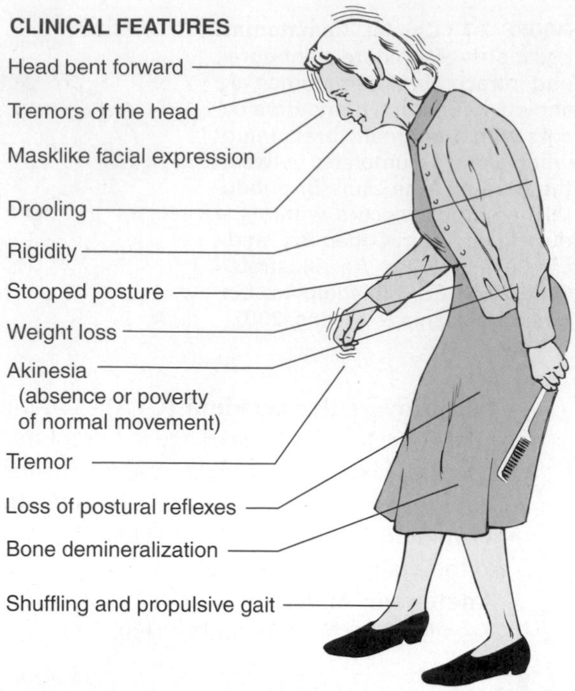

SEIZURE DISORDERS

A seizure occurs when there is an abnormal uncontrolled burst of electrical activity in the brain. Seizures may occur as a result of trauma, tumors, fevers, medications, or other causes. The end result may be unnoticed since it may be as subtle as experiencing weird odors or staring off into space; or it may be as obvious as the more well-known seizures in which the person loses consciousness and involuntarily moves his or her arms and legs. This last kind of seizure is commonly called a convulsion.

Epilepsy is a chronic disorder, characterized by recurrent seizures that result from the excessive discharge of neurons in the brain. It is usually accompanied by some alteration of consciousness. There are two basic types of epileptic seizures that should be mentioned, **grand mal seizures** and **petit mal seizures**. A grand mal seizure is severe and characterized by tonic-clonic convulsions, which are the alternating contraction and relaxation of muscles that produce jerking movements of the face, trunk, and/or extremities. A petit mal seizure is a milder form of seizure lasting only a few seconds and does not include convulsive movements.

BEHAVIORAL DISORDERS

A number of behavioral disorders are related to the nervous system. They may be caused by physical changes, substance abuse, medications, or any combination thereof. The categories include anxiety, mood, and psychotic disorders.

CLINICAL FEATURES

Head bent forward

Tremors of the head

Masklike facial expression

Drooling

Rigidity

Stooped posture

Weight loss

Akinesia
 (absence or poverty
 of normal movement)

Tremor

Loss of postural reflexes

Bone demineralization

Shuffling and propulsive gait

FIGURE 7-9   Parkinson's disease. Patients with Parkinson's disease may exhibit all or only a few of the clinical features identified here. Early signs may include weakness and decreased flexibility. As the disease advances, rigidity and lack of associated muscle movements may be seen. Modified from Rosdahl CB. Book of Basic Nursing, 7th Ed. Philadelphia: Lippincott-Raven, 1999:1063, Figure 77-3.

- **Anxiety disorders:** Anxiety disorders are characterized by feelings of apprehension or uneasiness, sometimes associated with the anticipation of danger. Common examples include **obsessive-compulsive disorder (OCD),** which often consist of repetitive behaviors; panic disorder; posttraumatic stress disorder (PTSD); and the various **phobias**, which are persistent and irrational fears of specific situations or things.
- **Mood disorders:** Mood disorders include **depression**, which results in prolonged periods of lost interest or pleasure in almost all activities, and **bipolar** (formerly called **manic-depressive) disorder,** which is characterized by manic and depressive episodes. A manic episode is one characterized by an atypically elated mood, inflated self-esteem, rapid speech, increased creativity, little need for sleep, and an inability to function normally as a result of these. Patients with bipolar disorders alternately exhibit both behaviors: mania and depression.
- **Psychotic disorders:** Psychotic disorders are more serious than anxiety or mood disorders because they feature a loss of contact with reality and a deterioration of normal social functioning. **Psychoses** (singular: **psychosis**; psych/o means "mind"; -osis means "an abnormal condition") are normally separated from **neuroses** (singular: **neurosis**; neur/o means "nerve"; -osis means "an abnormal condition"). An example of a psychosis is **schizophrenia** (schiz/o means "to split"; phren means "mind"; -ia is a suffix meaning "condition of"), which may manifest itself as paranoia, withdrawal, or psychotic symptoms, such as hallucinations and/or delusions.

Procedures and Practitioners

When evaluating the health of a person's nervous system, medical professionals may use various procedures. Sometimes, assessing a patient's level of consciousness may simply involve a qualified professional observing and talking with the patient. Other times, a medical professional may prescribe certain diagnostic tests to evaluate the condition of the brain and/or its activity. Some of these diagnostic procedures are listed below.

- **Computerized tomography (CT)** (tom/o means "to cut"; -graphy means "to write or record") is a noninvasive radiologic test that uses a computer to produce cross-sectional images of the soft tissue structures of the brain and spinal cord. This procedure can reveal problems such as brain tumors, aneurysms, herniations, and cerebral hemorrhages, to name a few.
- **Magnetic resonance imaging (MRI)** uses radio waves and a very strong magnetic field to produce images of the neural soft tissues. It is used to visualize disease-related changes in the brain or spinal cord when many conventional X-ray procedures would be unable to detect them. For example, MRIs are able to isolate damaged areas of the brain caused by multiple sclerosis.
- **Electroencephalography (EEG)** (electr/o means "electricity"; encephal/o means "brain"; -graphy means "the process of recording"): The electroencephalogram produced by EEG is a written record of the brain's electrical activity and is used to document increased electrical events of the brain seen with seizure activity in epilepsy.
- **Lumbar puncture (LP)** requires the insertion of a needle into the subarachnoid space between the third and fourth or fourth and fifth lumbar vertebrae to withdraw cerebrospinal fluid for analysis (Fig. 7-10).

The medical specialists who diagnose and treat the nervous system are **neurologists, neurosurgeons,** and **psychiatrists** (psych/o means "mind"; iatr/o means "physician"). Neurologists and neurosurgeons work with patients who experience disorders of the neuromuscular system, while psychiatrists treat behavioral and mental health disorders. The health care professional with an advanced academic degree who treats mental and behavioral disorders is a **psychologist.**

Pharmacology

Several major drug classifications are used to treat disorders of the nervous system. Pain control can be achieved using the same analgesics and narcotic analgesics discussed in earlier chapters. Sedatives (sedate comes from a Latin word meaning "to calm or relax") and **hypnotics** (hypn/o means "sleep") are used to produce a calming effect and sleep. **Anticonvulsants** (anti- means "against"; convulse refers to a violent shaking) are administered for seizure activity, and **antianxiety drugs** (anti- means "against"; anxiety refers to a state of apprehension) are given to patients for anxiety suppression and muscle relaxation.

For severe psychoses, **antipsychotic** (anti- means "against"; psych/o means "mind") medications are administered. It is important to note that some of these drugs must be taken for a period of several weeks before they become effective and that patient compliance may be difficult to achieve.

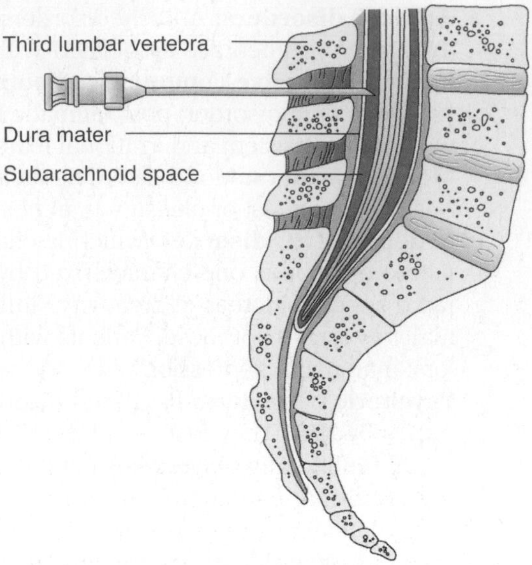

FIGURE 7-10   Lumbar puncture. Insertion of a needle between the third and fourth or fourth and fifth lumbar vertebrae to withdraw cerebrospinal fluid. From Cohen BJ. Medical Terminology: An Illustrated Guide, 5th Ed. Philadelphia: Lippincott Williams & Wilkins, 2007.

Serious side effects may occur when taking antipsychotic medications; these include low blood pressure, blurred vision, muscle rigidity, persistent muscle spasms, tremors, and arrhythmias. Some of the newer antipsychotic medications can have a negative effect on the immune system also and may cause diabetes and high cholesterol. Examples of traditional antipsychotic drugs include haloperidol (Haldol), chlorpromazine (Thorazine), and perphenazine (Etrafon, Trilafon).

Abbreviation Table • The Nervous System

ABBREVIATION	MEANING
ADHD	attention deficit hyperactivity disorder
CNS	central nervous system
CVA	cerebrovascular accident
ECT	electroconvulsive therapy
EEG	electroencephalography
ICP	intracranial pressure
IQ	intelligence quotient
LOC	level of consciousness

ABBREVIATION	MEANING
LP	lumbar puncture
MS	multiple sclerosis
OBS	organic brain syndrome
OCD	obsessive-compulsive disorder
PERRLA	pupils equal, round, and reactive to light and accommodation
PNS	peripheral nervous system
PTSD	posttraumatic stress disorder
SAD	seasonal affective disorder
TENS	transcutaneous electrical nerve stimulation
TIA	transient ischemic attack

Study Table • *The Nervous System*

TERM AND PRONUNCIATION	ANALYSIS	MEANING
Structure and Function		
autonomic nervous system (aw-to-NOM-ik) (ANS)	autonomy (self-sufficiency); *-ic* (adjective suffix)	the parts of the PNS that carry messages between the CNS and organs that function autonomously
arachnoid mater (ah-RAK-noyd MAY-turh)	from the Greek word *arachne* (spider, cobweb); *-oid* (resemblance)	delicate web-like layer of the meninges; middle layer
axon (AX-ohn)	*axo-* (axis); *-n* noun ending	the part of a neuron that conducts electrical impulses
brain stem	common English words	the part of the brain that controls functions including heart rate, breathing, and body temperature; includes midbrain, pons, and medulla oblongata
cell body	common English words	one of the three parts of a neuron cell; the other two are the axon and dendrites
central nervous system (CNS)	common English words	the subdivision of the nervous system that includes the brain and spinal cord
cerebellum (SERR-uh-bell-uhm)	*cerebr/o* (brain)	the part of the brain that controls the skeletal muscles

(continued)

TERM AND PRONUNCIATION	ANALYSIS	MEANING
cerebral cortex (seh-REE-bruhl KOR-tex)	*cerebr/o* (brain); *-al* (adjective suffix)	the gray matter surrounding the cerebrum
cerebrospinal fluid (seh-REE-bro-SPY-nuhl)	*cerebr/o* (brain); from Latin word *spina*; fluid (common English word)	the fluid in and around the brain and spinal cord
cerebrum (seh-REE-bruhm)	*cerebr/o* (brain)	the largest part of the brain; controls conscious thought and stores memories
dendrite (DEN-dryte)	from the Greek word *dendrites* (relating to a tree)	one of two processes extending from a neuron cell body; the other is the axon
diencephalon (dy-en-SEFF-uh-lohn)	*di-* (two); *encephal/o* (of or relating to the brain); *-on* (noun suffix)	the part of the brain containing both the thalamus and the hypothalamus
dura mater (DOO-ruh MAY-tuhr)	Latin words meaning "hard mother"	the outer meninges, the fibrous membrane protecting the CNS
frontal lobe (FRUN-tahl)	common English words	the front part of the brain from which voluntary muscle movements and other sensory and motor tasks are directed
ganglion (GANG-lee-ohn); plural: ganglia	a Greek word meaning swelling or knot	a group of neuron cell bodies grouped together in the PNS
hypothalamus (HY-po-thal-uh-muhs)	*hypo-* (below, deficient); from the Greek word *thalamus* (a bed, a bedroom)	the hormone and emotion center of the brain that controls autonomic functions
leptomeninx (LEPP-toh-ME-ninks)	*lepto-* (light, slender, thin frail); meninx is plural form of *mening/o* (membrane)	collective term for the arachnoid mater and pia mater
medulla oblongata (meh-DUH-luh ohb-lohng-GAH-tuh)	a Latin word (marrow); from the Latin *oblongatus* (oblong)	the part of the brain stem that sends sensory information to the thalamus to direct the autonomic functions of the heart, lungs, and other viscera
meninges (meh-NIHN-jees)	*mening/o* (membrane)	three layer membrane surrounding brain and spinal cord
mesencephalon (mez-ehn-SEFF-ah-lon)	*mes/o* (middle); *encephal/o* (brain); *-on* (noun suffix)	the middle part of the brain between the diencephalon and the pons; also called the midbrain

TERM AND PRONUNCIATION	ANALYSIS	MEANING
myelin sheath (MY-eh-lin sheeth)	*myel/o-* (bone marrow; spinal cord)	a fatty white envelope of cells providing protection and electrical insulation to neurons
nerve	common English word	a whitish, cordlike structure composed of one or more bundles of nerve fibers outside the CNS, together with their connective tissues and nourishing blood vessels
neuroglia (nuhr-o-GLEE-uh)	*neur/o* (nerve); from the Greek *glia* (glue)	cells within both the CNS and PNS, which, although they are external to neurons, form an essential part of nerve tissue
neuron (NUHR-ohn)	*neur/o* (nerve); *-on* (noun suffix)	a nerve cell, including the cell body and its axon
neurotransmitter (NOO-roh-TRANS-mitt-ehr)	*neur/o* (nerve); from the Latin *trans* (across); *mittere* (to send)	chemical released by the presynaptic cell that is then picked up by the postsynaptic cell to effect an action
nucleus (NEW-klee-uhs); plural: nuclei (NEW-klee-eye)	a Latin word meaning kernel	a group of neuron cell bodies grouped together in the CNS
occipital lobe (AWK-sihp-ih-tuhl lobe)	from Latin word *occiput* (back of the head)	the part of the brain that processes information from the sense of sight and other sensory and motor tasks
parietal lobe (pah-RY-uh-tuhl lobe)	from the Latin word *parietalis* (walls); *-al* (adjective suffix)	the part of the brain that processes information from the sense of touch and other sensory and motor tasks
peripheral nervous system (puh-RIFF-uh-ruhl) (PNS)	*peri-* (surrounding); from the Greek word *pherein* (to carry); nervous system (common English words)	made up of neurons, neuroglia, and associated tissue, including the cranial and spinal nerves and the sensory and motor nerves that extend throughout the body
pia mater (PEE-ah MAY-turh)	Latin words meaning "tender mother"	inner layer of the meninges
pons (POHNS)	a Latin word meaning "bridge"	the part of the brain stem that passes information to the cerebellum and the thalamus to regulate subconscious somatic activities

(continued)

TERM AND PRONUNCIATION	ANALYSIS	MEANING
psychomotor (SY-ko-mo-tuhr)	*psych/o* (of the mind); from the Latin *motor* (mover)	an adjective used to indicate the relation between activity psychic and muscular movement
somatic nervous system (so-MAT-ik)	*somat/o* (body, bodily); *-ic* (adjective suffix)	the parts of the PNS that carry impulses for conscious rather than habitual activity
spinal nerves (SPY-nahl)	from the Latin word *spina* (spine)	the 31 pairs of nerves located along the spinal column
synapse (SIH-naps)	*syn-* (together); from the Greek word *hapto* (clasp)	the connecting point between nerve cells or between a nerve cell and a receptor or effector cell
temporal lobe (TEM-puh-ruhl lobe)	from the Latin word *temporalis* (time, temple)	the part of the brain that processes information from the senses of hearing, smell, and taste, and other sensory and motor tasks
thalamus (THAL-uh-muhs)	from the Greek word *thalamus* (bed, bedroom)	part of the brain that processes sensory information
ventricles (VEN-trik-uhls)	from the Latin *ventriculus*, dim. of *venter* (belly)	cavities between the cerebrum and brain stem
Common Disorders		
Alzheimer disease (ALZ-hy-mur)	named after German physician Alois Alzheimer, who first described it in 1906	a disease that may begin in late middle life, characterized by progressive mental deterioration that includes loss of memory and visual and spatial orientation
amnesia (am-NEE-zah)	*a-* (without); *-mnesia* (memory)	loss of memory
aneurysm (AN-ur-izm)	from the Greek *ana* (up) and *eurys* (broad)	localized dilation of an artery, due to vessel wall weakness
anxiety disorder	common English words	a feeling of apprehension or uneasiness that results from anticipation of danger
aphasia (uh-FAY-jhah)	*a-* (absence of); from the Greek word *phases* (speech)	loss of speech
astrocytoma (A-stroh-sy-TOH-mah)	from the Greek word *astron* (star); *cyt/o* (cell); *-oma* (tumor)	star-shaped tumor that usually develops in the cerebrum; frequently in people younger than 20 years old

TERM AND PRONUNCIATION	ANALYSIS	MEANING
ataxia (ah-TAK-see-ah)	*a-* (without); from the Greek word *taxis* (order)	lack of muscular coordination
bipolar disorder	*bi-* (twice, double); from the Latin *polus* (the end of an axis)	clinical course characterized by manic episodes alternating with depressive episodes
cerebral thrombosis (seh-REE-bruhl throm-BO-sihs)	*cerebr/o* (brain); *-al* (adjective suffix); *thromb/o* (of or relating to a blood clot); *-sis* (abnormal condition)	blood clot in the brain
cerebrovascular accident (seh-REE-bro-VAS-ku-lahr) (CVA)	*cerebr/o* (brain); *vascul/o* (blood vessel); *-ar* (adjective suffix)	a synonym for *cerebral stroke,* an acute clinical event, related to impairment of cerebral circulation, lasting more than 24 hours
cerebrovascular disease (seh-REE-bro-VAS-ku-lahr)	*cerebr/o* (brain); *vascul/o* (blood vessel); *-ar* (adjective suffix)	brain disorder involving a blood vessel
delirium (duh-LEER-ee-uhm)	from the Latin word *deliro* (to be crazy)	impaired consciousness
delusion (deh-LOO-shun)	from the Latin word *ludere* (to play)	false belief or wrong judgment despite evidence to the contrary
dementia (duh-MEN-shah)	from Latin *de* (apart, away); *mens* (mind)	impaired intellectual function
depression	from the Latin *depressio*	prolonged period where there is a loss of interest or pleasure in almost all activities
dysphasia (DISS-fay-jhah)	*dys-* (bad, difficult); from the Greek word *phases* (speaking)	impaired speech
encephalitis (en-seff-uh-LY-tiss)	*encepal/o* (of or pertaining to the brain); *-itis* (inflammation)	inflammation of the brain
epidural hematoma (EH-pih-dur-ahl hee-mah-TOH-ma)	*epi-* (above); dural (relating to the dura mater); *hemat/o* (blood); *-oma* (tumor)	a collection of blood in the space between the skull and dura mater
epilepsy (EPP-ih-lepp-see)	from the Greek *epilepsia* (seizure)	CNS disorder often characterized by seizures
glioblastoma (GLY-oh-blass-TOH-mah)	*glio* (glue); from the Greek *blastos* (germ); *-oma* (tumor)	a cerebral tumor occurring most frequently in adults

(continued)

TERM AND PRONUNCIATION	ANALYSIS	MEANING
glioma (gly-OH-muh)	*glio-* (glue); *-oma* (tumor)	tumor of glial tissue
grand mal seizure (grahn-mahl SEEZ-yuhr)	French words meaning big illness	type of severe seizure with tonic-clonic convulsion
hallucination (hah-LOO-sih-nay-shun)	from the Latin *alucinor* (to wander in mind)	subjective perception of an object or voice when no such stimulus exists
hemiparesis (heh-mee-puh-REE-suhs)	*hemi-* (one-half); *-paresis* (slight paralysis)	partial paralysis of one side of the body
hemiplegia (hehm-ee-PLEE-jee-ah)	*hemi-* (one-half); *-plegia* (paralysis)	paralysis of one side of the body
Huntington disease (HUN-ting-tuhn)	named after American physician George Huntington who described the disorder in 1872	hereditary disorder of the CNS
hydrocephalus (hy-dro-SEFF-uh-lehs)	*hydro-* (water); *cephal/o* (of or pertaining to the head)	excessive cerebrospinal fluid in the brain
hyperesthesia (hy-per-ess-THEE-zyuh)	*hyper-* (extreme or beyond normal); *esthesi/o* (sensation)	abnormal sensitivity to touch
kleptomania (klep-toh-MAY-knee-yah)	from the Greek word *klepto-* (to steal); from the Latin *-mania* (insanity)	uncontrollable impulse to steal
meningioma (meh-nihn-jee-OH-muh)	*mening/o* (membrane); *-oma* (tumor)	benign tumor of the meninges
meningitis (meh-nihn-JY-tiss)	*mening/o* (membrane); *-itis* (inflammation)	inflamed meninges
multiple sclerosis (skleh-RO-sihs)	multiple (English word meaning many); *scler/o* (hardness); *-osis* (abnormal condition)	disease of the CNS characterized by the formation of plaques in the brain and spinal cord
myasthenia gravis (MY-ahs-THEE-nee-ah GRA-viss)	*my/o* (muscle); *astheneia* (weakness)	muscle weakness, lack of strength
myelitis (my-eh-LY-tiss)	*myel/o* (bone marrow or spine); *-itis* (inflammation)	inflammation of the spinal cord
myelomeningocele (MY-loh-mih-NIHN-gee-oh-seel)	*myel/o* (bone marrow or spine); *meningi/o* (membrane); *-cele* (hernia)	protrusion of the membranes of the brain or spinal cord through a defect in the cranium or vertebral column
neuralgia (nuh-RALL-jah)	*neur/o* (nerve); *-algia* (pain)	pain in a nerve
neuropathy (nuh-ROP-ah-thee)	*neur/o* (nerve); *-pathy* (disease)	a disease involving the cranial, central, or autonomic nervous systems

TERM AND PRONUNCIATION	ANALYSIS	MEANING
obsessive-compulsive disorder (OCD)	common English words	type of anxiety disorder characterized by persistent thoughts and impulses with repetitive responses that interfere with daily activities
paralysis (pah-RALL-ih-sihs)	*para-* (abnormal, alongside); *-lysis* (destruction)	loss of one or more muscle functions
paranoia (pahr-ah-NOY-ya)	*para-* (abnormal, alongside); from Greek word *noeo* (to think)	a serious mental disorder characterized by unreasonable suspicion or jealousy, along with a tendency to interpret everything others do as hostile
paraplegia (pahr-ah-PLEE-jee-ah)	*para-* (abnormal, alongside); *-plegia* (paralysis)	paralysis of the lower extremities and, often, the lower trunk of the body
paresthesia (per-ess-THEE-zyuh)	*para-* (abnormal); *esthesi/o* (sensation)	numbness
Parkinson disease (PAR-kin-suhn); also Parkinson's, parkinsonism	named for English physician James Parkinson, who described it in 1817	disease of the nerves in the brain due to an imbalance of dopamine
petit mal seizure (petty-mahl SEEZ-yuhr	French words meaning small illness	milder form of seizure lasting only a few seconds and does not include convulsive movements; also known as *absence seizures*
phobia (FOH-bee-ah)	*phob/o* (exaggerated fear); *-ia* (noun suffix)	a fear of something that is not a hazard from a statistical point of view
plegia (PLEE-jee-uh)	*-plegia* (paralysis)	paralysis
poliomyelitis (pohl-ee-oh-MY-eh-LY-tiss)	*polio-* (denoting gray color); *myel/o* (bone marrow or spine); *-itis* (inflammation)	inflamed gray matter of the spinal cord
psychosis (sy-KO-sihs)	*psych/o* (of or pertaining to the mind); *-sis* (condition of)	a serious disorder involving a marked distortion of, or sharp break from, reality; general term covering severe mental or emotional disorders
quadriplegia (kwad-rih-PLEE-jee-ah)	*quadr/i* (four); *-plegia* (paralysis)	paralysis of all four limbs

(continued)

TERM AND PRONUNCIATION	ANALYSIS	MEANING
schizophrenia (skits-oh-FREN-ee-ah)	*schiz/o* (denoting split or double sided); from the Greek word *phren* (mind)	a severe mental illness characterized by auditory hallucinations, paranoia, and an inability to distinguish reality from fiction
seizure (SEE-zhur)	common English word	sudden disturbance in brain function sometimes producing a convulsion
somnambulism (sahm-NAM-bu-lih-sm)	from Latin words *somnus* (sleep) and *ambulo* (walk); *-ism* (a medical condition)	sleep walking
subdural hematoma (SUB-dur-ahl hee-mah-TOH-ma)	*sub-* (beneath); *dura* (hard); *-al* (adjective suffix); *hemat/o* (blood); *-oma* (tumor)	a collection of blood trapped in the space beneath the dura mater, between the dura and arachnoid layers of the meninges
syncope (SIN-kuh-pee)	from the Greek word *syncope* (a cutting short, a swoon)	fainting
transient ischemic attack (TRANS-ee-ent IH-skee-mik)	from the Greek word *ischo* (to keep back) and *haima* (blood)	temporary interruption in the blood supply to the brain
vertigo (VER-tih-goh)	from the Latin word *verto* (turn)	dizziness

Practice and Practitioners

neurologist (nuhr-AWL-ih-gihst)	*neur/o* (nerve); *-logist* (practitioner)	a medical specialist who treats nervous system disorders
neurology (nuhr-AWL-uh-jee)	*neur/o* (nerve); *-logy* (the study of)	medical specialty dealing with the nervous system
neurosurgeon (NOO-roh-sur-juhn)	*neur/o* (nerve); from the Greek word *kheirourgos* (working or done by hand)	surgeon who specializes in operations on the nervous system
psychiatrist (sy-KY-ah-trist)	*psych/o* (of or pertaining to the mind); *iatr/o* (of or pertaining to medicine or a physician); *-ist* (one who specializes in)	a medical doctor who specializes in the diagnosis and treatment of psychological disorders
psychologist (sy-KOL-oh-jist)	*psych/o* (of or pertaining to the mind); *-logist* (one who studies a certain field)	a (nonmedical) doctor of psychology who specializes in the diagnosis and treatment of psychological disorders

TERM AND PRONUNCIATION	ANALYSIS	MEANING
Diagnosis and Treatments		
antianxiety agent	*anti-* (against); from the Greek word *angho* (to squeeze, embrace throttle)	drug used to suppress anxiousness and relax muscles
anticonvulsant agent	*anti-* (against); from the Latin *con* (with) and *vulsus* (to tear up)	drugs used to decrease seizure activity
antipsychotic agent	*anti-* (against); *psych/o* (of or pertaining to the mind); *-tic* (adjective suffix)	drug given to patients to affect behavior and treat psychiatric disorders
craniectomy (KRAY-nee-ek-tuh-mee)	*crani/o* (cranium); *-ectomy* (excision)	excision of part of the skull
craniotomy (KRAY-nee-aw-tuh-mee)	*crani/o* (cranium); *-tomy* (cutting operation)	incision into the skull
electroconvulsive therapy (ECT) or electroshock therapy (EST)	*electr/o* (electric); from the Latin words *con* (with) and *vulsus* (to tear up)	a controlled convulsion produced by passing an electric current through the brain
electroencephalography (ee-LEK-tro-en-sef-ah-LAH-grah-fee) (EEG)	*electr/o* (electric); *encephal/o* (brain); *-graphy* (process of recording)	record of the electrical potential of the brain
lobotomy (lo-BAWT-uh-mee)	*lob/o* (lobe); *-tomy* (cutting operation)	incision into a lobe
lumbar puncture (LP)	from the Latin word *lumbus* (lion)	insertion of a needle into the subarachnoid space between the third and fourth or fourth and fifth lumbar vertebrae to withdraw fluid for diagnosis
magnetic resonance imaging (MRI)	common English words	uses radio waves and a very strong magnetic field to produce images of the soft tissue
myelography (my-eh-LOG-rah-fee)	*myel/o* (bone marrow or spine); *-graphy* (process of recording)	radiography of the spinal cord and nerve roots
neuroplasty (NURR-oh-plass-tee)	*neur/o* (nerve); *-plasty* (repair)	surgery to repair a nerve
sedatives or hypnotics	from the Latin *sedeo* (sit); from the Greek word *hypnotikos* (causing one to sleep)	drugs used to induce calming effect or sleep

EXERCISES

EXERCISE 7-1   Figure Labeling: Neuron

Label the parts of the motor neuron. Select from the terms listed in the table.

axon branch	cell body	muscle	nucleus
axon covered with myelin sheath	dendrites	myelin sheath	

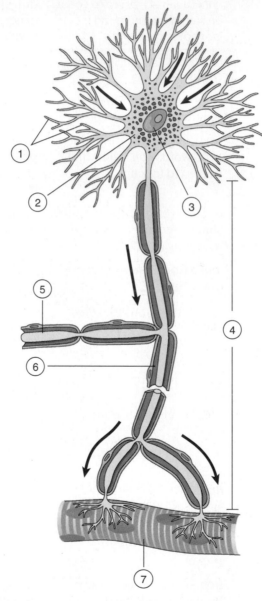

1. _____   4. _____   6. _____

2. _____   5. _____   7. _____

3. _____

EXERCISE 7-2   Case Study

Read the following excerpt from an Emergency Room record and answer the questions.

CHIEF COMPLAINT: Mental status changes and aphasia.

BRIEF HISTORY: J.D. is an 85-year-old female who presents to the Emergency Department with difficulty talking. Her daughter states that J.D. has had garbled speech for the past few days, repeatedly says "How do you do?" and answers the same to any questions asked. This has happened in the past, but the daughter says her mother has always "gotten better." This morning J.D. woke up and has weakness on the right side of her body. There are no other modifying factors or associated signs or symptoms.

ASSESSMENT: Probable history of TIA; now CVA with resulting dysphasia and right hemiparesis.

1. What is a TIA? _____

2. What does the acronym CVA represent? _____

3. Break up the medical term *dysphasia* and define its word elements. _____

   _____

4. What does the root word *paresis* mean? _____

5. What is the difference between *hemiparesis* and *hemiplegia*? _____

   _____

6. Break up the term *hemiplegia* and define the word elements. _____

   _____

EXERCISE 7-3   Word Parts

Fill in the blanks with the proper combining forms.

1. The combining form for "nerve" is _____.

2. The combining form for "spinal cord" is _____.

3. The suffix for "to cut" is _____.

4. The combining form for "head" is _____.

5. The suffix for "speech" is _____.

6. The combining form for "to split" is _____.

7. Name a root and a suffix for "mind": _____ and _____.

EXERCISE 7-4   Word Parts

Break the following into word components: R (root), P (prefix), S (suffix), and CV (combining vowel). Say the terms to a peer and then define each term.

Example   *cerebrospinal*

cerebr = R, o = CV, spin = R, al = S

pertaining to the brain and spinal cord

1. *psychosis*

2. *electroencephalography*

3. *astrocytoma* (astrocyte is a star-shaped brain cell)

4. *cerebrovascular*

5. *hemiplegia*

6. *hydrocephalus*

7. *encephalitis*

_____

_____

8. *epidural*

_____

_____

9. *psychiatrist*

_____

_____

10. *meningioma*

_____

_____

EXERCISE 7-5 Matching

Match the term in the first column with its definition in the second column.

1. ____ cerebrum

2. ____ cerebral cortex

3. ____ brain stem

4. ____ somatic nerves

5. ____ pons

6. ____ autonomic nerves

7. ____ meningomyelocele

8. ____ neuralgia

9. ____ convulsion

10. ____ syncope

A. accumulation of fluid on the brain

B. nerve pain

C. contains the mesencephalon (midbrain), pons and medulla oblongata

D. dizziness

E. hernia of the meninges and the spinal cord

F. outer layer of the cerebrum

G. fainting

H. smallest part of brain

I. contact point between two nerves

J. involuntary nerves

11. ____ vertigo   K. largest part of the brain

12. ____ hydrocephalus   L. inflammation of a nerve

13. ____ neuritis   M. seizure

14. ____ synapse   N. voluntary nerves

EXERCISE 7-6   Spell Check

Circle the correct spelling of the medical term.

1. _____ is the loss, due to brain damage, of the ability to speak or write or to comprehend the written or spoken word.

   Aphasia   Afasia   Aphazia   Aphesia

2. _____ is a type of psychosis that may manifest itself as paranoia, withdrawal, or psychotic symptoms.

   Skitzophrenia   Schizofrenia   Schizophrenia   Skizophrenia

3. _____ are the potent chemicals in the synaptic space between neurons.

   Nuerotransmiters Neurotransmiters Neurotransmitters Neuritransmitters

4. _____ _____ is a collection of blood in the subdural space.

   Subdaral hemitoma   Subdural hemitonia   Subdural henitoma   Subdural hematoma

EXERCISE 7-7   Crossword Puzzle: Nervous System

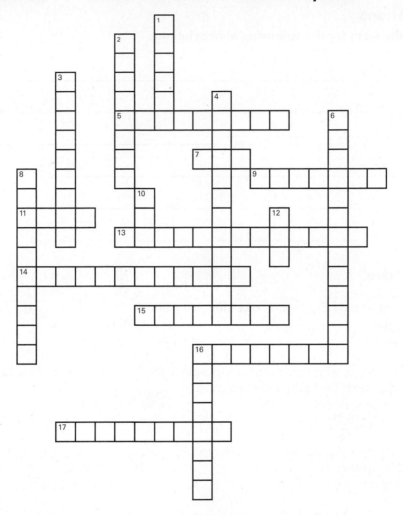

ACROSS

5. part of the NS containing the midbrain, pons, medulla oblongata
7. abbreviation for obsessive-compulsive disorder
9. manic-depressive
11. bridge
13. paranoia, withdrawal from reality, chronic psychosis
14. space between the arachnoid and pia mater
15. drug used to induce sleep
16. processes visual and audible sensory information in the brain
17. nerve glue

DOWN

1. extreme persistent and irrational fear
2. largest part of the brain
3. false beliefs
4. nonphysician who treats behavior disorders
6. perception in the absense of a stimulus; seeing and hearing things
8. prolonged period with a loss of interest
10. abbreviation for level of conciousness
12. abbreviation for magnetic resonance imaging
16. white fatty sheat covering nerves

CHAPTER 7 QUIZ

Abbreviations

Write out the term for the following abbreviations.

1. TIA = _____

2. PEERLA = _____

3. LP = _____

4. EEG = _____

5. MS = _____

6. OBS = _____

Multiple Choice

7. Which term means paralysis on **one side** of the body?
   a. diplegia
   b. paraplegia
   c. monoplegia
   d. hemiplegia

8. Which of the following terms means a disease of the CNS characterized by the formation of plaques in the brain and spinal cord?
   a. amyotrophic lateral sclerosis
   b. Parkinson's disease
   c. multiple sclerosis
   d. poliomyelitis

9. What does the term cerebrocranial refer to?
   a. brain and cranium
   b. cerebellum and cranium
   c. cerebrum and brain
   d. cerebrum and cerebellum

10. The axon is one of two processes that extend from a neuron cell body. What is the other?
    a. effector
    b. dendrite
    c. neurotransmitter
    d. ganglia

11. Which of the following means accumulation of blood under the outermost meningeal layer?
    a. epidural hematoma
    b. intracerebral hematoma
    c. subdural hematoma
    d. cerebral concussion

12. Which of the following means hardening of the brain?
    a. multiple sclerosis
    b. encephalosclerosis
    c. encephalomyelopathy
    d. epilepsy

13. What is cerebral meningitis?
    a. inflammation of the cerebellum
    b. inflammation of the medulla
    c. inflammation of the meninges of the brain
    d. inflammation of the meninges of the spinal cord

14. Which part of the nervous system conducts impulses to skeletal muscle and is under *conscious* control?
    a. autonomic
    b. central
    c. somatic
    d. afferent

15. _____ is the loss, due to brain damage, of the ability to comprehend written or spoken speech.
    a. aphazia
    b. aphesia
    c. aphasia
    d. apazia

Fill in the Blank: Disorders of the Nervous System
Use the terms listed below to fill in the blanks.

agnosia	epilepsy	myasthenia gravis	paraplegia
ataxia	hyperesthesia	myelitis	poliomyelitis
cerebral thrombosis	laminectomy	myelomeningocele	somnambulism
convulsion	meningitis	neuralgia	syncope
dementia	multiple sclerosis	neurosis	vertigo

16. Abnormal sensitivity to touch is called _____.

17. The name for "inflamed" gray matter of the spinal cord is _____.

18. Impaired intellectual function is called _____.

19. The demyelinization of the spinal cord nerves is called _____.

20. The protrusion of the meninges and spinal cord tissue through a spina bifida is called a/an _____.

21. The term for a blood clot in the brain is _____.

22. _____ is characterized by a lack of muscular coordination.

23. CNS disorder often characterized by seizures is termed _____.

24. _____ is synonymous with fainting.

25. Pain in a nerve is _____.

CHAPTER 8

The Endocrine System

LEARNING OBJECTIVES

Upon completion of this chapter, you should be able to:

- Interpret the word elements of the endocrine system.
- List the names of major glands of the endocrine system and their secretions.
- Build, spell, and pronounce medical terms that relate to the endocrine system.
- Identify selected endocrine system pathology terms.
- Identify selected endocrine system diagnostic and surgical procedure terms.
- Identify selected drug classifications and medications relating to the endocrine system.
- Recall and interpret selected abbreviations relating to the endocrine system.
- Analyze and define the new terms introduced in this chapter.

Word Elements • The Endocrine System

WORD ELEMENT	REFERS TO
acr/o	extremities
aden/o	gland
adren/o; adrenal/o	adrenal glands
calc/i	calcium
crin/o	to separate or secrete
endocrin/o	endocrine
gluc/o; glyc/o	sugar; glucose; glycogen
hypophys/o	pituitary gland
-ine	suffix used in the formation of names of chemical substances
-megaly	enlargement
-oma	tumor
pancreat/o	pancreas
parathyr/o; parathyroid/o	parathyroid gland
thyr/o; thyroid/o	thyroid gland
-tropin (from the Greek word *trophe*)	suffix meaning "nourishment" or "stimulation"

An Overview of the Endocrine System

The **endocrine system** (end/o means "within"; crin/o means "to separate or secrete") consists of glands that produce special chemicals called **hormones**. This system is responsible for maintaining homeostasis, a balance or stable condition within the body. Unlike the nervous system, the endocrine system responds more slowly to internal changes in the body. Its release of hormones is regulated by the nervous system, which is either stimulated or delayed according to an intricate feedback mechanism. This feedback system in the body strives to maintain the homeostatic environment through a coordination of the two systems. The nervous system plays a vital role in regulating endocrine functions as it directs the release of hormones that influence other tissues in the body.

    Endocrinology is the medical practice of treating **endocrine** and hormonal disorders. The practitioner, an **endocrinologist** (end/o means "within"; crin/o means "to separate or secrete"; -logy means "to study"; -ist means "specialist") specializes in caring for patients with endocrine diseases and hormonal dysfunctions that may involve sexual development, body growth, or other body functions.

Structure and Function

There are nine primary glands in the endocrine system (Fig. 8-1); this chapter covers seven of the more common glands: **pituitary**, **thyroid**, **parathyroid**, **adrenal**, **pancreas**, **ovaries**, and

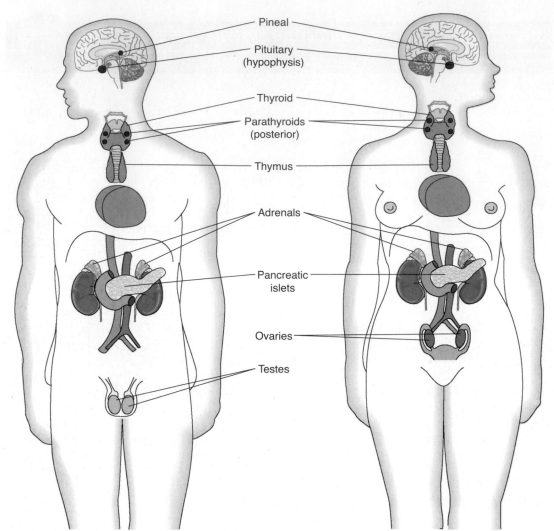

FIGURE 8-1   The endocrine glands. From Cohen BJ. Medical Terminology: An Illustrated Guide, 5th Ed. Philadelphia: Lippincott Williams & Wilkins, 2007.

testes. The other two primary endocrine glands are the pineal and thymus glands. The hormonal secretions and primary functions of each gland are described in Table 8-1.

ENDOCRINE GLANDS

The endocrine glands are ductless glands that secrete their hormones directly into the bloodstream. A hormone is a chemical messenger that is released by an endocrine gland and is transported by the circulatory system to other parts of the body called target organs. The word hormone comes from the Greek language and means "to urge on or set in motion." When the hormone reaches the target organ, the organ reacts or responds to the hormone. Let's look at some of the primary endocrine glands.

Pituitary Gland

The pituitary gland, also known as the master gland or **hypophysis** (hypo- means "below" or "under"; physis means "growth"), is located at the base of the brain below the hypothalamus (hypo- means "below"; thalamus refers to the thalamus gland). It is called the master gland because it

Table 8-1 Summary of the Endocrine Glands, Hormones, and Hormone Functions

Gland	Hormone	Hormone Function
pituitary		master gland; regulates activities of other glands
anterior lobe	growth hormone (GH)	growth and development of bones, muscles, other organs
	thyroid-stimulating hormone (TSH)	growth and development of thyroid gland
	adrenocorticotropin hormone (ACTH)	growth and development of adrenal cortex
	follicle-stimulating hormone (FSH)	stimulates production of sperm in the male and growth of ovarian follicles in the female
	luteinizing hormone (LH)	stimulates the production of testosterone in the male and secretion of estrogen and progesterone in the female
	prolactin hormone (PRL)	stimulates milk secretion in the mammary glands
	melanocyte-stimulating hormone (MSH)	regulates skin pigmentation
posterior lobe	antidiuretic hormone (ADH)	stimulates the reabsorption of water by the kidney tubules
	oxytocin	stimulates the uterus to contract during labor and delivery
thyroid	thyroxine (T_4)	influences growth and development, both physical and mental
	triiodothyronine (T_3)	maintenance and regulation of metabolism
	calcitonin	decreases the blood level of calcium
parathyroid	parathormone (PTH)	increases the blood level of calcium
adrenal		consists of outer portion (cortex) and inner portion (medulla)
cortex	cortisol (hydrocortisone)	regulates carbohydrates, proteins, fat metabolism; anti-inflammatory effect; helps the body cope during stress
	aldosterone	regulates water and electrolyte balance
	androgen (sex hormone)	development of secondary male sex characteristics
medulla	epinephrine (adrenaline)	acts as a vasoconstrictor, cardiac stimulant (increases heart rate and cardiac output), and antispasmodic; releases glucose into the blood (giving the body a spurt of energy)
	norepinephrine (noradrenaline)	acts as a vasoconstrictor; elevates blood pressure and heart rate
pancreas (islets of Langerhans)	insulin	transports glucose into the cells; decreases blood glucose levels
	glucagon	promotes release of glucose by liver; increases blood glucose levels
ovaries	estrogen	promotes growth, development, and maintenance of female sex organs
	progesterone	prepares uterus for pregnancy; promotes development of mammary glands
testes	testosterone	promotes growth, development, and maintenance of male sex organs

controls the activities of the other endocrine glands by releasing special hormones that regulate glandular functions. The pituitary gland is divided into the anterior lobe, or **adenohypophysis** (aden/o refers to gland; so this part of the pituitary is composed of glandular tissue), and the posterior lobe, or **neurohypophysis** (neur/o refers to nerve or nerve tissue; so this part of the pituitary is composed of nerve tissue).

The adenohypophysis secretes several hormones essential for the development of the sex glands, muscles, bones, thyroid gland, and other organs. The neurohypophysis secretes two hormones that are produced in the hypothalamus, the **antidiuretic** (anti- means "against"; diuresis means "to promote urination") **hormone (ADH)** and **oxytocin**. The antidiuretic hormone helps our bodies regulate fluid balance by reducing urination. The latter hormone, oxytocin, stimulates labor during childbirth and promotes milk release during lactation. Its chief function in males is not yet known (see Table 8-1). Figure 8-2 indicates the hormones secreted by the pituitary gland and their target organs. Although the names of most stimulating hormones are not pertinent to a terminology text, their inclusion in the diagram emphasizes the importance of the pituitary or "master" gland.

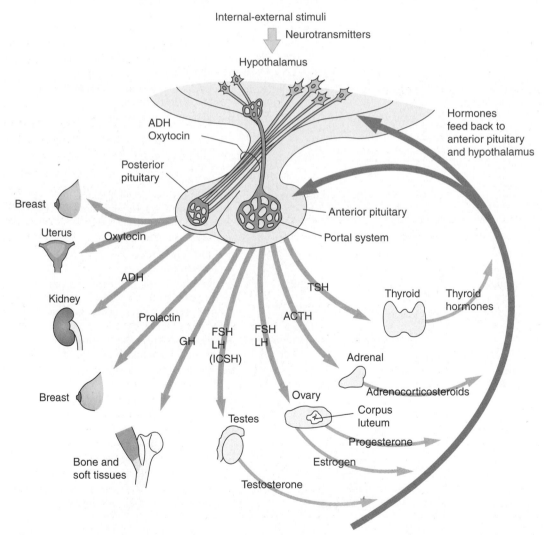

FIGURE 8-2   Hormone secretions from the pituitary gland. The anterior and posterior pituitary glands secrete their hormones, which are transported to the specific target tissues or organs where the regulatory effects stimulate a functional response from the target tissue or organ. From Cohen BJ, Wood DL. Memmler's The Human Body in Health and Disease, 9th Ed. Philadelphia: Lippincott Williams & Wilkins, 2000.

Thyroid Gland

The thyroid is a butterfly-shaped gland that wraps around the larynx (Fig. 8-3). Its main functions are to regulate the body's metabolism and calcium levels. The thyroid produces **triiodothyronine (T₃), thyroxine (T₄)**, and **calcitonin**. T_3 and T_4 regulate cellular metabolism and can accelerate metabolic processes. Calcitonin maintains calcium homeostasis by lowering the amount of calcium in the blood when levels become too high.

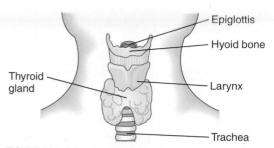

FIGURE 8-3 The thyroid gland. The thyroid gland is a two-lobed, butterfly-shaped gland that is located on the anterior surface of the upper trachea. It secretes a number of hormones that affect both metabolism and calcium levels in the blood. Modified from Cohen BJ. Medical Terminology: An Illustrated Guide, 5th Ed. Philadelphia: Lippincott Williams & Wilkins, 2007.

Parathyroid Gland

There are four **parathyroid glands** consisting of a superior and inferior pair, which are located on the dorsal surface of the thyroid gland (Fig. 8-4). The hormone **parathormone (PTH)**, or parathyroid hormone, produced by the parathyroid gland, is essential for the maintenance of correct calcium and phosphate levels in the blood. Parathormone works with the thyroid hormone calcitonin to maintain homeostasis of calcium in the blood.

Adrenal Glands

The **adrenal glands** (ad- means "in addition to"; ren- means "kidney"; -al is an adjective suffix) consist of two triangular-shaped glands, each one located on the top of a kidney. Their position on top of the kidneys has also earned them the name **suprarenal glands** (supra- means "above"; ren- means "kidney"; -al is an adjective suffix). Each gland is divided into an outer portion called the **adrenal cortex** (*cortex* is the Latin word for "bark" or "husk") and an inner part called the **adrenal medulla** (*medulla* is the Latin word for "marrow" or "middle") (Fig. 8-5). Each secretes its own hormones that are involved in the body's response to stress. The cortex secretes the steroid hormones **cortisol** and **aldosterone**. Cortisol regulates various body functions and has

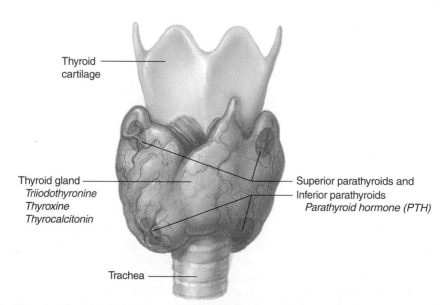

FIGURE 8-4 The parathyroid glands. The parathyroid (para- meaning "adjacent" or "near to") glands consists of four glands, a superior and inferior pair. These are located on the posterior surface of the thyroid gland. Their hormone secretion helps to regulate calcium balance.

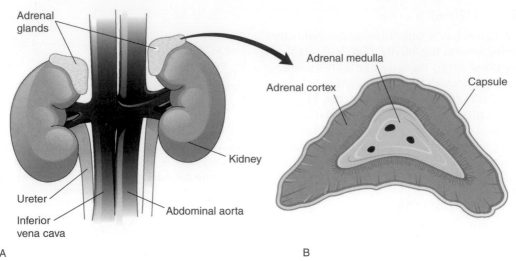

A   B

FIGURE 8-5   The adrenal glands. The adrenal (ad- means "increase" or "move toward") or suprarenal (supra- means "above") glands are situated on top of the kidneys. They have two distinct regions, the cortex and medulla. Each secretes their own hormones. From Cohen BJ. Medical Terminology: An Illustrated Guide, 5th Ed. Philadelphia: Lippincott Williams & Wilkins, 2007.

an anti-inflammatory effect (anti- means "against"; inflammatory means "inflammation"), which helps the body cope with stress. Aldosterone is essential in maintaining the body's electrolyte balance. **Androgens** (andr/o means "male"), which are adrenal cortex hormones, contribute to the development of male sex characteristics.

The adrenal medulla secretes hormones that include **adrenaline** (the suffix -ine means "of"), also known as **epinephrine** (epi- means "upon" or "above"; nephr/o means "kidneys"; -ine means "of"), which stimulates the sympathetic nervous system. This stimulation causes an increase in heart and respiratory rate, along with other changes associated with stress.

Pancreas

The pancreas is a feather-shaped organ that lies posterior to the stomach. The pancreas has clusters of specialized cells called the **islets of Langerhans**, which produce two hormones, **insulin** and **glucagon** (gluc/o means "sugar" or "sweet"). The function of the islet cells is to control blood sugar levels and glucose metabolism throughout the body. Insulin promotes the use of glucose in the cells, thereby lowering blood sugar levels, and it is vital in carbohydrate, protein, and fat metabolism. The hormone glucagon is released in response to low blood sugar levels or hypoglycemia, (hypo- means "below"; glyc/o means "sugar"; -emia means "blood"). It facilitates the breakdown of glycogen to glucose, causing a rise in blood sugar level.

Gonads

The ovaries and testes are the female and male gonads. They receive stimulating hormones from the pituitary gland and respond by producing the female and male hormones that allow for the secondary sex characteristics to develop.

The ovaries (ovary comes from the Latin word *ovarius* meaning "egg holder") are two oval-shaped glands located in the pelvic cavity on either side of the uterus. The ovaries produce the female egg as well as two important hormones: **estrogen** and **progesterone**. These hormones are responsible for the development of female sex characteristics, regulating the menstrual cycle, and preparing the uterus for and maintaining pregnancy.

The male gonads, or testes, are two oval organs that lie in the scrotum. They produce the male hormone **testosterone** (testost/o means "testis" or "male gonad"; -one is a suffix for a chemical compound), which controls the male sexual development and reproductive function.

Disorders and Treatments

Disorders of the endocrine system are almost always the result of either an excess or a deficit in hormone production. That means that either too much or too little of a hormone will cause a problem. The serum or blood level of a hormone may be assessed by means of a laboratory examination, scans, magnetic resonance imaging (MRIs), and/or ultrasonic examinations to detect abnormalities. A biopsy may be used to determine whether lesions detected during testing are benign or malignant.

The treatment of the disorder depends on its cause. If there is a deficit in hormone production, then replacement therapy would be the normal treatment. If there is an overproduction of a hormone, then surgical or radiation intervention may be used. Table 8-2 is a summary of some of the more common disorders of the endocrine system. Brief discussions of the major ones follow.

DISORDERS OF THE PITUITARY GLAND

One of the most common causes of pituitary disorders is a benign (nonmalignant or noninvasive) adenoma (aden/o means "gland"; -oma means "tumor"). The hormonal effects of the tumor may cause an excessive amount of hormone to be secreted, or the tumor may destroy pituitary cells, causing a deficit in hormone production. It is important to determine the cause of the hormonal imbalance—whether it is in the pituitary gland or the target gland. As mentioned earlier, the treatment will usually be hormone replacement or surgical excision (ex- means "outside, out"; -cise means "to cut out"); the decision depends on whether the problem is overproduction or underproduction of a hormone.

Diabetes Insipidus

Diabetes insipidus is caused by an insufficient production of the antidiuretic (anti- means "against"; diuresis means "excessive urination") hormone (ADH). An excess amount of fluid is excreted by the kidneys, resulting in extreme thirst and excessive urination (**polyuria:** poly- means "many" or "a lot"; ur/o means "urine"; -ia is an adjective suffix meaning "pertaining to"). Treatment usually consists of administration of a form of the antidiuretic hormone to replace the deficit.

Table 8-2   Endocrine Disorders

Gland	Hormone	↓	↑	Disorder
pituitary	growth hormone	↓		dwarfism
	antidiuretic hormone	↓		diabetes insipidus
	growth hormone		↑	gigantism in children; acromegaly in adults
thyroid	T_3, T_4	↓		hypothyroidism; a deficiency in adults
	T_3, T_4	↓		Hashimoto, Graves, Addison, and Cushing thyroiditis
	T_3, T_4		↑	Graves disease; usually characterized by goiter and exophthalmos
	T_3, T_4		↑	goiter or thyromegaly
	T_3, T_4		↑	hyperthyroidism
adrenal	cortisol	↓		Addison disease
	cortisol		↑	Cushing syndrome
	epinephrine		↑	pheochromocytoma
pancreas	insulin	↓		hypoglycemia
	insulin	↓		diabetes mellitus; type 1, type 2
gonads	estrogen		↑	gynecomastia (males only)
	testosterone		↑	hirsutism (females only)

Gigantism and Acromegaly

Gigantism is an abnormal overgrowth of the body or any of its parts. It is caused by excessive secretion of the growth hormone before puberty. **Acromegaly** is enlargement of the extremities (mostly hands and feet) caused by excessive secretion of the growth hormone after puberty (Fig. 8-6). Treatment for these two conditions is similar. Surgery and radiation of a tumor that is the cause of the excess hormone production is frequently used, along with a medication regimen to decrease the hormone.

DISORDERS OF THE THYROID GLAND

As with other endocrine disorders, an excess or deficient amount of thyroid hormone production creates an imbalance in our body. It affects the physical growth and function of many of the body's tissues. A few of the hyperthyroid and hypothyroid conditions will be discussed here.

Hypothyroidism

Hypothyroidism (hypo- means "below"; thyroid refers to the thyroid gland; -ism means "state of, characteristic quality") is characterized by a decrease in thyroid function. It is usually caused by removal of or other loss of thyroid tissue and produces slowed mental processes, hoarse speech, loss of hair, and muscle weakness. Treatment with hormone replacement medication usually produces positive results in about two weeks but must be continued for the remainder of the person's life.

   Hashimoto thyroiditis (thyroid refers to the thyroid gland; -itis means "inflammation of") is an autoimmune disorder in which lymphocytes (lymph refers to lymph or fluid containing white cells; -cyte means "cell") invade the thyroid gland, causing an inflammation that eventually destroys the thyroid gland and produces hypothyroidism.

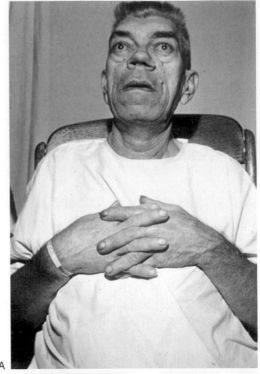

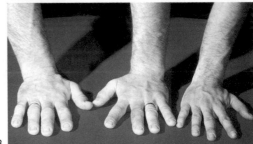

FIGURE 8-6 Person with acromegaly. Notice the wide forehead, wide-set eyes, square chin, and enlarged wide hands. **A.** Note coarse facial features. **B.** Note the patient's large hands at left and single normal hand at right. From McConnell TH. The Nature Of Disease Pathology for the Health Professions. Philadelphia: Lippincott Williams & Wilkins, 2007.

Hyperthyroidism

One of the common types of **hyperthyroidism** (hyper- means "above"; thyroid refers to the thyroid gland; -ism means "state of, characteristic quality") is called **Graves disease**, which is caused by an increase in thyroid hormone secretion. This is also known as a toxic goiter and is marked by diffuse hyperplasia (hyper- means "excess"; -plasia means "growth") of the thyroid gland. Toxic usually refers to a substance that can impair health and is sometimes used synonymously with poison. In this case, the thyroid gland is producing too much hormone, causing health problems. Goiter (from Latin *gutter* meaning "throat"), also called **thyromegaly** (thyr/o means "thyroid"; -megaly means "enlargement"), is a visible enlargement of the thyroid gland on the front of the neck. It is caused by a deficiency of iodine in the diet. Figure 8-7 depicts a person with a pronounced goiter.

DISORDERS OF THE ADRENAL GLAND

Inflammatory conditions and viral infections that involve the adrenal glands can cause a decrease in hormone production because they destroy glandular tissue. On the other hand, benign tumors are frequent causes of increased hormone production from the adrenal glands.

Addison Disease

Addison disease is a progressive disorder caused by an insufficient amount of cortisol production in the adrenal gland. It may also be caused by a failure of the pituitary gland to produce one of its stimulating hormones targeting the adrenal gland. Symptoms include low blood pressure, weakness, nausea, and an increase in brown pigmentation of the skin. Treatment includes replacing the necessary hormones.

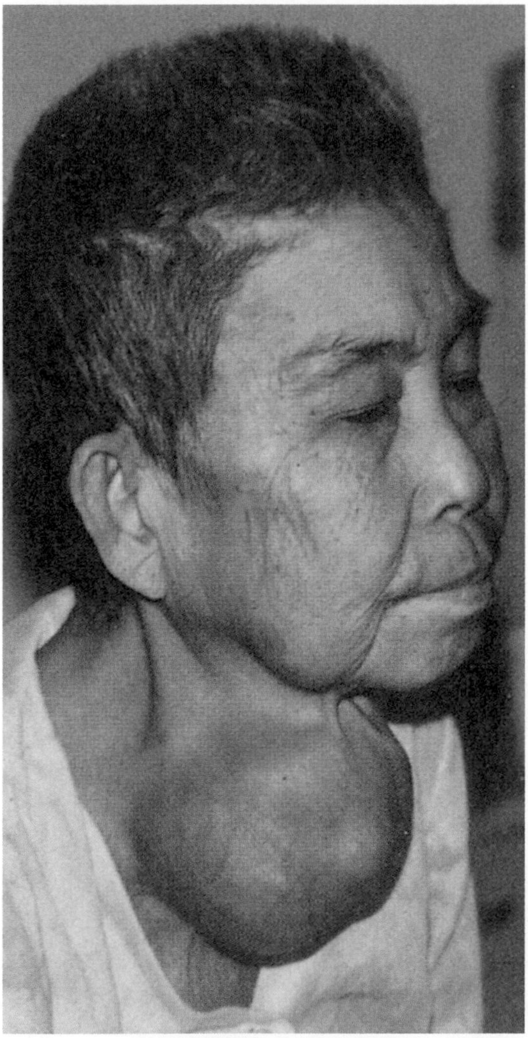

Cushing Syndrome

Cushing syndrome is caused by an excessive amount of adrenal hormone secretion and is characterized by obesity localized in the trunk, a "moon-shaped" face, and excess fat at the back of the neck (colloquially called a "buffalo hump"). It can also be attributed to taking steroids such as prednisone for other conditions. Treatment is usually aimed at treating the symptoms but also involves decreasing the steroid medication when possible. Figure 8-8 illustrates a person exhibiting symptoms of Cushing syndrome.

DISORDERS OF THE PANCREAS

One of the most common endocrine disorders involves the pancreas and how it responds to the body's need for glucose. This condition,

FIGURE 8-7 Goiter. Goiter, which means "gullet or throat," is the term given for an enlarged thyroid. Goiter is visibly seen in the anterior neck and is more often found in people from specific geographic locations where there is low iodine levels. Iodine is necessary for thyroid hormone production, so without it, the thyroid compensates and becomes enlarged. From Rubin E. Essential Pathology, 3rd Ed. Philadelphia: Lippincott Williams & Wilkins, 2000.

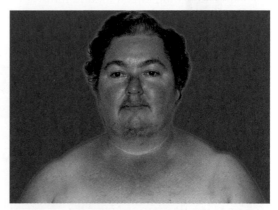

FIGURE 8-8 Cushing syndrome. The woman has a moon face, buffalo hump, increased facial hair, and thinning of the scalp hair. From Cohen BJ. Medical Terminology: An Illustrated Guide, 5th Ed. Philadelphia: Lippincott Williams & Wilkins, 2007.

called diabetes mellitus, is a major health problem that can have lifelong effects. There are two main types of diabetes, type 1 and type 2, each of which is discussed here.

Type 1 diabetes mellitus (DM) is a metabolic disorder caused by insufficient production of insulin from the islet cells of the pancreas. Symptoms in the early stages include **glycosuria** (sugar in the urine; glyc/o means "sugar" or "sweet"; uria is from *ouron*, a Greek word meaning "urine"); **hyperglycemia** (excess sugar in the blood; hyper- means "excess"; glyc/o means "sugar" or "sweet"; -emia means "blood"), frequent urination, and weight loss. Fatigue and slow healing processes may be noted later on, along with multiple organ complications if the disease remains uncontrolled and untreated. Replacement therapy with insulin injections, diet, and exercise make up the usual course of therapy.

Type 2 diabetes mellitus is an insulin-resistant disorder. The islet cells produce insulin, but the body fails to use it effectively. Symptoms may not be noted for several years. Treatment usually consists of a change in diet, exercise, and medications called **hypoglycemics** (hypo- means "below"; glyc/o means "sugar" or "sweet"; -emic means "blood"; adjective form of term referring to a medication taken to reduce sugar in the blood) to lower blood sugar.

Pharmacology

As mentioned earlier, the endocrine system secretes a variety of hormones that affect the entire body. When these hormones are deficient, the body responds with characteristic disease states. Hormone replacement therapy is often used to correct these disorders. Examples of disorders treatable by hormone replacement are hypothyroidism and diabetes mellitus. Medications for hypothyroidism include Synthroid, Levothroid, and Levoxyl. Some of the more common medications given for diabetes mellitus are insulin (Humulin, Lente, NPH) and the oral hypoglycemic agents Orinase, Diabinese, Glucophage, metformin, Avandamet, and Avandia. Oral hypoglycemic drugs are prescribed for patients who have some insulin production by the pancreas but not enough to sustain proper blood sugar levels. The ultimate goal in prescribing replacement hormones is to maintain the body at an optimal homeostatic balance.

As mentioned earlier, the adrenal glands secrete corticosteroids, which act on the immune system to relieve inflammation and swelling and suppress the body's response to infection or trauma. Corticosteroids may be administered as a replacement therapy or for their immunosuppressant and anti-inflammatory properties. They usually are used as a supportive therapy as opposed to being curative. Corticosteroids have a variety of preparations including creams (topical), inhalants, oral, injection, and intravenous. Some examples include Decadron, Solu-Cortef, Kenalog, Aristocort, Rhinocort, Prelone, and Solu-Medrol, to name a few.

Abbreviation Table • *The Endocrine System*

ABBREVIATION	MEANING
ACTH	adrenocorticotrophic hormone
ADH	antidiuretic hormone
BS	blood sugar
DM	diabetes mellitus
FBS	fasting blood sugar
FSH	follicle-stimulating hormone
GH	growth hormone

ABBREVIATION	MEANING
HbA1c	hemoglobin A1c (reflects average long-term glucose levels for 2–3 months before glucose blood level is drawn)
IDDM	insulin-dependent diabetes mellitus
LH	luteinizing hormone
MSH	melanocyte-stimulating hormone
NIDDM	non–insulin-dependent diabetes mellitus
PRL	prolactin
TSH	thyroid-stimulating hormone

Study Table • The Endocrine System

TERM AND PRONUNCIATION	ANALYSIS	MEANING
Structure and Function		
adenogenous (ad-eh-NAW-jeh-nuhs)	*aden/o* (gland); *-genous* (originating)	originating in a gland
adenohypophysis (AD-eh-noh-hy-POFF-ih-sihs)	*aden/o* (gland); *hypophys/o* (pituitary gland)	the anterior pituitary gland
adrenal glands (ah-DREE-nahl); adrenal cortex, adrenal medulla	*adren/o* (adrenal glands); *cortex* (a Latin word meaning "bark"); *medulla* (a Latin word meaning "marrow, innermost part")	two glands, one located at the top of each kidney; adrenal cortex is the outer portion, adrenal medulla is the inner portion
adrenaline (ah-DREN-ah-lihn)	*adren/o* (adrenal glands); *-ine* (a suffix used to form names of chemical substances)	synonym for epinephrine, secreted from the adrenal medulla
adrenocorticotropic (ACTH) (ah-DREE-oh-KOR-tih-ko-TROH-pik)	*cortic/o* (from *cortex* [bark]); from the Greek word *trophe* (nourishment); *-in* (a suffix used to form names of biochemical substances)	pituitary secretion that stimulates the adrenal glands
androgen (AN-droh-jen)	*andro-* (masculine); *-gen* (suffix meaning "precursor of")	male hormone secreted by the adrenal cortex
aldosterone (al-DOSS-teh-rone)	ald (ehyd) + ster(ol) + -one (chemical suffix)	one of the corticosteroids, hormones produced by the adrenal glands
antidiuretic hormone (AN-tee-dy-uh-RET-ik) (ADH)	*anti-* (against); from the Greek *dia* (through); *-uresis* (urination)	hormone secreted by the posterior pituitary gland to prevent the kidneys from expelling too much water

(continued)

TERM AND PRONUNCIATION	ANALYSIS	MEANING
calcitonin (kal-sih-TOH-nihn) (CT)	*calci-* (calcium); from the Greek *tonos* (to stretch); *-in* (suffix used to form names of biochemical substances)	hormone secreted by the thyroid to prevent too much calcium from absorbing into the bones
corticosteroids (KOR-tih-ko-STEHR-oyds)	*cortic/o* (from Latin word *cortex* [bark]); from *Steros* (solid); *-oid* (resemblance to)	steroid produced by the cortices of the adrenal glands, cortisol
endocrine (EN-doh-krin)	*endo-* (within, inner); from the Greek word *krino* (to separate)	adjective describing a gland that delivers its secretions directly into blood stream
epinephrine (EP-ih-NEFF-rihn)	*epi-* (upon); *nephr/o* (kidney); *-ine* (suffix used to form the names of chemical substances)	synonym for adrenaline, secreted from the adrenal medulla
estrogen (EHS-troh-jen)	from the Greek word *oistrus* (estrus); *-gen* (producing)	one of two hormones secreted by the ovaries
exocrine (EX-oh-krihn)	*exo-* (outside of); from the Greek word *krino* (to separate)	adjective describing a gland that delivers its secretions through a duct onto the skin or other epithelial surface
glucagon (GLOO-ka-guhn)	*gluc/o* (glucose); from the Greek word *ago* (to lead)	hormone secreted by the pancreas
gonadotropin (FSH) (GO-nad-oh-TROH-pin)	from the Greek word *gone* (seed); from the Greek word *trophe* (nourishment); *-in* (suffix used to form names of biochemical substances)	follicle-stimulating hormone; hormone promoting gonadal growth
gonadotropin (ICSH) (GO-nad-oh-TROH-pin)	from the Greek word *gone* (seed); from the Greek word *trophe* (nourishment); *-in* (suffix used to form names of biochemical substances)	interstitial cell-stimulating hormone; hormone promoting gonadal growth in the male
gonadotropin (LH) (GO-nad-oh-TROH-pin)	from the Greek word *gone* (seed); from the Greek word *trophe* (nourishment); *-in* (suffix used to form names of biochemical substances)	luteinizing hormone; stimulates ovulation

TERM AND PRONUNCIATION	ANALYSIS	MEANING
hormone (HOHR-mohn)	from the Greek word *hormao* (to rouse or set in motion)	chemical messenger that is secreted by an endocrine gland directly into the bloodstream
hydrocortisone (hy-droh-KOR-tih-sone)	*hydro-* (water); *cortic/o* (from the Greek word *cortex* meaning "bark"); *-one* (chemical suffix)	an adrenal gland hormone secretion
hypophysis (hy-POFF-ih-sihs)	*hypophys/o* (pituitary gland)	synonym for pituitary gland
insulin (IN-soo-lihn)	from the Latin word *insula* (island)	one of two hormones produced in the pancreas
islets of Langerhans (EYE-lets LAN-gehr-hans)	after German pathologist Paul Langerhans, who described it in 1869; islets are the regions of the pancreas that contain its hormone-producing cells	clusters of specialized cells in the pancreas that secrete insulin
melanocyte-stimulating hormone (MEL-an-oh-syte) (MSH)	*melan/o* (black); *-cyte* (cell); from the Greek word *hormao* (to rouse or set in motion)	hormone secreted from the anterior pituitary gland
melatonin (mel-ah-TONE-ihn)	melanophore + Greek *tonos* (to stretch); *-in* (suffix used to form names of biochemical substances)	hormone secreted by the pineal gland
neurohypophysis (NUHR-oh-hy-POFF-ih-sihs)	*neur/o* (nerve); *hypophys/o* (pituitary gland)	synonym for posterior pituitary gland
noradrenaline (nor-ah-DREN-ah-lihn)	*nor-* (chemical prefix); *adrenal/o* (adrenal glands); *-ine* (a suffix used to denote chemical substances)	synonym for norepinephrine; secreted from the adrenal medulla
norepinephrine (NOR-ehp-ih-NEFF-rihn)	*nor-* (chemical prefix); *epi-* (upon); from the Greek word *nephros* (kidney); *-ine* (a suffix used to denote chemical substances)	synonym for noradrenaline; secreted from the adrenal medulla
ovaries (OH-vayr-ees)	from the Latin word *ovum* (egg)	female gonads; two oval-shaped glands that are located in the pelvic cavity
oxytocin (ox-ih-TOH-sihn) (OT)	from the Greek word *oxytokos* (swift birth); *-in* (suffix used to form names of biochemical substances)	hormone secreted by the posterior pituitary gland

(continued)

TERM AND PRONUNCIATION	ANALYSIS	MEANING
pancreas (PAN-kree-uhs)	from the Greek word *pancreas* (sweetbread)	feather-shaped organ that lies posterior to the stomach
parathyroid gland (pahr-ah-THY-royd)	*para-* (prefix denoting involvement of two like parts; also denoting adjacent, alongside, near); *thyr/o* (thyroid gland)	secretes parathyroid hormone (PTH)
parathyroid hormone (pahr-ah-THY-royd), parathormone (PTH)	*para-* (prefix denoting involvement of two like parts; also denoting adjacent, alongside, near); *thyr/o* (thyroid gland); from the Greek word *hormao* (to set in motion)	a hormone secreted by the parathyroid gland
pineal gland (PIHN-ee-ahl)	from the Latin word *pinus* (pine); *-al* (adjective ending)	gland that secretes melatonin, an antioxidant that is otherwise not well understood
pituitary gland (pih-TOO-ih-tahr-ee)	from the Latin word *pituita*	synonym for hypophysis; master gland
progesterone (proh-JES-ter-ohn)	from the Latin *pro* (for); from the Latin *gestare* (to carry about)	one of two female hormones secreted by the ovary
prolactin (PRL) (pro-LAK-tihn)	from the Latin *pro* (for); from the Latin *lacteus* (milky)	a secretion of the anterior pituitary gland
suprarenal glands (SOO-prah-REEN-ahl)	*supra-* (above); *ren-* (kidney); *-al* (pertaining to)	another name for the adrenal glands
testes (TES-tees)	from the plural form of the Latin *testis* (testicle)	male gonads; two oval organs that lie in the scrotum
testosterone (teh-STAH-steh-rone)	from the Latin *testis* (testicle); ster(ol); *-one* (chemical suffix)	male hormone secreted by the testes
thyroid gland (THY-royd)	*thyr/o* (thyroid gland)	one of the four glands belonging solely to the endocrine system; located in the throat area
thyrotropin (TSH) (thy-ROT-roh-pihn)	*thyr/o* (thyroid gland); from the Greek *trophe* (nourishment); *-in* (suffix used to form names of biochemical substances)	thyroid-stimulating hormone

TERM AND PRONUNCIATION	ANALYSIS	MEANING
thyroxine (thy-ROK-sihn) (T_4)	*thyr/o* (thyroid gland); *-ine* (suffix used to form names of biochemical substances)	a secretion of the thyroid gland
triiodothyronine (try-EYE-oh-doh-THY-roh-neen) (T_3)	*tri-* (three); *iodo* (iodine); *thyr/o* (thyroid gland); *-ine* (a suffix used to form names of chemical substances)	another secretion of the thyroid gland that is often synthesized from thyroxine (T_4) by bodily organs

Common Disorders

TERM AND PRONUNCIATION	ANALYSIS	MEANING
acromegaly (AK-roh-mehg-alee)	from the Greek *akron* (extremity); *-megaly* (enlargement)	enlargement of the extremities (mostly hands and feet) caused by excessive secretion of the growth hormone *after* puberty
Addison (or Addison's) disease	after the British physician, Thomas Addison, who first described the condition in 1855	a disorder characterized by a failure of the adrenal glands to produce hydrocortisone and, in some cases, aldosterone
adenitis (ad-eh-NY-tihs)	*aden/o* (gland); *-itis* (inflammation)	inflammation of a gland
adenohypophysitis (AD-eh-noh-hy-poff-ih-SY-tihs)	*aden/o* (gland); *hypophys/o* (pituitary gland); *-itis* (inflammation)	inflammation of the hypophysis
adrenalitis (ah-dree-nah-LY-tiss)	*adrenal/o* (adrenal glands); *-itis* (inflammation)	inflammation of an adrenal gland
adrenalopathy (ah-dree-nah-LOP-ah-thee); sometimes also adrenopathy (ah-dree-NOP-ah-thee)	*adrenal/o* (adrenal glands); *-pathy* (disease)	any disease of the adrenal glands
adrenomegaly (ah-dree-noh-MEG-ah-lee)	*adren/o* (adrenal gland); *-megaly* (enlargement)	enlargement of the adrenal glands
Cushing (or Cushing's) syndrome	named after Harvey Cushing, American physician, who described the disorder in 1932	a hormonal disorder caused by too much hydrocortisone
diabetes insipidus (DY-ah-BEET-ehs ihn-SIP-ih-duhs)	*diabetes*, a Greek word meaning a compass, a siphon; *insipidus* (lacking flavor or zest)	condition brought about by the posterior pituitary's failure to produce enough ADH (antidiuretic hormone)

(continued)

TERM AND PRONUNCIATION	ANALYSIS	MEANING
diabetes mellitus, Type 1 and Type 2 (DY-ah-BEET-ehs meh-LY-tuhs)	*diabetes*, a Greek word meaning "a compass, a siphon"; *mellitus*, a Latin word meaning "sweetened with honey" or "honey-sweet"	condition brought about by insufficient production of insulin in the pancreas (type 1) or the failure of the body's cells to absorb glucose (type 2)
gigantism (JEYE-gan-tizm)	*giant* (common English word); *-ism* (condition)	abnormal overgrowth of the body due to excessive secretion of the growth hormone *before* puberty
glycosuria (GLY-koh-SYUR-ee-ah)	*glyc/o/s* (sugar); *-uria* (urine)	sugar in the urine
goiter (GOY-tuhr)	from the Latin word *gutter* (throat)	chronic enlargement of the thyroid gland
Graves (or Graves') disease	named after Robert James Graves (1796–1853), an Irish physician who first described exophthalmic goiter in 1835	a common form of hyperthyroidism resulting from overproduction of thyroxine; caused by a false immune system response
Hashimoto (or Hashimoto's) thyroiditis (Hah-shee-moh-toh)	Hashimoto (Japanese surgeon, 1881–1934); *thyr/o* (thyroid gland); *-itis* (inflammation)	an autoimmune disorder that attacks the thyroid gland causing hypothyroidism
hyperglycemia (hy-puhr-gly-SEEM-ee-ah)	*hyper-* (above normal); *glyc/o* (sugar); *-ia* (condition)	excessive sugar in the blood
hyperpituitarism (HY-puhr-pih-TOO-iht-ahr-izm)	*hyper-* (above normal); from the Latin word *pituita*	excessive hormone secretion by the pituitary gland
hyperthyroidism (HY-puhr-THY-royd-izm)	*hyper-* (above normal); *thyr/o* (thyroid); *-ism* (condition)	condition caused by an overactive thyroid; usually caused by an immune system disorder known as Graves' disease
hypophysitis (hy-poh-fih-SY-tihs)	*hypophys/o* (pituitary gland); *-itis* (inflammation)	inflammation of the pituitary gland
hypopituitarism (hy-poh-pih-TOO-ih-tahr-izm)	*hypo-* (below normal); from the Latin word *pituita*; *-ism* (condition)	condition of diminished hormone secretion from the anterior pituitary gland
hypothyroidism	*hypo-* (below normal); thyroid refers to the thyroid gland; *-ism* (state of)	a decrease in thyroid function

TERM AND PRONUNCIATION	ANALYSIS	MEANING
pituitarism (pih-TOO-iht-ahr-izm)	from the Latin word *pituita*; *-ism* (condition)	any pituitary dysfunction
thyroaplasia (THY-roh-a-PLAY-zee-ah)	*thyr/o* (thyroid gland); aplasia from the Greek *a plassien* (not to form)	congenital condition characterized by low thyroid output
thyroiditis (thy-roy-DY-tihs)	*thyr/o* (thyroid gland); *-itis* (inflammation)	inflammation of the thyroid gland
thyromegaly (thy-roh-MEG-ah lee)	*thyr/o* (thyroid gland); *-megaly* (enlargement)	enlargement of the thyroid gland

Practice and Practitioners

endocrinologist (en-do-krih-NOL-oh-jist)	*endocrin/o* (endocrine); *-logist* (one who specializes)	medical specialist in endocrinology
endocrinology	*endocrin/o* (endocrine); *-logy* (study of)	medical specialty of the endocrine system

Diagnosis and Treatments

adenectomy (ad-eh-NEK-toh-mee)	*aden/o* (gland); *-ectomy* (excision)	excision of a gland
adenotomy (ad-eh-NOT-oh-mee)	*aden/o* (gland); *-tomy* (cutting operation)	incision of a gland
adrenalectomy (ah-dree-nah-LEK-toh-mee)	*adrenal/o* (adrenal glands); *-ectomy* (excision)	surgical removal of one or both adrenal glands
hypoglycemic (HY-poh-gly-SEE-mik)	*hypo-* (below normal); *glyc/o* (sugar); *-ic* (pertaining to)	drug used to lower blood sugar
hypophysectomy (HY-poh-fih-SEK-toh-mee)	*hypophys/o* (pituitary gland); *-ectomy* (excision)	surgical removal of the hypophysis (pituitary gland)
parathyroidectomy (PAHR-ahthy-royd-EK-toh-mee)	*parathyr/o* (parathyroid gland); *-ectomy* (excision)	surgical excision of the parathyroid gland
thyroidectomy (THY-royd-EK-toh-mee)	*thyr/o* (thyroid gland); *-ectomy* (excision)	excision of the thyroid gland
thyroparathyroidectomy (THY-roh-pehr-ah-THY-roy-DEK-toh-mee)	*thyr/o* (thyroid gland); *parathyr/o* (parathyroid gland); *-ectomy* (excision)	excision of the thyroid and parathyroid glands
thyrotomy (thy-ROT-oh-mee)	*thyr/o* (thyroid gland); *-tomy* (cutting operation)	surgery performed on the thyroid gland

EXERCISES

EXERCISE 8-1   Figure Labeling: The Endocrine System

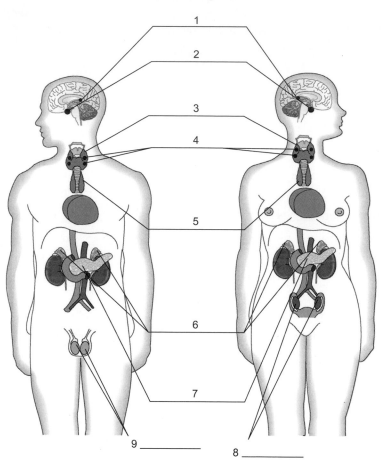

The endocrine glands

Select the endocrine gland from the list and place it by the corresponding number.

1. _____   adrenals

2. _____   ovaries

3. _____   parathyroids

4. _____   pancreatic islets

5. _____   pineal

6. _____   pituitary (hypophysis)

7. _____   testes

8. _____   thymus

9. _____   thyroid

EXERCISE 8-2   Case Study

ENDOCRINOLOGY OFFICE CONSULTATION

After reading the case study, answer the following questions:

OFFICE NOTE: This 59-year-old woman has previously been in good health. On a routine physical examination, she was noted to have a thyroid nodule on the right lobe of the thyroid. She complained of hoarseness, dysphasia, local tenderness, and a slight enlargement on the right side of her neck. She also admits to an increase in activity and inability to sleep throughout the night.

On physical examination, the right side of the neck was visibly enlarged, and a nodule was felt; it was noted that the patient's eyes were bulging outward. A blood test to check her thyroid hormone blood levels indicated a high value of TSH. No other modifying factors or associated signs or symptoms were present.

1. What is another name for hyperthyroidism? _____

2. What does dysphasia mean? _____

3. What is the medical term for an "enlargement of the thyroid gland"? _____

4. What is TSH? _____

5. What is the medical term for bulging of the eyes? Define the word elements of this term.

_____

EXERCISE 8-3   Spell Check

Circle the correct spelling of the medical term.

1. An _____ is a physician who specializes in caring for patients with endocrine diseases and hormonal dysfunctions.

   enocreenologist   endokrineologist   endocrineologist   endocrinologist

2. A medication that can be taken orally to lower the blood sugar is called a

    _____.

    hypogysemic   hyperglycemic   hypoglycemic   hyperglysemik

3. _____ is one of the hormones produced in the pancreas that
    regulates blood sugar.

    insullin   insulin   insalin   insulen

4. One of the main disorders of the pancreas is called _____.

    diabetes mellitus   diabetis mellitus   diabetis melletes   diabetes melitus

---

EXERCISE 8-4   Disorders and Symptoms of the Endocrine System

Match the terms listed with the definitions below.

acromegaly	endogenous	polyuria
Cushing syndrome	glycosuria	thyromegaly
diabetes mellitus (DM)	hyperglycemia	

1. _____   enlarged thyroid gland, also referred to as goiter

2. _____   lack of or insufficient insulin production from the pancreas

3. _____   excessive and frequent urination

4. _____   abnormally high levels of glucose in the blood

5. _____   originating from within the body

6. _____   enlargement of extremities caused by overproduction of the
                        growth hormone in adults

7. _____   sugar in the urine

8. _____   excessive amount of adrenal hormone secreted; characterized
                        by moon-shaped face and a "buffalo hump"

EXERCISE 8-5   Word Building: The Endocrine System

Use *adren/o* to build the medical words meaning:

1. enlargement of the adrenal gland _____

2. surgical removal of an adrenal gland _____

3. disease of the adrenal glands _____

Use *thyr/o* or *thyroid/o* to build the medical words meaning:

4. condition of minimal functioning of the thyroid gland _____

5. inflammation of the thyroid gland _____

6. incision of the thyroid gland _____

7. enlargement of the thyroid gland _____

Use *pancreat/o* to build the medical words meaning:

8. tumor of the pancreas _____

9. inflammation of the pancreas _____

10. originating in the pancreas _____

EXERCISE 8-6 Crossword Puzzle: The Endocrine System

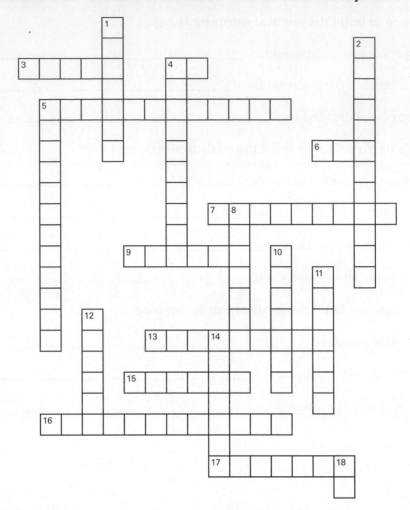

ACROSS

3. Female gonad
4. abbreviation for growth hormone
5. oral medication used to treat type 2 diabetes
6. abbreviation for fasting blood sugar
7. master gland
9. autommmune disorder resulting in hyperthyroidism; exophthalmos and goiter
13. condition caused by excess growth hormone in children
15. male gonads
16. located on the dorsal surface of the the thyroid gland
17. gland located on the top of the kidney

DOWN

1. T_3 and T_4 are secreted from which gland?
2. hormone secreted by the male gonad
4. excess sugar in the urine
5. low blood sugar
8. hormone not produced in type 1 diabetes
10. a syndrome resulting from excess secretion of adrenal cortex; obesity, hirsutism, weakness
11. chemical secreted by an endocrine gland
12. enlarged thyroid
14. tumor of a gland
18. abbreviation for luteinizing hormone

CHAPTER 8 QUIZ

Multiple Choice

1. The master gland is known as the:
    a. pituitary gland
    b. thymus gland
    c. thyroid gland
    d. pineal gland

2. The ovaries produce which two hormones?
    a. insulin and glucagon
    b. estrogen and progesterone
    c. testosterone and thymosin
    d. T_3 and T_4

3. Endocrine means:
    a. to cringe from within
    b. to secrete within
    c. to cry inside
    d. a disease of the gland

4. Oversecretion of the pituitary growth hormone in an adult produces a condition called:
    a. hyperthyroidism
    b. Simmond's disease
    c. acromegaly
    d. tetany

5. _____ is an enlargement of the thyroid gland.
    a. hypothyroidism
    b. goiter
    c. thyroidectomy
    d. Addison's disease

6. A chemical secreted from an endocrine gland is called a/an:
    a. hormone
    b. lymph
    c. neurotransmitter
    d. insulin

7. Hypersecretion of the *growth hormone* may cause:
    a. insulin
    b. cretinism
    c. hypothyroidism
    d. gigantism

8. _____ is associated with excessive hormone secretion from the adrenal cortex.
    a. Cushing's disease
    b. Conn's syndrome
    c. goiter
    d. gigantism

9. The two-lobed gland in the neck is called the:
    a. Adam's apple
    b. thymus
    c. pituitary
    d. thyroid

Matching

Select the best definition from Column 2 to match the term in Column 1.

TERM	DEFINITION
10. _____ adrenalopathy	A. synonym for epinephrine, which is an adrenal hormone secreted when immediate physical action may be needed by the body
11. _____ hyperpituitarism	B. thyroid-stimulating hormone, secreted by the anterior pituitary
12. _____ adenogenous	C. enlargement of the thyroid gland
13. _____ antidiuretic hormone	D. disease of the adrenal glands
14. _____ adrenaline	E. synonym for pituitary gland
15. _____ master gland, hypophysis	F. hormone secreted by the thyroid to prevent excessive calcium absorption into the bones
16. _____ calcitonin	G. originating in a gland
17. _____ goiter	H. excision of the thyroid and parathyroid glands
18. _____ parathyroid gland	I. hormone secreted by the posterior pituitary to prevent the kidneys from expelling too much water
19. _____ thyrotropin (TSH)	J. secretes PTH (parathyroid hormone), which slows the loss of calcium from bone
20. _____ thyromegaly	K. excessive pituitary secretion
21. _____ adenohypophysitis	L. inflammation of the anterior pituitary gland
22. _____ thyroparathyroidectomy	M. chronic enlargement of the thyroid, caused by insufficient iodine in the diet

CHAPTER 9

The Cardiovascular System

LEARNING OBJECTIVES

Upon completion of this chapter, you should be able to:

- Identify the major components of the cardiovascular system and the medical terms associated with their functions.
- Define selected terms associated with disorders, procedures, and treatments relating to the cardiovascular and blood systems.
- Recognize and write the word elements for the cardiovascular and blood systems introduced in this chapter.
- Identify and interpret selected abbreviations relating to the cardiovascular and blood systems.
- Build, spell, and pronounce medical terms that relate to blood and the cardiovascular system.
- Analyze and define the new terms introduced in this chapter.

Word Elements • The Cardiovascular System

WORD OR WORD ELEMENT	REFERS TO
angi/o	vessel
aort/o	aorta
arteri/o	artery
ather/o	fatty
atri/o	atrium
brady-	slow
cardi/o	heart
coron/o	crown; encircling, such as in the coronary blood vessels encircling the heart
-ectasis	dilation
electr/o	electrical
-emia	blood
endo-	inner, inside
-gram	written record
hem/o; hemat/o	blood
my/o	muscle
peri-	around, surrounding
phleb/o	vein
-stenosis	a narrowing
tachy-	fast
tens-	pressure (hyper/tens/ion)
thromb/o	clot
valv/o, valvul/o	valve
varic/o	dilated; from the Latin word *varix* ("a dilated vein")
vas/o	vessel
veno-	vein
ventricul/o	ventricle

An Overview of the Cardiovascular System

The **cardiovascular system** (cardi/o means "heart"; vascul/o means "blood vessel") comprises the heart, the blood, and the blood vessels that carry blood to all parts of the body (Fig. 9-1). As such, the system includes all the arteries, veins, and capillaries, which together form a closed delivery system for delivering oxygen and nutrients to all the cells of the body. The cardiovascular system also helps to regulate body temperature and collect waste products from the cells and

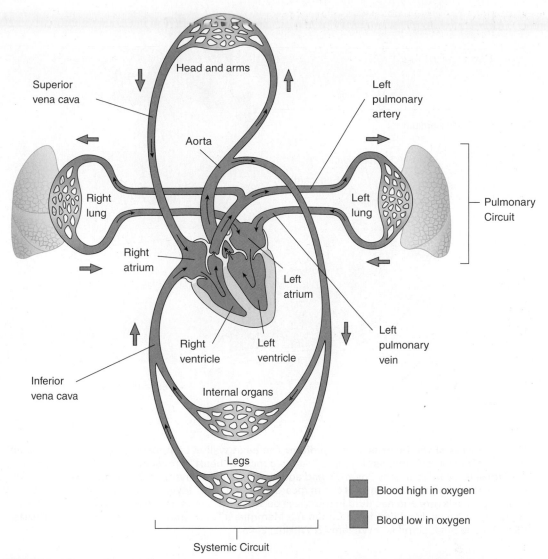

FIGURE 9-1   The cardiovascular system. The cardiovascular system consists of blood flow in a closed system of vessels. Oxygen content is exchanged in the pulmonary circuit, and blood rich in oxygen (red vessels) is returned to the left side of the heart. The pulmonary circuit carries blood to and from the lungs, and the systemic circuit carries blood to and from all other parts of the body. The vessels depicted in "red" signify blood that is high in oxygen; the vessels depicted in "blue" signify blood that is low in oxygen. From Cohen BJ. Medical Terminology: An Illustrated Guide, 5th Ed. Philadelphia: Lippincott Williams & Wilkins, 2007.

transport them to other parts of the body for elimination. This chapter covers the basic medical terms associated with the anatomical components of the cardiovascular system, terms naming its major functions, and terms related to its disorders, treatments, and procedures.

Structure and Function

THE HEART

The heart is a four-chambered hollow organ with three layers. The innermost layer is called the **endocardium** (endo- means "within"; cardi/o means "heart"). The middle layer, the heart muscle, is the thickest of the three layers and is called the **myocardium** (my/o means "muscle").

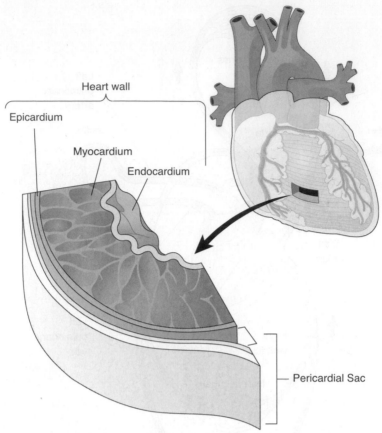

FIGURE 9-2   Layers of the heart and pericardium. The heart wall is composed of three layers: the epi-cardium (outer layer; epi- means "on top of"; cardi/o means "heart"), myocardium (heart muscle; my/o means "muscle"; cardi/o means "heart"), and endocardium (inner layer; endo- means "within"; cardi/o means "heart"). Note the thickness of the myocardial or "muscle" layer. The pericardial sac is actually composed of two layers and has fluid in the space between the layers. This fluid helps to reduce friction when the heart beats. Modified from Cohen BJ. Memmler's The Human Body in Health and Disease, 10th Ed. Philadelphia: Lippincott Williams & Wilkins, 2005.

The outer layer of the heart is called the **epicardium** (epi- means "upon"), which is actual-ly the inner layer of the **pericardium** (peri- means "around"), a sac that surrounds the heart (Fig. 9-2).

The heart acts as a double pump separated by a wall or **septum.** The right side pumps deoxygenated blood to the **pulmonary circuit** (lungs) where it picks up oxygen, and the left side of the heart pumps the oxygenated blood to all other parts of the body through the **systemic circuit** (systemic referring the entire body as opposed to one part). This delivery system oper-ates through the four chambers of the heart. The four chambers are as follows:

- **Right atrium:** Thin-walled, upper right chamber that receives blood from all body parts except the lungs; the interatrial (inter- is a prefix meaning "between"; so interatrial means "between the atria") septum separates the right and left atria.
- **Right ventricle:** Lower right chamber that receives blood from the right atrium and pumps it to the lungs (the interventricular septum separates the right and left ventricles).
- **Left atrium:** Upper left chamber that receives oxygen-rich blood as it returns from the lungs.
- **Left ventricle:** The lower left chamber with the thickest wall pumps blood to all parts of the body.

Heart Circulation

Blood flow through the heart is directed by one-way valves located at the entrance and exit to each of the ventricles. The atrioventricular (atri/o means "atria"; ventricul/o means "ventricle"; -ar is an adjective suffix) (AV) valves are found at the entrance to the ventricles and are so named because they come between the atria and ventricles. The right atrioventricular valve is also known as the **tricuspid valve** because it has three cusps or flaps that open and close. It controls the opening between the right atrium and right ventricle. The left atrioventricular valve is located between the left atrium and left ventricle and is called the **bicuspid** or **mitral valve**. It has two cusps or flaps that control blood flow.

> ✳ *Mitral is a substitute word for bicuspid in the name of the bicuspid valve. It comes from the Greek word mitra, which refers to a belt or turban. Its use in connection with the bicuspid valve is by way of the miter, an English word (British: mitre), meaning "a tall ceremonial hat," which the bicuspid valve resembles. The miter is worn by some clergymen as a symbol of their office.*

The exit valves are named **semilunar** (semi- means "half"; lunar means "moon") because the flaps resemble half moons. The exit point for leaving the right ventricle is called the **pulmonary** (pulmon/o means "lung or air"; -ary is an adjective suffix) **semilunar valve**, and it is located between the right ventricle and the pulmonary artery. The **aortic** (aort/o means "aorta"; -ic is an adjective suffix) **semilunar valve** is located between the left ventricle and the aorta.

> ✳ *Use the adjective "ventricular" only when you are absolutely sure of the meaning of the phrase you are uttering. The reason for caution is that the brain, as well as the heart, contains ventricles. Be careful, likewise, when combining the root "ventricul/o" with other word elements.*

The pathway of blood through the heart is illustrated in Figure 9-3.

The Heartbeat

To pump blood effectively throughout the body, the heart must contract and relax in a rhythmic cycle. Electrical nerve impulses stimulate the myocardium and the chambers of the heart to contract and relax in sequence. The electrical conduction system of the heart includes the following (Fig. 9-4):

- **Sinoatrial (SA) node:** Located in the upper posterior wall of the right atrium; sets the heartbeat; also called the *pacemaker* of the heart.
- **Atrioventricular (AV) node:** Located on the bottom of the right atrium near the ventricle; transmits electrical impulses to the bundle of His.
- **Bundle of His:** Located at the top of the interventricular septum and travels down along either side of the septum; transmits impulses to the Purkinje fibers.
- **Purkinje fibers:** Peripheral fibers that end in the right and left ventricles; stimulation from the bundle of His causes excitation of the ventricular muscles, resulting in contraction.

The *SA node*, or pacemaker, initiates the electrical impulse that begins the heartbeat. The impulse causes the atria to contract and simultaneously travels directly to the AV node. The electrical excitation travels through the bundle of His and through the ventricular walls by way of the Purkinje fibers, causing the ventricles to contract almost at the same time. Each contraction, called **systole**, is followed by **diastole**, or relaxation phase, during which the heart chambers fill with blood. These two phases make up the cardiac cycle and are illustrated in Figure 9-5.

The **heart rate** is determined by how many times the heart beats per minute. The blood that is forced through the vessels by contraction creates an increase in the artery pressure that can be measured by palpating a peripheral artery. The radial artery (located on the palm side of the wrist) is a common place to palpate or count the **pulse**, the rhythmic contraction of the heart.

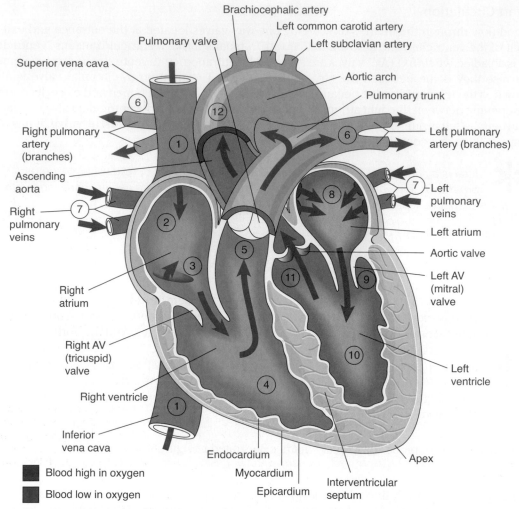

FIGURE 9-3 **The heart and pathway of blood flow.** Deoxygenated blood returns from the body into the heart through the superior and inferior venae cavae. The pathway of the blood through the heart begins when blood is returned to the vena cava (#1) and exits the heart through the aorta (#12) to the rest of the body. Note: The right side of the heart is colored in blue, signifying deoxygenated blood. The left side of the heart is colored in red because it carries oxygenated blood. From Cohen BJ. Medical Terminology: An Illustrated Guide, 5th Ed. Philadelphia: Lippincott Williams & Wilkins, 2007.

The electrical activity of the heart can be visualized and recorded on an **electrocardiogram (ECG or EKG)** (electr/o means "electricity"; cardi/o means "heart"; -gram means "a recording"). The electrical recording is obtained by placing electrodes (leads) on various parts of the body to detect electrical signals. These signals are displayed as waveforms and tracings by an electrocardiograph machine (electr/o means "electricity"; cardi/o means "heart"; -graph means "a recording instrument"). The waveforms are labeled with letters that represent different parts of the cardiac cycle. These waveforms have normal values and can provide valuable information for diagnosing cardiac abnormalities when the measured values lie outside normal limits. A **normal** or **sinus rhythm** originates in the SA node and has a normal rate of 60 to 100 beats per minute (BPM). A recording from an electrocardiograph machine is shown in Figure 9-6.

THE BLOOD AND BLOOD VESSELS

The blood vessels include the arteries, capillaries, and veins. Blood brings oxygen and nutrients to body cells and removes waste products. Blood itself is divisible into two main components: plasma,

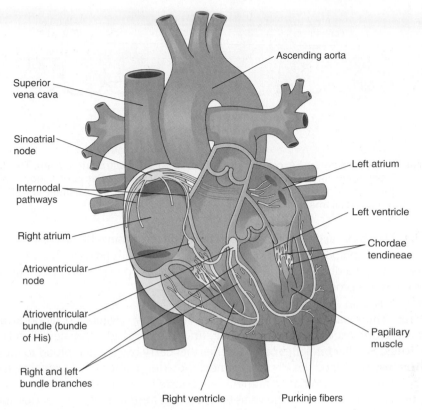

FIGURE 9-4 **Electrical conduction system of the heart.** The electrical stimulus begins in the sinoatrial (SA) node, also known as the pacemaker of the heart. The electrical stimulus moves from the SA node to the atrioventricular (AV) node, through the atrioventricular bundle of His, through the right and left bundle branches, and terminates in the Purkinje fibers where excitation of the ventricles occurs. Modified from Cohen BJ. Memmler's The Human Body in Health and Disease, 10th Ed. Philadelphia: Lippincott Williams & Wilkins, 2005.

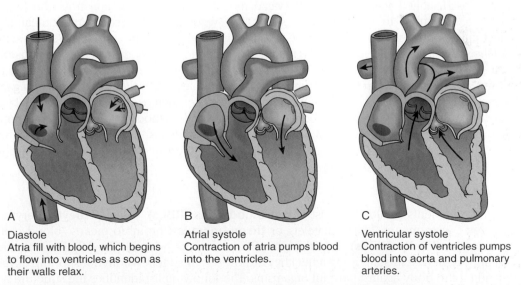

Diastole
Atria fill with blood, which begins to flow into ventricles as soon as their walls relax.

Atrial systole
Contraction of atria pumps blood into the ventricles.

Ventricular systole
Contraction of ventricles pumps blood into aorta and pulmonary arteries.

FIGURE 9-5 **The cardiac cycle. A.** Diastole: Ventricles relax as blood flows into the chambers. **B.** Atrial systole: Atria contract, pushing blood into the ventricles. **C.** Ventricular systole: Ventricles contract and pump blood into the pulmonary arteries and aorta. From Cohen BJ. Memmler's The Human Body in Health and Disease, 10th Ed. Philadelphia: Lippincott Williams & Wilkins, 2005.

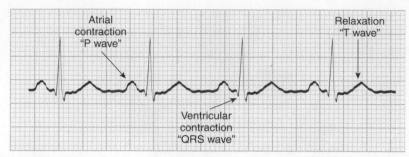

FIGURE 9-6   An electrocardiogram. A normal rhythm strip of an electrocardiogram. The three waves are illustrated: "P wave" or atrial contraction; "QRS wave" or ventricular contraction; and "T wave" or relaxation of the heart. Modified from Cohen BJ. Medical Terminology: An Illustrated Guide, 5th Ed. Philadelphia: Lippincott Williams & Wilkins, 2007.

which is the liquid portion, and the formed elements within the plasma. Blood plasma, which is clear and straw-colored, is composed mostly of water (91%), along with proteins and other nutrients in solution. Plasma is the medium for circulating blood cells. It also provides nourishment to body cells and removes the waste products from cellular metabolism.

The blood vessels in the cardiovascular system are:

- **Arteries:** Thick-walled elastic blood vessels that carry oxygenated blood away from the heart (note one exception: the pulmonary arteries carry unoxygenated blood).
- **Arterioles:** Smaller branches of the arteries that carry oxygenated blood to the capillaries.
- **Capillaries:** The blood vessels that connect the arterial and venous systems; they are one cell in thickness and exchange nutrients and waste material.
- **Venules:** Smaller braches of the veins that receive blood from the capillaries and transport it to the veins.
- **Veins:** The blood vessels that return deoxygenated blood to the heart; veins have valves that permit one-directional flow (note one exception: the pulmonary veins carry oxygenated blood).

The **lumen** of a blood vessel is the opening through which blood flows. The nervous system can stimulate the lumen to be more open, called **vasodilation** (sometimes vasodilatation) (vas/o means "vessel"; dilation from the English verb *dilate*, meaning "to open up a hollow structure"), or more closed, called **vasoconstriction** (vas/o means "vessel"; constriction from the English verb *constrict*, meaning "to narrow a hollow structure"). Vasodilation or vasoconstriction can have an effect on blood pressure. Blood pressure is a measurement of the amount of pressure exerted against the walls of the blood vessels and is recorded as a fractional number: **systolic** over **diastolic**. Systolic pressure occurs when the ventricles contract (the highest pressure is exerted against the vessel walls), and diastolic pressure occurs when the ventricles relax (the lowest pressure against the vessel walls). Other factors also influence blood pressure, such as blood volume and elasticity of vessel walls. Blood pressure can be measured by several methods, but the most common is with an instrument called a **sphygmomanometer** (sphygm/o means "pulse"; man/o means "thin"; -meter means "measuring device"), commonly called a blood pressure cuff (Fig. 9-7). A normal adult blood pressure is about 120/80 mmHg.

Elements of Blood

The formed elements in blood consist of **red blood cells (RBCs)**, or **erythrocytes** (erythr/o means "red"; -cyte means "cell"); platelets, or **thrombocytes** (thromb/o means "blood clot"); and **white blood cells (WBCs)**, or **leukocytes** (leuk/o means "white") (Fig. 9-8). Each element has an important role in supporting a healthy cardiovascular system—from transporting oxygen to defending the body against harmful organisms. The following list identifies the structure and function of each element:

- Erythrocytes: The main function of erythrocytes is to transport oxygen. The oxygen binds to **hemoglobin (Hb)** (hem/o means "blood"; -globin means "protein"), a protein in the

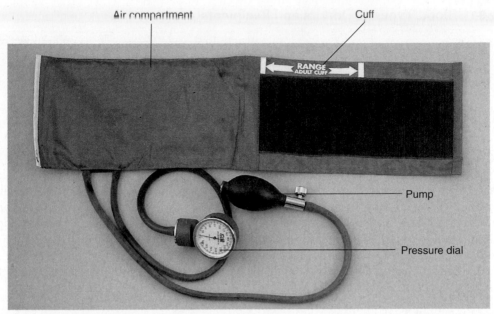

FIGURE 9-7 Sphygmomanometer (blood pressure cuff). From Cohen BJ. Medical Terminology: An Illustrated Guide, 5th Ed. Philadelphia: Lippincott Williams & Wilkins, 2007.

cell. Erythrocytes are disk-shaped bodies with a depression on both sides. They have a life span of approximately 120 days and are continually produced in bone marrow.

- Thrombocytes: Thrombocytes (thromb/o means "thrombus" or "clot"; -cyte means "cell"), also known as platelets, play an important role in the blood-clotting process. Thrombocytes are the smallest of the formed elements, roughly half the size of erythrocytes. When damage to a tissue occurs, thrombocytes are activated and stick together to form a plug or clot.
- Leukocytes (leuk/o means "white"; -cyte means "cell"): There are five types of leukocytes: neutrophils, eosinophils, basophils, lymphocytes, and monocytes. Leukocytes are the body's main defense against harmful organisms. Some destroy bacteria by means of **phagocytosis** (phag/o means "to ingest"). Their numbers usually increase during an infection.

Blood Groups

The four major blood groups (types) are A, AB, B, and O. Care must be taken to ensure blood type compatibility when transferring or transfusing blood from one person to another. Table 9-1 lists the blood type compatibilities for donors and recipients.

The presence of a substance in the red blood cell is responsible for what is known as the **Rh factor**. The Rh factor was first discovered in the blood of rhesus monkeys, for which species it was named. A person whose blood contains this substance is Rh positive. People with blood that does not contain the Rh factor are Rh negative.

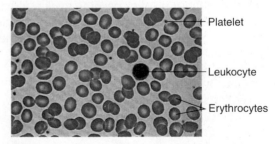

FIGURE 9-8 Blood cells. The three types of blood cells are indicated in this figure: leukocytes, platelets or thrombocytes, and erythrocytes. Leukocytes (leuk/o means "white"; -cyte means "cell") are the body's main defense against harmful organisms. Thrombocytes (thromb/o means "thrombus" or "clot"; -cyte means "cell"), also known as platelets, play an important role in the blood-clotting process. Erythrocytes (erythr/o means "red"; -cyte means "cell"), or red blood cells, transport oxygen. From Cohen BJ. Medical Terminology: An Illustrated Guide, 5th Ed. Philadelphia: Lippincott Williams & Wilkins, 2007.

Table 9-1   Blood Types as Donors and Recipients

Blood Type	Can Donate To	Can Receive From
A	A or AB only	A or O only
B	B or AB only	B or O only
AB (universal recipient)	AB only	A, B, AB, O
O (universal donor)	A, B, AB, O	O only

Practice and Practitioners

The specialists who treat disorders of the cardiovascular system include **cardiologists** (cardi/o means "heart"; -logy means "study of"; -ist means "one who specializes"), cardiovascular (cardi/o means "heart"; vascul/o means "vessel"; -ar means "pertaining to") surgeons, and **hematologists** (hemat/o means "blood"; logy means "study of"; -ist means "one who specializes"). Each one specializes in a different area. Cardiologists diagnose and treat heart disorders medically or non-surgically. **Cardiovascular surgeons** surgically correct disorders of the cardiovascular system. Hematologists treat disorders of the blood.

Disorders and Treatments

There are numerous disorders of the cardiovascular system, many of which involve the heart directly, such as coronary artery disease and thrombosis, because they develop from diseased vessels. Additionally, **anemia** (an- means "without"; -emia is a suffix meaning "blood") and **leukemia** (leuk/o means "white"; -emia means "blood") are blood disorders that affect the cardiovascular system. These disorders and others are described in more detail in the following sections.

CORONARY ARTERY DISEASE

One of the main causes of coronary artery disease (CAD) is **atherosclerosis** (ather/o means "fatty"; scler/o means "hardening"; -osis means "abnormal condition"), which is a progressive build-up of plaque that can cause the lumen of the coronary arteries, which nourish the myocardium, to narrow. When these plaques become thick and hard, they may also cause a loss of elasticity in the artery and impede blood flow to the heart muscle (Fig. 9-9). A deficiency of blood flow and oxygen to the myocardium is called **ischemia** (from the Greek word *isch/o*, meaning "to keep back").

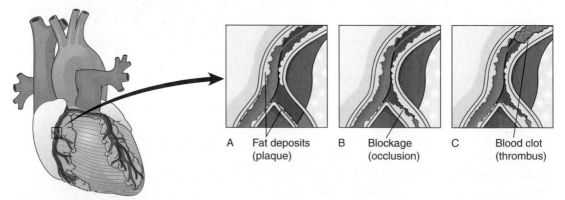

| A | Fat deposits (plaque) | B | Blockage (occlusion) | C | Blood clot (thrombus) |

FIGURE 9-9   Coronary atherosclerosis. Atherosclerosis (ather/o means "fatty"; scler/o means "hardening") is a progressive build-up of plaque that can cause the lumen of the coronary arteries, which nourish the myocardium, to narrow. The formation of thrombi (plural for thrombus or clot) may occur as plaque accumulates in the lumen. From Cohen BJ. Medical Terminology: An Illustrated Guide, 5th Ed. Philadelphia: Lippincott Williams & Wilkins, 2007.

One of the major causes of plaque build-up in the coronary arteries is a condition called **hyperlipidemia** (hyper- means "excessive"; lipid means "fatty"; -emia means "blood"). These deposits can cause degenerative changes on the interior wall of the artery and lead to a roughened surface that may promote blood clot formation.

Treatment for atherosclerosis may consist of nonpharmaceutical interventions and lifestyle changes such as cessation of smoking, moderation of diet, and a program of regular exercise. If these measures fail to improve the patient's **lipid panel** (blood tests that determine the levels of lipoproteins and both low-density lipoprotein [LDL] and high-density lipoprotein [HDL] cholesterol), then medications may need to be used. Such medications can include **statins** and other **antihyperlipidemic agents**. (Details on these types of medications are in the Pharmacology section later in this chapter.)

If nonpharmaceutical and/or pharmaceutical interventions fail, a number of surgical procedures may be done. These include:

- **Percutaneous transluminal coronary angioplasty (PTCA)** (per- means "through"; cutane/o means "skin"; -ous means "pertaining to"; angi/o means "vessel"; -plasty means "surgical repair"): Involves the insertion of a balloon-tipped catheter to open the blocked coronary artery. The balloon is inflated and deflated to flatten the plaque against the arterial wall. This process is repeated until there is optimal flow through the artery, at which time the catheter is removed (Fig. 9-10).
- **Arterial stent:** Another type of angioplasty includes the implantation of an arterial stent. A stent is a mesh tube that is implanted into an artery to provide support and prevent restenosis (the term that describes an artery that closes again after angioplasty) (Fig. 9-11).
- **Coronary artery bypass graft (CABG):** An open thoracic surgical procedure to graft another blood vessel (usually a saphenous vein or internal mammary artery [IMA]) to a

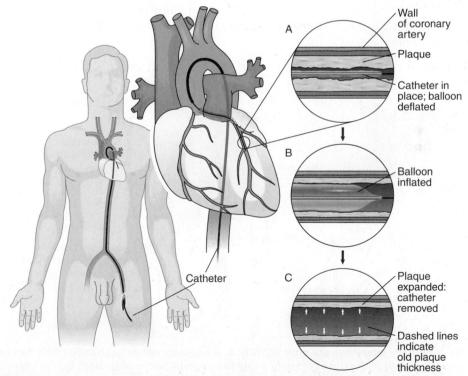

FIGURE 9-10   Percutaneous transluminal coronary angioplasty (PTCA). A. Plaque deposits in the artery. **B.** Plaque build-up narrows the coronary vessel, impeding blood flow to the myocardium. **C.** The rough interior edges encourage clot formation in the artery. From Cohen BJ. Medical Terminology: An Illustrated Guide, 5th Ed. Philadelphia: Lippincott Williams & Wilkins, 2007.

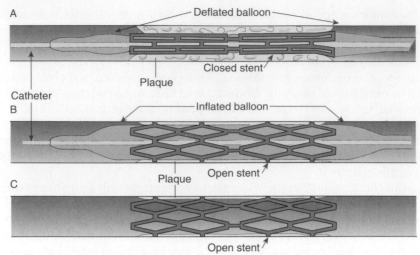

FIGURE 9-11   Arterial stent. A. A balloon-tipped catheter is placed into the artery with the balloon deflated and the stent closed. **B.** When the stent is in the proper position of the narrowed artery, the balloon is inflated, causing the stent to open. **C.** The catheter is removed, and the stent remains in place. From Cohen BJ. Medical Terminology: An Illustrated Guide, 5th Ed. Philadelphia: Lippincott Williams & Wilkins, 2007.

diseased coronary artery. As seen in Figure 9-12A and B, the vein graft and the IMA graft "bypass" the blocked arteries and provide blood flow to the coronary arteries distal to the blockages.

- **Endarterectomy** (end- means "within, inner"; arter/o means "artery"; -ectomy means "surgical removal"): Surgical removal of the inner lining of an artery that is blocked with atheromatous plaques (**atheroma** is a plaque of fatty tissue; ather/o means "fatty"; -oma means "tumor").

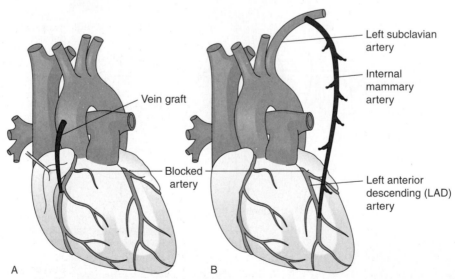

FIGURE 9-12   Coronary artery bypass graft (CABG). A. A segment of the saphenous vein carries blood from the aorta to a part of the right coronary artery that is distal to the occlusion. **B.** The internal mammary artery is used to bypass an obstruction in the left anterior descending coronary artery. The graft redirects the blood flow or "bypasses" the blocked artery. Modified from Cohen BJ. Medical Terminology: An Illustrated Guide, 5th Ed. Philadelphia: Lippincott Williams & Wilkins, 2007.

THROMBOSIS

Thrombosis (thromb/o means "blood clot") is a formation of a blood clot, or **thrombus**, in a blood vessel (see Fig. 9-9C). A thrombus can impede blood flow to the myocardium and cause ischemia. If the clot ruptures and totally occludes the vessel, then an **infarction** occurs. An infarction is "death to the tissue."

Treatment consists of the prevention of hyperlipidemia and atherosclerosis, which may predispose a person to thrombi formation (see treatment for atherosclerosis).

MYOCARDIAL INFARCTION

A **myocardial infarction (MI)**, or heart attack, results from a lack of oxygen supply to the myocardium. The heart muscle dies (becomes **necrotic**; necr/o means "death"; necrosis) (Fig. 9-13). Symptoms include sudden severe chest pain that may be located in common areas such as the chest, left arm, neck, and shoulder blade. Other signs include profuse sweating, nausea, vomiting, weakness, and cool, clammy skin.

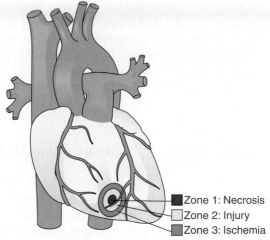

Zone 1: Necrosis
Zone 2: Injury
Zone 3: Ischemia

FIGURE 9-13 Myocardial infarction. The three zones depict the level of injury due to a lack of blood flow to the myocardium. Zone 3 indicates a lack of oxygen to the tissue, or ischemia. Zone 2 indicates injury to the tissue. Zone 1 illustrates death to the tissue from a lack of oxygen, or necrosis. From Cohen BJ. Medical Terminology: An Illustrated Guide, 5th Ed. Philadelphia: Lippincott Williams & Wilkins, 2007.

Various diagnostic tests can detect abnormal cardiac function. Electrocardiogram (ECG), **echocardiography** (an ultrasonic evaluation of the motion of the heart), **cardiac catheterization** (insertion of a catheter and contrast dye into the coronary arteries to detect blockage), and stress test (ECG monitoring during exercise on a treadmill) are all frequently used. A **nuclear stress test** (also sometimes called a thallium stress test) may also be ordered to assess the blood flow through the heart during a dictated activity.

When an MI occurs, treatment should begin immediately. Initial supportive care includes pain medication and oxygen to improve heart muscle function. **Thrombolytic** (-lysis means "destroy") agents may be administered directly into the coronary artery to dissolve the clot, open up the artery, and restore blood flow. The outcome depends on the amount of damage to the myocardium, which may be limited if treatment is initiated promptly. A simple blood test to discover whether troponin, a protein released into the bloodstream when an MI occurs, is present may be used to confirm a diagnosis of MI.

> *The acronym MONA is sometimes used to refer to standard emergency treatment for a suspected heart attack. M stands for morphine, O for oxygen, N for nitroglycerin, and A for aspirin.*

ARRHYTHMIAS

An arrhythmia (a- means "without" or "loss"; rhythm means "regular recurrence") is any irregularity of the heart's rhythm, such as a slow or fast rate or extra beats. **Bradycardia** (brady- means "slow") is a slower than average heart rate, and **tachycardia** (tachy- means "fast" or "rapid") is a faster than average rate. **Fibrillation** describes rapid, random, and ineffective contractions of the heart. Some arrhythmias are more serious than others. **Atrial fibrillation (A-fib)** occurs when the atria beat faster than the ventricles. This condition causes a quivering motion of the atria, which is usually not life threatening. Atrial fibrillation can predispose the atria to thrombi formation due to ineffective emptying. It affects many people and can often be controlled with drugs, such as beta-blockers. On the other hand, sustained **ventricular fibrillation**, in which the ventricles ineffectively pump blood, can be fatal.

Cardioversion, a method of treatment for fibrillation, involves the application of an electric current to restore a normal heart rhythm. **Ablation therapy**, applying radiofrequency waves to the heart, is used to cure a variety of cardiac arrhythmias, such as some tachycardias and atrial fibrillation.

HYPERTENSION

High blood pressure, or **hypertension (HTN)**, occurs when the systolic blood pressure exceeds 140 mmHg or the diastolic pressure is greater than 90 mmHg. In primary or essential hypertension, the cause of high blood pressure is unknown. When the hypertension is related to another medical problem, such as a kidney disorder, it is called secondary hypertension.

Over time, an increase in blood pressure can cause the arterial walls to become hard and thick, resulting in **arteriosclerosis** (arteri/o means "artery"; scler/o means "hardening"; -osis means "abnormal condition of"). The arterial lumen becomes narrowed, and the vessel becomes hard and loses its elasticity, thereby creating a greater resistance to the heart's attempt to pump blood. The extra workload can cause the left ventricle of the heart to become enlarged (**hypertrophy:** hyper- means "over" or "above"; -trophy means "growth").

Many factors can predispose a person to hypertension, including obesity, prolonged exposure to stress, or excessive alcohol or sodium intake. Age, familial trends, and ethnicity may also contribute to the development of hypertension. Treatment usually includes a sequence of steps beginning with lifestyle changes, including a reduction in salt intake and regular exercise. Diuretics (medications to reduce fluid volume), followed by other antihypertensive agents, may be added in a medical regimen to reduce blood pressure.

CONGESTIVE HEART FAILURE

Congestive heart failure (CHF) is diagnosed when the heart cannot effectively pump enough blood to meet the body's needs for oxygen and nutrients. In response to the decreased cardiac output, the kidneys attempt to increase blood flow to the organs through a feedback mechanism, which results in an increase in blood pressure and retention of more fluid. The result is frequently swollen ankles and legs. Treatment includes rest, restriction of salt intake, and medications to reduce fluid volume and improve cardiac contractions.

BLOOD DISORDERS

A blood **dyscrasia** (dys- means "bad"; -crasia means "blending" or "mixture") is any abnormality of the blood. There are three major types of abnormalities involving the blood: **anemia**, **leukemia**, and **clotting disorders**.

- **Anemia:** An abnormally low level of hemoglobin or low level of RBCs, caused by excessive bleeding or **hemorrhage**, other conditions causing blood cells to rupture, or failure of bone marrow to produce RBCs.
- **Leukemia:** Characterized by an excessive increase in the number of WBCs.
- **Clotting disorders:** Disorders caused by a disruption of the clotting mechanism, including **hemophilia** (hereditary bleeding disorder caused by a deficiency of a special clotting factor), **thrombocytopenia** (-penia is a suffix meaning "a deficiency"; insufficient number of thrombocytes caused by insufficient production or increased destruction), and **disseminated intravascular coagulation** (extreme clotting or coagulation caused by massive burns, trauma, cancer, or infection).

Treatment of blood disorders depends on the cause of the disorder. For example, anemias can be treated with iron supplements or blood transfusions. Leukemias are treated with chemotherapy and radiation. Treatments for clotting disorders are specific to the cause.

Pharmacology

As discussed earlier, the heart is a muscle that moves blood through the blood vessels in the cardiovascular system. Occasionally, efficient cardiac function becomes impaired and requires therapeutic intervention. Several classes of drugs can alleviate many of the cardiac conditions:

- **Cardiac glycosides** are drugs that increase the force of the myocardial contractions without causing an increase in oxygen consumption; they are used in CHF and sometimes atrial fibrillation.
- **Antiarrhythmics** (anti- means "against"; a- means "without"; rhythm means "regular recurrence"; -ic is an adjective suffix meaning "pertaining to") restore heart rhythm to normal. There are different classes (I to IV) of antiarrhythmics, each of which has its own mechanism of action. For example, class I antiarrhythmics decrease the excitability of the heart, whereas class IV drugs have electrophysiologic properties and interfere with the ion movement within the cell membranes.
- **Diuretics** remove water or fluid from the body, thus decreasing blood pressure and workload of the heart.
- **Vasodilators** (vas/o means "vessel"; dilate means "open up a hollow structure") increase the lumen of the blood vessels (dilate the vessels). This action increases blood flow and also treats hypertension (high blood pressure).
- **Vasoconstrictors** (vas/o means "vessel"; constriction means "narrow the opening of a hollow structure") decrease the inside diameter of the blood vessels, causing an increase in blood pressure. Vasoconstrictors are used to treat hypotension (low blood pressure) and shock.
- **Antianginal** (anti- means "against"; angina is constricting chest pain) drugs are used to treat angina or chest pain. They frequently are part of the drug group, nitrates, and cause vasodilation by relaxing the vascular smooth muscle.
- **Statins** block the production of cholesterol in the liver. They lower LDL ("bad" cholesterol) and triglycerides and have a mild effect in raising HDL ("good" cholesterol). Because of the job they do, statins are part of a group called **antihyperlipidemic** (anti- means "against"; hyper- "above, over"; lipid means "lipids or fats"; -emic means "pertaining to the blood") drugs.

Abbreviation Table • The Cardiovascular System

ABBREVIATION	MEANING
A-fib	atrial fibrillation
AV	atrioventricular
BP	blood pressure
CABG	coronary artery bypass graft (open heart surgery)
CAD	coronary artery disease
CCU	cardiac care unit
CHF	congestive heart failure
CP	chest pain
DIC	disseminated intravascular coagulation
EKG or ECG	electrocardiogram; electrocardiograph; electrocardiography; cardiogram

(continued)

ABBREVIATION	MEANING
Hb	hemoglobin (protein in the blood that carries oxygen)
HDL	high-density lipoprotein
HR	heart rate
HTN	hypertension
ICU	intensive care unit
LDL	low-density lipoprotein
MI	myocardial infarction
P	pulse
PTCA	percutaneous transluminal coronary angioplasty
RBC	red blood cell
SA	sinoatrial
SOB	shortness of breath
WBC	white blood cell

Study Table • The Cardiovascular System

TERM AND PRONUNCIATION	ANALYSIS	MEANING
Structure and Function		
aorta (ay-OR-tah)	from the Greek word *aeirein* (to lift up or to be hung)	the main trunk of the systemic arterial system
aortic valve (ay-ORT-ik)	from the Greek word *aeirein* (to lift up or to be hung); from the Latin word *valva* (that which turns)	connects the left ventricle to the aorta
arteries (AR-tuh-rees)	from the Greek word *arteria* (windpipe)	the largest of the blood vessels that carry blood away from the heart
arterioles (ar-TEER-ee-oles)	from the Greek word *arteria* (windpipe)	the smallest arteries that connect with the capillaries
atria (singular: atrium) (AY-tree-ah; AY-tree-uhm)	a Latin word meaning entry hall	upper two of the four heart chambers, composed of the right atrium and left atrium
atrioventricular node (AY-tree-oh-ven-TRIK-u-lahr)	from the Latin word meaning entry hall; from the Latin *venter* (belly)	fibers located at the base of the right atrium near the ventricle that carry electrical stimulation to the bundle

TERM AND PRONUNCIATION	ANALYSIS	MEANING
basophil (BAY-soh-fil)	from the Greek *basis* and *philein* (to love)	a white blood cell with granules that stain with basic dyes
bicuspid or mitral valve (by-KUSS-pihd; MY-trahl)	*bi-* (two); from the Latin *cuspidem* (cusp or point); from the Latin *mitra* (turban); from the Latin word *valva* (that which turns)	connects the left atrium to the left ventricle
bundle of His	named for Swiss cardiologist Wilhelm His, Jr., who discovered the function of these cells in 1893	located at the top of the interventricular septum; carries electrical impulses from the atrioventricular node to Purkinje fibers
capillaries (KAP-ih-layr-ees)	from the Latin word *capillus* (hair)	the smallest of the blood vessels
cardiac cycle	*cardi/o* (heart); *-ac* (adjective ending)	a complete round of systole and diastole
diastole (dye-AS-toh-lee)	from the Greek word *diastole* (dilation)	relaxation phase of the heart
endocardium (en-doh-KAR-dee-uhm)	*endo-* (within); *cardi/o* (heart)	the inner surface of the heart
eosinophil (ee-oh-SIHN-oh-fil)	from the Greek words *eos* (dawn); *philein* (to love)	a white blood cell that stains with certain dyes
epicardium (ep-ih-KAR-dee-uhm)	*epi-* (on, upon); *cardi/o* (heart)	the outer covering of the heart
erythrocytes (er-RITH-ro-sites)	*erythr/o* (red); *-cyte* (cell)	red blood cells; abbreviated RBC
heart rate	common English words	the number of times per minute the heart contracts
hemoglobin (hee-mo-GLO-bihn)	*hem-* (blood); from the Latin *globus* (globe)	the protein that gives blood its red color; abbreviated Hb
inferior vena cava (VEE-nah KAV-ah)	*inferior*, a Latin word meaning lower; from the Latin words *vena* (vein); *cava* (hollow)	large vein that collects blood from the smaller veins of the lower body
left atrium (AY-tree-uhm)	a Latin word meaning entry hall	upper left heart chamber
left ventricle (VEN-trik-al)	from the Latin word *venter* (belly)	lower left heart chamber
leukocytes (LUKE-o-sytes)	*leuk/o* (white); *-cyte* (cell)	white blood cells; abbreviated WBC

(continued)

TERM AND PRONUNCIATION	ANALYSIS	MEANING
mitral or bicuspid valve (MY-trahl; by-KUSS-pihd)	from the Latin word *mitra* (turban); from the Latin word *valva* (that which turns); *bi-* (two); from the Latin *cuspidem* (cusp or point)	connects the left atrium to the left ventricle
monocyte (MON-oh-site)	*mon/o* (single); *-cyte* (cell)	a relatively large white blood cell
myocardium (my-oh-KAR-dee-uhm)	*my/o* (muscle); *cardi/o* (heart)	the heart muscle, which includes nerves and blood vessels
neutrophil (NU-troh-fil)	from the Latin word *neuter* (neither); from the Greek word *philein* (to love)	a mature white blood cell normally constituting more than half of the total number of leukocytes
pericardial sac (pehr-ih-KAR-dee-ahl)	*peri-* (surrounding); *cardi/o* (heart); *-al* (adjective suffix)	another lining of the pericardium closest to the heart
pericardium (pehr-ih-KAR-dee-uhm)	*peri-* (surrounding); *cardi/o* (heart)	serous membrane lining the pericardial cavity
phagocyte (FAG-oh-site)	*phag/o* (eating, desiring); *-cyte* (cell)	a white blood cell capable of ingesting bacteria and other foreign matter
plasma (PLAZ-muh)	a Greek word meaning something molded or created	as differentiated from its nonmedical context, the yellow fluid that makes up a bit more than half of whole blood by volume
platelets (PLATE-lets); also called thrombocytes (THROM-boh-sytes)	from the English word plate and the diminutive suffix *-let*	smallest of the formed elements; important in the coagulation process
pulmonary artery (PULL-moh-nahr-ee)	*pulmon/o* (lung); from the Greek word *arteria* (windpipe)	vessel that carries deoxygenated blood from the right ventricle to the lungs
pulmonary valve (PULL-moh-nahr-ee)	*pulmon/o* (lung); from the Latin word *valva* (that which turns)	valve connecting the right ventricle and lungs
pulmonary veins (PULL-moh-nahr-ee vayns)	*pulmon/o* (lung); from the Latin word *vena* (blood vessel)	vessels that carry oxygenated blood from the lungs to the left atrium

TERM AND PRONUNCIATION	ANALYSIS	MEANING
pulse	from the Latin word *pulsum* (push, knock, drive)	rhythmic expansion and contraction of an artery produced by pressure of the blood moving through the artery
Purkinje fibers	named after Jan Evangelista Purkinje, who discovered them in 1839	fibers that carry stimulation throughout the ventricles
red bood cells	common English words	see erythrocyte
Rh factor	from rh(esus), so called because the blood group was discovered in rhesus monkeys	an antigen, first discovered in the rhesus monkey; a person is either Rh positive or negative
right atrium	a Latin word meaning entry hall	upper right heart chamber
right ventricle	from the Latin word *venter* (belly)	lower right heart chamber
septa (singular: septum) (SEPP-tah; SEPP-tuhm)	from the Latin word *saeptum* (a fence)	thin wall that separates cavities or masses; in the heart, septa separate the right atrium from the left atrium and the right ventricle from the left ventricle
sinoatrial node (SYE-noh-AY-tree-ahl)	from the Latin words *sinus* (bend, fold, curve) and *atrium* (entry hall)	known as the pacemaker of the heart; electrical impulse originates here
sinus rhythm (SYE-nus)	*sinus*, a Latin word meaning bend, fold, curve; from the Greek word *rhythmos* (measured flow or movement)	normal rhythm of the heartbeat
superior vena cava (VEE-nah KAV-ah)	*superior*, a Latin word meaning higher; from the Latin words *vena* (vein) and *cava* (hollow)	large vein that collects blood from the smaller veins of the upper body
systole (SIS-toh-lee)	a Greek word meaning contraction	contraction phase of the heart
tricuspid valve (try-KUSS-pihd)	*tri-* (three); from the Latin *cuspidem* (cusp or point)	valve connecting the right atrium to the right ventricle (right atrioventricular valve)
troponin (TROH-poh-nihn)	from the Greek word *trepein* (to turn)	a protein that is released into the bloodstream when a heart attack occurs

(continued)

TERM AND PRONUNCIATION	ANALYSIS	MEANING
vascular (VASS-cue-lahr)	*vascul/o* (blood vessel); *-ar* (adjective suffix)	adjectival form of *vessel*
vasoconstriction (vaz-oh-CON-strik-shun)	*vas/o* (duct, blood vessel); from the Latin word *constringere* (to draw tight)	narrowing of the blood vessels
vasodilation (vaz-oh-DYE-lay-shun)	*vas/o* (duct, blood vessel); from the Latin word *dilatare* (to make wider, enlarge)	widening of the blood vessels
veins (VAYNS)	from the Latin word *vena* (vein)	the blood vessels that return blood from the tissues to the heart
venous (VEE-nuhs)	from the Latin word *vena* (vein)	adjectival form of *vein*
venules (VEE-nuhls)	from the Latin *venula* (diminutive form of *vena* [vein])	small veins
ventricle (VEN-trik-uhl)	from the Latin word *venter* (belly)	lower two of the four heart chambers, composed of the right ventricle and left ventricle
white blood cells	common English words	formed element in the blood that protects the body against harmful bacteria

Common Disorders

anemia (ah-NEE-mee-a)	from the Greek word *anaimia* (without blood)	abnormally low red blood cell count
aneurysm (AN-yur-iz-um)	from the Greek word *aneurysmos* (to dilate)	a localized dilation of an artery, cardiac chamber, or other vessel
angina pectoris (an JY-nah-pek-TOR-ihs)	from the Greek word *agkhone* (a strangling); also *angere* (anguish); *pectoris*, a Latin word meaning chest	pain in the chest due to ischemia
angiospasm (AN-jee-o-spaz-uhm)	*angi/o* (blood vessel); from the Greek word *spasmos* (spasm)	spasm in blood vessels
angiostenosis (AN-jee-o-steh-NO-siss)	*angi/o* (blood vessel); *-stenosis* (a narrowing)	narrowing of a blood vessel
arrhythmia (ah-RITH-mee-ah)	*a-* (without); from the Greek word *rhythmos* (measured flow or movement); *-ia* (condition)	abnormal rhythm; irregular heartbeat

TERM AND PRONUNCIATION	ANALYSIS	MEANING
arteriosclerosis (ar-TEER-ee-o-sklu-RO-sis)	from the Greek word *arteria* (windpipe); *scler/o* (hardness); *-osis* (abnormal condition of)	hardening of the arteries
arteriospasm (ar-TEER-ee-o-spaz-uhm)	from the Greek word *arteria* (windpipe); from the Greek word *spastikos* (afflicted with spasms)	spasm of an artery
arteriostenosis (ar-TEER-ee-oh-steh-NO-sihs)	from the Greek word *arteria* (windpipe); *-steno* (narrow); *-osis* (abnormal condition)	narrowing of an artery
arteritis (ar-tur-EYE-tihs)	from the Greek word *arteria* (windpipe); *-itis* (inflammation)	inflammation of an artery or arteries
atheroma (ath-er-OH-mah)	from the Greek word *ather* (groats, porridge); *-oma* (tumor)	fatty deposit or plaque within the arterial wall
atherosclerosis (ath-er-oh-skleh-ROH-sis)	from the Greek word *ather* (groats, porridge); *scler/o* (hardening); *-osis* (abnormal condition of)	hardening and narrowing of the arteries
atrial fibrillation (fih-brih-LAY-shun)	from the Latin word *atrium* (entry hall) *-al* (adjective suffix); from the Latin word *fibra* (fiber, string, thread)	rapid, random, ineffective contractions of the atrium
atriomegaly (AY-tree-oh-MEG-ah-lee)	from the Latin word *atrim* (hall); *-megaly* (enlargement)	enlargement of an atrium
bradycardia (bray-dee-KAR-dee-ah)	*brady-* (slow); *cardi/o* (heart); *-ia* (condition)	abnormally slow heartbeat
cardiac arrest (KAR-dee-ak)	*cardi/o* (heart); from the Latin words *ad* and *restare* (to stop; remain behind)	cessation of heart activity
cardiodynia (kar-dee-oh-DIN-ee-ah)	*cardi/o* (heart); *-dynia* (pain)	heart pain
cardiomalacia (kar-dee-oh-mah-LASH-ee-ah)	*cardi/o* (heart); *-malacia* (softening)	softening of the heart
cardiomegaly (kar-dee-oh-MEG-ah-lee)	*cardi/o* (heart); *-megaly* (enlargement)	enlargement of the heart
cardiomyopathy (kar-dee-oh-my-AWP-uh-thee)	*cardi/o* (heart); *my/o* (muscle); *-pathy* (disease)	disease of the heart muscle (myocardium)
cardiopathy (kar-dee-AWP-uh-thee)	*cardi/o* (heart); *-pathy* (disease)	any heart disease

(continued)

TERM AND PRONUNCIATION	ANALYSIS	MEANING
cardiorrhexis (kar-dee-oh-REX-ihs)	*cardi/o* (heart); *-rrhexis* (rupture)	rupture in the wall of the heart
carditis (kar-DY-tiss)	*cardi/o* (heart); *-itis* (inflammation)	inflammation of the heart
congestive heart failure	from the Latin word *congerere* (to bring together, pile up)	syndrome where the heart is unable to pump enough blood to meet the body's needs for oxygen and nutrients; as a result, fluid is retained and accumulates in the ankles and legs
disseminated intravascular coagulation (DIC) (dih-SEMM-ihn-ayted ihn-tra-VASS-kyu-lahr koh-AG-yu-LAY-shun)	from the Latin *dis-* (in every direction); *seminare* (to plant, propagate); *intra-* (within); *vascul/o* (vessel); *-ar* (adjective suffix); coagulation (from the Latin verb *coagulo* [curdle])	widespread clotting in the blood vessels causing obstruction to the tissues
dyscrasia (dys-KRAY-sha)	*dys-* (bad, difficult); from the Greek word *krasis* (mingling)	general term for a blood disorder
endocarditis (en-doh-kar-DY-tiss)	*endo-* (within); *cardi/o* (heart); *-itis* (inflammation)	inflammation of the endocardium
hemolysis (hee-MAWL-ih-sihs)	*hem/o* (blood); *-lysis* (destruction)	change or destruction of red blood cells
hemophilia (hee-mo-FEEL-ee-ya)	*hem/o* (blood); *-phil(ia)* (attraction)	congenital disorder affecting the coagulation process
hemorrhage (HEM-o-rij)	*hem/o* (blood); *-rrhage* (burst forth)	discharge of blood
hyperlipidemia (high-per-LIP-ih-DEE-mee-ah)	*hyper-* (above normal); *lip/o* (fat); *-demia* (from hema [blood])	elevated cholesterol, triglycerides, and lipoproteins in the blood
hypertension	*hyper-* (above normal); from the Latin word *tendere* (to stretch)	elevated blood pressure (>140/90)
ischemia (is-KEEmee-ah)	from the Greek word *iskhaimos* (a stopping of the blood); *-ia* (condition)	deficiency in blood supply to the tissues
myocardial infarction (my-oh-KAR-dee-ahl in-FARK-shun) (MI) (Note: MI is an abbreviation, not an acronym.)	*my/o* (muscle); *cardi/o* (heart); *-al* (adjective suffix); from the Latin word *infractionem* (a breaking)	heart attack
myocarditis (my-oh-kar-DY-tiss)	*my/o* (muscle); *cardi/o* (heart); *-itis* (inflammation)	inflammation of the heart muscle

TERM AND PRONUNCIATION	ANALYSIS	MEANING
pericarditis (pehr-ih-kar-DY-tiss)	*peri-* (surrounding); *cardi/o* (heart); *-itis* (inflammation)	inflammation of the pericardium
tachycardia (tak-ih-KAR-dee-ah)	*tachy-* (fast); *cardi/o* (heart); *-ia* (condition)	abnormally rapid heartbeat
thrombocytopenia (THROM-boh-sigh-toh-PEE-nee-ah)	*thromb/o* (blood clot); *cyt/o* (cell); *-penia* (deficiency)	abnormal decrease in the number of thrombocytes or platelets
thrombus (THROM-bus)	*thromb/o* (blood clot)	blood clot attached to an interior wall of a vein or artery
valvulitis (valv-yu-LY-tiss)	from the Latin word *valva* (that which turns); *-itis* (inflammation)	inflammation of a heart valve
vasculitis (also angiitis)	*vascul/o* (blood vessel); *-itis* (inflammation)	inflammation of a vessel
vasoconstriction (VAZE-o-kon-STRIK-shun)	*vas/o* (duct, blood vessel); from the Latin word *constingere* (to draw tight)	narrowing of the arteries
vasodilation (VAZE-o-dy-LAY-shun) (also sometimes vasodilatation)	*vas/o* (vessel); from the Latin word *dilitare* (to make wider)	the widening of the arteries

Diagnosis and Treatment

ablation (ah-BLAY-shun)	from the Latin words *ab-* (away); and *latus* (brought)	partial destruction of the pathway of the electrical conduction system of the heart to treat irregular heart rhythms
angiogram (AN-jee-o-gram)	*angi/o* (blood vessel); *-gram* (record or picture)	printed record obtained through angiography
angiography (an-jee-AWG-ruff-ee)	*angi/o* (blood vessel); *-graphy* (process of recording)	radiography of a blood vessel after injection of a contrast medium
antianginals	*anti-* (against); *angi/o* (blood vessel); *-al* (adjective suffix)	drugs used to treat chest pain
antiarrhythmics	*anti-* (against); *a-* (without); from the Greek word *rhythmos* (measured flow or movement)	drug used to treat rhythm abnormalities
cardiac catheterization (KATH-eh-ter-eye-zay-shun)	*cardi/o* (heart); *-ac* (pertaining to); from the Greek word *kathienai* (to let down, thrust in)	procedure where a catheter is inserted into an artery and guided into the heart; may be used for diagnosis of blockages or treatment

(continued)

TERM AND PRONUNCIATION	ANALYSIS	MEANING
cardiac glycosides	*cardi/o* (heart); -ac (pertaining to); *glyc/o* (sugar) + -ide	drugs used to improve heart output by increasing the muscular contraction
cardiogram (KAR-dee-oh-gram) (Note: Associated terms are electrocardiogram [ee-LEK-troh-KAR-dee-oh-gram] and electrocardiograph [ee-LEK-troh-KAR-dee-oh-graf]; the abbreviation for any of them can be either EKG or ECG.)	*cardi/o* (heart); -*gram* (record or picture)	a graphic trace of electrical activity in the heart
cardioversion (KAR-dee-oh-VER-zhun)	*cardi/o* (heart); from the Latin word *vertere* (to turn)	use of electrical shock to restore the heart's normal rhythm
diuretic (DYE-ur-eh-tik)	from the Greek word *diouretikos* (prompting urine)	a drug used to increase urine production or urination
echocardiography (EK-oh-KAR-dee-AH-grah-fee)	from the Greek word *ekhe* (sound); *cardi/o* (heart); -*graphy* (process of recording)	ultrasonic procedure used to evaluate the structure and motion of the heart
nuclear stress test	common English words	assessment of blood flow through the heart through the use of a nuclear element injection while the patient exercises
sphygmomanometer (SFIG-moh-mah-NOM-eh-ter)	from the Greek words *sphygmos* (pulse), *manos* (thin), *metros* (measure)	instrument used to measure blood pressure
statins	from lovastatin, from *lo* + *vastatin* (stuff)	a type of cholesterol-lowering drug
stent	English word *stenting* refers to the process of stiffening	a device implanted into an artery to open and provide support to the arterial wall
ventricular fibrillation (ven-TRIK-yu-lahr fih-brih-LAY-shun)	from the Latin *ventriculus* (little belly); -*ar* (adjective suffix); from the Latin word *fibra* (fiber, string, thread)	irregular contractions of the ventricles; may be fatal unless reversed

Practice and Practitioners

cardiologist (kar-dee-AWL-oh-jist)	*cardi/o* (heart); -*logist* (one who specializes)	heart specialist
cardiology (kar-dee-AWL-oh-jee)	*cardi/o* (heart); -*logy* (study of)	medical specialty dealing with the heart

TERM AND PRONUNCIATION	ANALYSIS	MEANING
hematologist (HEE-mah-tah-lo-gist)	*hemat/o* (blood); *-logist* (one who specializes)	blood specialist
hematology (HEE-mah-TAH-lo-jee)	*hemat/o* (blood); *-logy* (study of)	medical specialty dealing with blood
Surgical Procedures		
angioplasty (AN-jee-o-plass-tee)	*angi/o* (blood vessel); *-plasty* (surgical repair)	surgical repair of a blood vessel
atrioseptoplasty (AY-tree-o-SEP-toh-plass-tee)	from the Latin words *atrium* (entry hall) and *saeptum* (fence); *-plasty* (surgical repair)	surgical repair of an atrial septum
cardiotomy (kar-dee-AW-tuh-mee)	*cardi/o* (heart); *-tomy* (cutting operation)	incision into the heart or incision into the cardia of the stomach
coronary artery bypass graft (CABG)	from the Latin *cor* (heart); common English words	through an open chest, a graft (piece of vein or other heart artery) is implanted on the heart to bypass a blockage
endarterectomy (end-art-er-ECK-toh-mee)	*endo-* (within); *arteri/o* (artery); *-ectomy* (excision)	surgical removal of the lining of an artery
pericardiotomy (PEHR-ih-car-dee-AW-toh-mee)	*peri-* (surrounding); *cardi/o* (heart); *-tomy* (cutting operation)	incision into the pericardium
valvoplasty (VALV-oh-plass-tee); also valvuloplasty (VALV-yu-loh-plass-tee)	from the Latin word *valva* (that which turns); *-plasty* (surgical repair)	surgical repair of a heart valve
valvotomy (valv-AW-toh-mee); also valvulotomy (valv-yu-LAWT-oh-mee)	from the Latin word *valva* (that which turns); *-tomy* (cutting operation)	surgical removal of a blocked heart valve (stenosis of a heart valve) by cutting into it

EXERCISES

EXERCISE 9-1   Figure Labeling: The Blood Flow Through the Heart

Label the parts of the heart using the terms listed.

aorta	left atrium	pulmonary valve	right ventricle
aortic valve	left ventricle	pulmonary veins	superior and inferior vena cavae
mitral or bicuspid valve	pulmonary arteries	right atrium	tricuspid valve

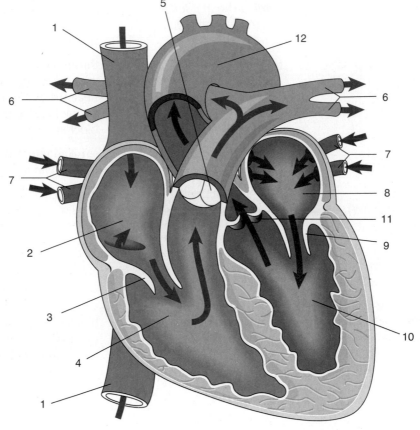

1. _____

2. _____

3. _____

4. _____

5. _____

6. _____

7. _____

8. _____

9. _____

10. _____

11. _____

12. _____

EXERCISE 9-2   Case Study

BRIEF HISTORY: The patient is a 56-year-old male who had been complaining of recurrent chest pain when performing mild activities at home. The chest pain subsides when he lies down. He also has experienced shortness of breath (SOB) when carrying in the groceries and climbing up one set of stairs. He has a history of high blood pressure.

EMERGENCY ROOM VISIT: The patient arrives at the emergency room with angina pectoris that is relieved by rest, a blood pressure of 180/110, and SOB. An EKG is performed that indicates the patient is having atrial arrhythmias and a myocardial infarction. He is given aspirin and started on antiarrhythmics, diuretics, vasodilators, and oxygen. He is admitted to the CCU for observation and treatment.

DIAGNOSIS: Hypertension, a myocardial infarction, and atrial fibrillation.

Answer the following questions using information learned in this chapter and found in the chapter tables.

1. Define angina pectoris. _____

2. What does the acronym SOB stand for? _____

3. What is hypertension? _____

4. What is an EKG? _____

5. What type of pharmacologic intervention is used with this patient? Define each drug classification. _____
   _____

6. What is a myocardial infarction? What are the two combining forms in myocardial, and what do they mean? _____
   _____

7. Define atrial fibrillation. _____

EXERCISE 9-3   Word Building: The Cardiovascular System

Using this chapter and the knowledge you've gained from the previous chapters, complete this exercise. The word elements are provided in the table for you.

a-, an-	-ectomy	-lysis	-spasm
angio/o	-emia	-megaly	-stenosis
arteri/o	erythr/o	my/o	thromb/o
ather/o	-genic	-oma	-tomy

atri/o	hem/o; hemat/o	-penia	valv/o
cardi/o	-ic, -ia, -ac, -al, -ar, -ary, -ous, -um	peri-	vas/o
-cyte	inter-	-philia	ven/o
-dilation	leuk/o	-rhythm	ventricul/o

1. originating in the heart _____

2. an incision into the atrium _____

3. a red blood cell _____

4. hereditary bleeding disorder caused by a deficiency of a clotting factor _____

5. spasm of a vein _____

6. removal of a blood clot _____

7. dilation of a vessel _____

8. enlargement of the heart _____

9. narrowing of an artery _____

10. fatty plaque _____

11. a white blood cell _____

12. the surgical removal of a valve _____

13. pertaining to the heart _____

14. destruction of red blood cells _____

15. between the ventricles _____

16. an abnormally low level of hemoglobin _____

17. heart muscle _____

18. removal of a fatty plaque _____

19. abnormal heart rhythm _____

EXERCISE 9-4   Spelling

In the space provided, write the correct spelling of the misspelled terms.

1. throbcytpenia _____

2. oyxgen _____

3. mycardial _____

4. iscemia _____

5. artrectomy _____

6. atriventrcular _____

7. lukemia _____

8. athrosclersis _____

9. semiluner _____

10. distolic _____

EXERCISES 9-5   Matching

Match the term in Column B with the correct definition in Column A.

COLUMN A

1. _____ pacemaker of the heart

2. _____ electric current used to restore normal sinus rhythm

3. _____ surgical removal of the inner lining of an artery

4. _____ abnormality of the blood

5. _____ thrombocytes

6. _____ a protein in the RBC

7. _____ deficiency of blood flow to an organ

8. _____ vessels are narrowed

9. _____ low level of oxygen in the blood

10. _____ between the right atrium and right ventricle

COLUMN B

A. ischemia

B. anemia

C. cardioversion

D. SA node

E. hemoglobin

F. vasoconstriction

G. tricuspid valve

H. endarterectomy

I. platelets

J. dyscrasia

EXERCISE 9-6   Crossword Puzzle: Cardiovascular System

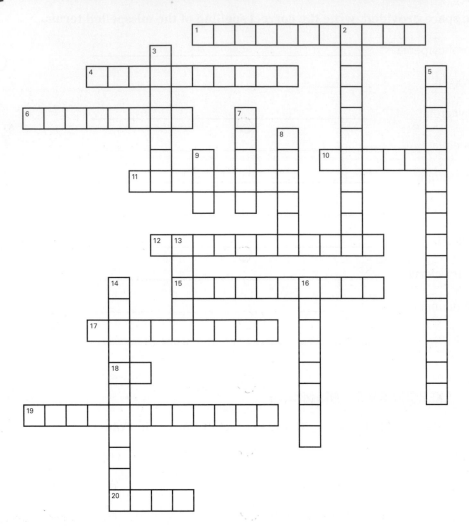

ACROSS
1. process of blood clotting
4. small arteries
6. blood clot
10. valve between the left ventricle and aorta
11. deficiency of oxygen to the tissues
12. smallest blood vessels
15. study of blood
17. any abnormality of the blood
18. abbreviation for hemoglobin
19. white cells ingest bacteria
20. suffix for blood

DOWN
2. another term for platelet
3. small veins
5. narrowing of blood vessels
7. swelling due to excessive fluid
8. fluid portion of the blood
9. abbreviation for congestive heart failure
13. root for "fatty"
14. red blood cell
16. malignant overgrowth of immature white blood cells

CHAPTER 9 QUIZ

Multiple Choice

1. A reduction in white blood cells is called:
   a. eosinophil
   b. polycythemia
   c. leukopenia
   d. anemia

2. An increase in red blood cells is called:
   a. eosinophil
   b. sickle cell
   c. polycythemia
   d. erythrocytopenia

3. Which of the following is a type of white blood cell?
   a. thrombocyte
   b. eosinophil
   c. erythrocyte
   d. platelet

4. What is the term that describes the destruction of bacteria by special white blood cells?
   a. phagocytosis
   B. leukocytosis
   c. erythrocytosis
   d. neutrophilosis

5. Platelets are also referred to as:
   a. erythrocytes
   b. thrombocytes
   c. basophils
   d. neutrophils

6. Oxygen-carrying pigment of red blood cells is called:
   a. hematocrit
   b. hemoglobin
   c. leukemia
   d. gamma globulin

7. The "universal recipient" is what blood type?
   a. O
   b. A
   c. B
   d. AB

8. Which of the following is a malignant disease of the hematopoietic organs (blood)?
   A. leukemia
   b. leukopenia
   c. erythropenia
   d. thrombosis

9. Which of the following terms describes hardened tissue?
   a. sclerotic
   b. thrombotic
   c. occluded
   d. fibrillated

10. What is the name of the artery that carries blood out of the heart to the lung?
    A. jugular
    b. venous
    c. pulmonary
    d. aorta

11. The study of the heart and heart conditions is called:
    a. cardiology
    b. cardiopathology
    c. cardiopathy
    d. myocardiology

12. An incision into a vein is called:
    a. phlebitis
    (b.) phlebotomy
    c. phlebostomy
    d. venitis

13. The heart muscle is supplied with blood vessels called:
    a. capillaries
    (b.) coronaries
    c. corpuscles
    d. carpals

14. The term for low blood pressure is:
    a. tachycardia
    b. bradycardia
    c. hypertension
    (d.) hypotension

15. The term for a rapid pulse rate is:
    a. hypertension
    (b.) tachycardia
    c. hypotension
    d. brachypnea

16. What is the function of a leukocyte?
    a. transports O_2
    b. manufactures Hgb
    c. initiates coagulation
    (d.) defends against disease

17. Which of the following means "one who studies cells"?
    a. hematology
    b. hematologist
    c. cytology
    (d.) cytologist

18. Which is the smallest blood vessel?
    a. artery
    b. arteriole
    c. vein
    (d.) capillary

19. Which of the following is characteristic of the artery in arteriostenosis?
    a. hardened
    b. soft
    c. dilated
    (d.) narrowed

20. What is the term for the area between the ventricles?
    a. intraventricular
    b. interdermal
    c intracranial
    (d.) interventricular

CHAPTER 10

The Lymphatic System and Immunity

LEARNING OBJECTIVES

Upon completion of this chapter, you should be able to:

- Define the terms associated with the structures and functions of the lymphatic system.
- Define immunity and the major sources of immunity in the body.
- Define the terms associated with the disorders and treatments of the lymphatic system.
- Build, spell, and pronounce medical terms that relate to the lymphatic system and immunity.
- Analyze and define the new terms introduced in this chapter.

Word Elements • The Lymphatic System and Immunity

WORD ELEMENT	REFERS TO
an-	without
immun/o	immune system
lymphaden/o	lymph nodes
lymphangi/o	lymph vessels
lymph/o; lymphat/o	lymph or lymphatic system
-megaly	enlargement
phag/o	ingest or engulf
-phylaxis	protection
splen/o	spleen
thym/o	thymus
tonsill/o	lymph node, usually palatine tonsil

An Overview of the Lymphatic System and Immunity

The lymphatic system is a network of tissues and vessels that is widespread throughout the body. The lymphatic system and the cardiovascular system are closely related body systems that are joined by a capillary network. The lymphatic system circulates fluid called **lymph** through a one-way system as opposed to the closed circuit of the cardiovascular system. Lymph is similar to blood in that it is composed of special cells and fluid. **Lymphocytes** (lymph/o means "lymph"; -cyte means "cell") are a type of white blood cell that work in the lymph system to fight disease and infection. Therefore, the lymph system is an integral part of the body's defense against disease. **Immunity** (from a Latin word meaning "exemption or free from service") means protection against disease. In other words, one of the major functions of the lymphatic system is immunity or to protect the body from infection. The other two major functions of the lymphatic system are to maintain a balance of fluid and to absorb fats that are broken down in the digestive tract.

> *Like blood plasma,* lymph *is a fluid that consists mostly of water. It also contains a low concentration of proteins in solution and, of course, lymphocytes. The word* lymph *is also used as an adjective in naming lymph vessels, lymph nodes, and so on. A second adjective,* lymphatic, *is most often used when referring to the whole system and some specific parts of the system, such as the* right lymphatic duct. *Either adjective, however, is acceptable in any context.*

Structure and Function

The lymph system consists of lymph vessels, lymph, special lymphoid (lymph/o means "lymph"; -oid means "like" or "resembling") tissues called lymph nodes, and lymph organs. All of these structures play an important role in the body's immune responses. As mentioned earlier, one of the other major functions of the lymphatic system is to maintain fluid balance.

This function is accomplished through a complex network of vessels and tissues. These structures are discussed first.

LYMPHATIC STRUCTURES

The lymph capillaries (comes from the Latin word *capillus* meaning "hair") are similar to blood capillaries in that they are thin-walled tubes that carry fluid (lymph) to larger vessels (Fig. 10-1). Lymph is a clear yellowish liquid that is collected from tissues as it seeps out of capillaries from the cardiovascular system. It contains lymphocytes (lymph/o means "lymph"; -cyte means "cell") that attack and destroy foreign organisms. Lymph is picked up by the lymph vessels, filtered by the lymph nodes, and propelled back into the venules and, subsequently, into the veins (Fig. 10-2). Lymph nodes are small bean-shaped structures that filter the lymph

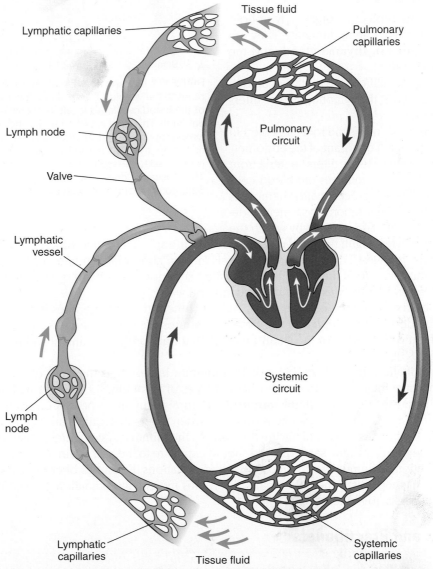

FIGURE 10-1   The lymphatic system in relation to the cardiovascular system. The lymphatic capillaries pick up the fluid in the tissues that exits from the blood capillaries. The fluid circulates in the lymph system and is returned to the blood vessels near the heart. Modified from Cohen BJ, Taylor J. Memmler's Structure and Function of the Human Body, 8th Ed. Baltimore: Lippincott Williams & Wilkins, 2005.

to remove harmful substances such as bacteria and viruses. When disease or infection is present, lymph nodes swell with lymph fluid, indicating that the lymphatic system is at work defending against the invading organism. Swollen lymph nodes can be felt in the cervical (neck), axillary (armpit), and inguinal (groin) regions, where the main nodal groups are located. This is why a physician often feels for swollen lymph nodes as part of an examination—to determine whether infection may be present.

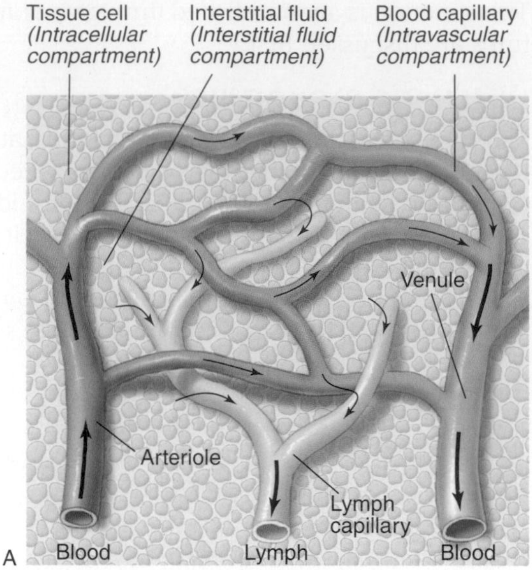

LYMPHATIC ORGANS

There are four protective organs (lymphoid tissues) that play a role in immunity. They are the **tonsils, spleen, thymus gland,** and the **appendix** (Fig 10-3).

- Tonsils (tonsill/o is the root): Located in the pharynx, this lymphoid tissue filters bacteria.
- Spleen (splen/o is the root): Located in the upper left quadrant of the abdomen, this lymphatic tissue filters bacteria from the blood and removes old blood cells by means of a process called hemolysis (hem/o means "blood"; -lysis means "destruction of"). The process by which the

FIGURE 10-2   Lymph flow. Fluid travels from the arterioles to the venules. Some of the fluid that leaks out of the blood capillaries is left in the tissues (interstitial fluid). This fluid is picked up by the open-ended lymph capillaries and circulates in the lymph system as lymph. It travels in the lymphatic system until it is returned to the bloodstream. From Premkumar K. The Massage Connection Anatomy and Physiology. Baltimore: Lippincott Williams & Wilkins, 2004.

lymphocytes engulf the bacteria and debris in the spleen is called **phagocytosis** (phag/o means "to ingest"; cyt/o means "cell"; -osis means "abnormal condition of").

- Thymus (thym/o is the root) gland: Located superior to the heart, this endocrine gland processes lymphocytes and stimulates immunity.
- Appendix (appendic/o is the root): An attachment to the large intestine, it contributes to the development of immunity. **Peyer's patches** are small bundles of lymphoid tissue located on the walls of the small intestine that help protect against invading organisms (Fig. 10-3).

The lymphatic organs play a big role in immunity. Immunity is the state of not being susceptible to a specific disease. There are different types of immunity, such as **natural immunity, acquired immunity,** and **artificial immunity.** Natural immunity is passed on from mother to child before birth. Acquired immunity is obtained when a person acquires an infectious disease, such as chickenpox. As a result of having the disease, the immune system retains a special "memory" that defends against the same disease should exposure to it occur again. Artificial immunity, or immunization, is immunity acquired through vaccinations. Examples of current vaccines are influenza (flu), hepatitis B (hepat/o means "liver"; -itis means "inflammation"), measles, meningitis, and pertussis, to name a few.

Practice and Practitioners

A number of medical specialists treat disorders of immunity and of the lymph system. **Allergists** specialize in diagnosing and treating altered immunologic and allergic conditions. **Hematologists** (hemat/o means "blood"; -logy means "study of"; -ist means "one who specializes") diagnose and treat disorders of the blood and blood-forming tissue. Lymph is frequently included in this specialty. An **immunologist** is a specialist who studies, diagnoses, and treats problems with immunity. At times, an **oncologist** (onc/o means "tumor"; -logy means "study of"; -ist means "one who specializes") is also involved in the care of some of these patients when tumors are diagnosed.

Disorders and Treatments

One of the primary functions of the lymphatic system is to filter out harmful organisms. When bacteria spread to the lymphatic system or when an injury to the body is not treated effectively, an infection can occur and may result in **lymphadenitis** (lymph/o means "lymph"; aden/o means "gland"; -itis means "inflammation"). Tissue swelling or **lymphedema** (lymph/o means "lymph"; edema means "accumulation of excess fluid") can result from an infection or an obstruction of the lymph vessels resulting from tumors or surgical excision of nodes. **Lymphadenopathy**, or enlarged lymph nodes (lymph/o means "lymph"; aden/o means "gland"; -pathy means "disease"), is a common symptom of infections and cancerous conditions. Lymph and immune disorders include the following:

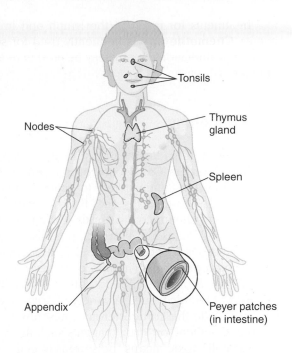

FIGURE 10-3 Location of lymphoid tissues and protective organs. Lymph tissues and organs. Peyer's patches are found in the lining of the intestine and help to protect against invading organisms. Modified from Cohen BJ. Medical Terminology: An Illustrated Guide, 5th Ed. Philadelphia: Lippincott Williams & Wilkins, 2007.

- Acquired immunodeficiency syndrome (AIDS): This is an advanced stage of human immunodeficiency virus (HIV), an infectious process characterized by swollen lymph glands or lymphadenopathy (lymph/o means "lymph"; aden/o means "gland"; -pathy means "disease").
- Infectious mononucleosis: An acute infection also caused by a virus and noted by enlarged cervical lymph nodes and an increase in monocytes (a type of white blood cell [WBC]; mono means "one"; -cyte means "cell").
- Splenomegaly (splen/o means "spleen"; -megaly means "large") of the lymphatic system: Enlargement of the spleen seen with other infectious diseases.
- Anaphylaxis (an- means "without"; -phylaxis means "protection"): Life-threatening reaction to a foreign substance; symptoms include blockage of air passages, decreased blood pressure, and generalized edema.
- Hodgkin lymphoma: Chronic malignant disease of the lymph nodes diagnosed on biopsy of the lymph node; symptoms include lymphadenopathy (lymphaden/o means "lymph gland"; -pathy means "disease") and splenomegaly (splen/o means "spleen"; -megaly means "enlargement") of the lymphatic system.
- Rheumatoid (rheumat/o means "flux" or "flow"; -oid means "resembling") arthritis (arthr/o means "joint"; -itis means "inflammation"): An autoimmune disorder (an abnormal reaction to one's own tissues) that progressively destroys joints (see Chapter 5).
- Systemic (adjective: relating to an anatomical system or, as in this case, the entire body) lupus (Latin for wolf) erythematosus (erythematosus means "redness"): Chronic inflammatory disorder that affects multiple body systems; characterized by a "butterfly rash" over the face. Systemic lupus erythematosus is abbreviated SLE.

Treatments for many of the lymph and immune disorders involve pharmacotherapeutic agents. **Chemotherapy** is frequently used for some of the cancers, as is bone marrow transplantation. Radiation therapy may be used in treating some tumors such as those occurring with Hodgkin's disease.

Pharmacology

A number of drug classifications are used as part of a therapeutic regimen in lymphatic and immune disorders. **Corticosteroids** (cortic/o means "cortex," which is the outer part of an organ) may be administered to relieve inflammatory conditions. Corticosteroid medications are used to treat diseases that can cause inflammation such as systemic lupus erythematosus and rheumatoid arthritis. Examples of common prescription medications include prednisone (Deltasone, Flovent), prednisolone (Delta-Cortef), methylprednisone (Medrol), dexamethasone (Decadron), and hydrocortisone (Solu-Cortef, Cortef, Cortisporin cream). **Immunosuppressants** (immun/o means "immune system"; suppressant means "to prevent or lessen") are drugs prescribed to prevent or reduce the body's normal reactions to invasion of diseases of foreign tissues. A variety of drug classifications fall under the immunosuppressants. These include the corticosteroids (described earlier) and some chemotherapeutic (chem/o means "chemical" or "drug") agents such as Cytoxan and Imuran that have a cytotoxic (cyt/o means "cell"; toxic means "poisonous to cell") effect. **Immunizations,** or **vaccinations,** provide an artificially acquired immunity. (*Vacca* is Latin for "cow." The word vaccination originated from the technique of injecting a cowpox medicine to prevent smallpox.) A few examples of vaccines include hepatitis B vaccine (prevents hepatitis B), Tripedia (tri- means "three"; ped/o means "child"; diphtheria, tetanus toxoids, and pertussis used to prevent these three diseases), and the meningitis vaccine. Another drug classification called **antiviral agents** (anti- means "against"; viral is an adjective form of virus) may be used to treat diseases such as HIV and other viral infections. These drugs are used to treat and halt specific diseases caused by a virus. Examples of antiviral medications include amantadine (Symmetrel) used for flu or influenza illnesses; acyclovir (Zovirax) used for genital herpes and herpes zoster; raltegravir (Isentress) used for infections associated with HIV; and didanosine (Videx), indinavir (Crixivan), and nelfinavir (Viracept) given in management of HIV.

Abbreviation Table • *The Lymphatic System and Immunity*

ABBREVIATION	MEANING
AIDS	acquired immunodeficiency syndrome
CBC	complete blood count
HIV	human immunodeficiency virus
HLA	human leukocyte antigen
RA	rheumatoid arthritis
RIA	radioimmunoassay
SLE	systemic lupus erythematosus (usually shortened to lupus), an autoimmune disorder

Study Table • The Lymphatic System and Immunity

TERM AND PRONUNCIATION	ANALYSIS	MEANING
Structure and Function		
acquired immunity	common English words	resistance resulting from previous exposure to an infectious agent
allergen (AL-ur-jehn)	from the Greek word *allos* (other); *-gen* (producing)	an allergy-producing substance
antibody	*anti-* (against) + body	a molecule generated in specific opposition to an antigen
antigen (AN-tih-jehn)	*anti-* (against); *-gen* (producing)	substance that induces sensitivity or an immune response in the form of antibodies
appendix (ah-PEN-dicks)	from the Latin verb *appendum* (attach)	worm-like dead-end projection that is attached to the intestine
artificial immunity	Common English words	immunization; immunity acquired from a vaccination
autoimmunity (aw-toh-ih-MYUN-iht-ee)	*auto-* (self) + immunity	literally, immune to oneself
inflammation (in-flah-MAAY-shun)	common English word	redness and irritation caused by injury or abnormal stimulation by a physical, chemical, or biologic agent
leukocyte (LUKE-oh-site)	*leuk/o* (white); *-cyte* (cell)	white blood cell
lymph (limf)	from the Latin word *lympha* (water, clear water, goddess of water)	fluid that flows through the lymphatic system; adjective synonymous with *lymphatic*
lymphatic system (lihm-FAT-tik)	*lymph/o* (lymph); *-atic* (adjective suffix)	collectively, the vessels, nodes, and capillaries that carry the lymph and its disease-fighting cells to the areas in which they are needed
lymphocyte (LIHM-foh-syte)	*lymph/o* (lymph); *-cyte* (cell)	white blood cell in the lymphatic system
macrophage (MAK-roh-fayj)	*macro-* (large); *phag/o* (ingest or engulf)	large phagocyte
microphage (MIKE-roh-fayj)	*micro-* (small); *phag/o* (ingest or engulf)	small phagocyte

(continued)

TERM AND PRONUNCIATION	ANALYSIS	MEANING
monocyte (MON-oh-site)	*mono-* (single); *-cyte* (cell)	a type of white blood cell
natural immunity	common English words	resistance manifested by an individual who has not been immunized; immunity passed on from mother to fetus
neutrophil (NU-troh-fil)	*neutr/o* (neutral); *-phil* (love)	a granulocyte that is the chief phagocytic white blood cell
pathogen (PATH-oh-jehn)	*path/o* (disease); *-gen* (produce)	substance that produces disease
phagocyte (FAG-oh-syte)	*phag/o* (ingest or engulf); *-cyte* (cell)	white blood cell that clears away pathogens and debris
phagocytosis (FAG-oh-sy-	*phag/o* (ingest or engulf); *cyt/o* (cell); *-sis* (condition of)	process of white blood cells
reaction (ree-AK-shun)	common English word	an action of an antibody on a specific antigen; also, in reference to immune responses, an abnormal or unwanted reaction
spleen (SPLEEN)	*splen/o* (spleen)	immune system organ that gets rid of damaged red blood cells and reclaims and stores iron
T cell	T (stands for thymus) + cell	cells that make up about 80% of lymphocytes; the T denotes their work with the thymus
thymus (THY-muhs)	*thym/o* (thymus)	immune system gland located behind the sternum
tonsil (TON-sihl)	*tonsill/o* (tonsil)	collection of lymph tissue; in common understanding, the lingual, pharyngeal, and (especially) palatine tonsils

Common Disorders

anaphylaxis (an-ah-FIL-ax-ihs)	*ana-* (without); from the Greek word *phylaxis* (protection)	life-threatening reaction to a foreign substance; symptoms include blockage of air passages, decreased blood pressure, generalized edema
hemolysis (hee-MAWL-ih-sihs)	*hem/o* (blood); *-lysis* (destruction)	change or destruction of red blood cells

TERM AND PRONUNCIATION	ANALYSIS	MEANING
Hodgkin lymphoma (HODJ-kin lim-FOH-mah)	named after English physician Thomas Hodgkin (1798–1866) who first described it; *lymph/o* (lymph or lymphatic system); *-oma* (tumor)	chronic malignant disease of the lymph nodes
immunodeficiency (IM-yu-noh-dee-FISH-ehn-see)	*immun/o* (immune system) + deficiency	impairment of the immune system
lymphadenitis (LIM-FAD-eh-NY-tiss)	*lymph/o* (lymph or lymphatic system); *aden/o* (gland); *-itis* (inflammation)	inflammation of a lymph node (or nodes)
lymphadenopathy (lim-fah-deh-NOP-ah-thee)	*lymph/o* (lymph or lymphatic system); *aden/o* (gland); *-pathy* (disease)	chronic or excessively swollen lymph nodes; any disease of the lymph nodes
lymphangitis (lim-fan-JY-tihs); also sometimes lymphangiitis (lim-FAN-jee-EYE-tihs); see also lymphatitis	*lymphangi/o* (lymph vessel); *-itis* (inflammation)	inflammation of lymph vessels
lymphatitis (lim-fah-TY-tihs)	*lymph/o* (lymph or lymphatic system); *-itis* (inflammation)	inflammation of the lymph vessels or nodes
lymphedema (lim-feh-DEE-mah)	*lymph/o* (lymph or lymphatic system); from the Greek word *oidema* (a swelling tumor)	swelling of the subcutaneous tissues due to obstruction of lymph vessels or nodes
lymphoma (lim-FOH-mah)	*lymph/o* (lymph or lymphatic system); *-oma* (tumor)	tumor of lymph tissue
lymphopathy (lim-FOP-ah-thee)	*lymph/o* (lymph or lymph gland); *-pathy* (disease)	disease of the lymph vessels or nodes
splenitis (splee-NY-tihs)	*splen/o* (spleen); *-itis* (inflammation)	inflammation of the spleen
splenomegaly (splee-noh-MEG-ah-lee)	*splen/o* (spleen); *-megaly* (enlargement)	enlargement of the spleen
splenopathy (splee-NOP-ah-thee)	*splen/o* (spleen); *-pathy* (disease)	any disease of the spleen
systemic lupus erythematosus (sis-TEM-ik LOO-pahs er-RITH-ee-mah-TOH-suhs)	adjective form of the English word *system*; *lupus* (a Latin word meaning wolf); *erythematous* (from the Greek word *erythema* meaning flush)	an inflammatory connective tissue disorder with variable features; diffuse erythematous (red) butterfly rash on face
thymitis (thy-MY-tihs)	*thym/o* (thymus); *-itis* (inflammation)	inflammation of the thymus

(continued)

TERM AND PRONUNCIATION	ANALYSIS	MEANING
tonsillitis (TAWN-sih-LY-tihs)	*tonsill/o* (tonsils); *-itis* (inflammation)	inflammation of a tonsil (commonly the palatine tonsil)

Diagnosis and Treatment

antiviral (an-ty-VIR-al)	*anti-* (against); from the Latin word *virus* (poison, sap of plants, slimy liquid)	drugs used to treat various viral infections or conditions
chemotherapy (KEE-moh-ther-ah-pee)	*chem/o* (chemical) + therapy, a common English word	treatment of malignancies using chemical agents and drugs (usually reserved for treatment of cancer)
corticosteroids (kor-tih-ko-STER-oyds)	from the Latin word *cortex* (bark); from the Greek *steros* (solid, stable)	hormone-like preparations used as anti-inflammatory agents; topical agents used for their immunosuppressive and anti-inflammatory properties
immunization (IM-u-ny-zay-shun)	*immun/o* (immune system); *-ization* (noun suffix)	process by which resistance to an infectious disease is induced
immunosuppressant (IM-yu-no-suh-PRESS-ant)	*immun/o* (immune system) + suppressant	something that interferes with the immune system
lymphangiography (lim-FAN-jee-OG-rah-fee)	*lymphangi/o* (lymph vessel); *-graphy* (process of recording)	radiography of the lymph vessels

Practice and Practitioners

allergist	from the Greek words *allos* (other, different, strange) and *ergon* (activity); *-ist* (one who specializes)	a medical practitioner who specializes in the diagnosis and treatment of allergies
hematologist (hee-mah-TAHL-oh-jist)	*hemat/o* (blood); *-logist* (one who specializes)	a medical practitioner who specializes in the diagnosis and treatment of blood disorders
immunologist (im-yu-NOL-oh-jist)	*immun/o* (immune system); *-logist* (one who specializes)	a medical practitioner specializing in the immune system
immunology (IM-yu-NOL-oh-jee)	*immun/o* (immune system); *-logy* (study of)	the medical specialty dealing with the immune system

TERM AND PRONUNCIATION	ANALYSIS	MEANING
oncologist (on-KOL-oh-jist)	from the Greek word *onkos* (mass, bulk); *-logist* (one who specializes)	a medical practitioner who specializes in the diagnosis and treatment of malignant tumors
Surgical Procedures		
lymphadenectomy (lim-fah- deh-NEK-toh-mee)	*lymphaden/o* (lymph gland); *-ectomy* (excision)	excision of lymph nodes
lymphangiectomy (lim-FAN-jee-EK-tah-mee)	*lymphangi/o* (lymph vessel); *-ectomy* (excision)	excision of a lymph vessel
lymphangiotomy (lim-FAN-jee-OT-oh-mee)	*lymphangi/o* (lymph vessel); *-tomy* (cutting operation)	incision of a lymph vessel
splenectomy (splee-NEK-toh-mee)	*splen/o* (spleen); *-ectomy* (excision)	excision of the spleen
splenorrhaphy (splee-NOR-ah-fee)	*splen/o* (spleen); *-rraphy* (rupture)	suture of a ruptured spleen
splenotomy (splee-NOT-oh-mee)	*splen/o* (spleen); *-tomy* (cutting operation)	incision of the spleen
thymectomy (thy-MEK-toh-me)	*thym/o* (thymus); *-ectomy* (excision)	excision of the thymus
tonsillectomy (TAWN-sih-LEK-toh-mee)	*tonsill/o* (tonsil); *-ectomy* (excision)	excision of a tonsil

EXERCISES

EXERCISE 10-1   Case Study

BRIEF HISTORY: A 16-year-old male complained to his parents of being extremely fatigued. He wasn't able to keep up with his school schedule or after-school sport activities. His throat was sore and he noticed "lumps" in his neck and groin. He had a fever and loss of appetite. He recently began to complain of pain in his "upper left belly."

OFFICE VISIT: A physician examined the patient and ordered blood tests. He noted lymphadenopathy in the cervical, axillary, and inguinal areas. He also observed an erythematous throat and determined that the spleen was enlarged.

DIAGNOSIS AND TREATMENT PLAN: The diagnosis was mononucleosis, an infectious disease caused by a virus. The prescribed treatment consisted of over-the-counter analgesics to reduce the abdominal pain, along with fluids and rest. Throat lozenges were prescribed to ease sore throat discomfort.

Answer the following questions using information learned in this chapter and found in the chapter tables. You may also need to draw on knowledge learned in previous chapters.

1. Define "lymphadenopathy." _____

2. What are "analgesics"? Give an example. _____

3. What is the medical term for an "enlarged spleen"? _____

EXERCISE 10-2   Matching

Match the term in Column B with the correct definition in Column A.

COLUMN A

1. _____ enlarged spleen

2. _____ specialty that deals with immune disorders

3. _____ artificially acquired immunity

4. _____ life-threatening allergic reaction to a foreign substance

5. _____ disease of the lymph glands

6. _____ accumulation of fluid in the intercellular tissues

7. _____ the process of engulfing foreign materials

COLUMN B

A. lymphadenopathy

B. lymphedema

C. phagocytosis

D. autoimmune

E. splenomegaly

F. lymphocyte

G. immunology

8. _____ protective lymph organ that is attached to the proximal end of the large intestine

H. anaphylaxis

9. _____ the body reacts to its own tissues

I. appendix

10. _____ specialized WBC of the immune system

J. immunization

EXERCISE 10-3   Word Building: The Lymphatic System and Immunity

Use the following word elements to build the terms defined below.

aden/o	-graphy	-logist	-oma	thym/o
angi/o	immun/o	lymph/o	-pathy	
-cytosis	-itis	-megaly	phag/o	

1. inflammation of a lymph gland _____

2. tumor of a lymph gland _____

3. enlargement of the thymus _____

4. inflammation of a lymph vessel _____

5. disease of a lymph gland _____

6. specialist who studies and treats the immune system _____

7. radiographic procedure of the lymphatic system _____

8. process of a WBC engulfing a harmful organism _____

EXERCISE 10-4   Crossword Puzzle: The Lymphatic System and Immunity

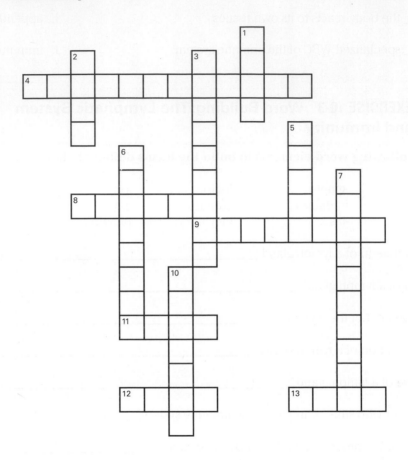

ACROSS

4. use of drug agents to treat malignancies
8. gland located in the chest that produces lymphocytes
9. protection against disease
11. acronym for acquired immunodeficiency syndrome
12. suffix meaning "blood"
13. root word for "gland"

DOWN

1. root word meaning "to ingest" or "engulf"
2. root word for "white"
3. destruction of red blood cells
5. root word for spleen
6. redness
7. disorder that results from an immune response to one's own tissues
10. disease of the lymphatic system that may spread

CHAPTER 10 QUIZ

True or False
Circle the best answer.

1. True   False   Hodgkin's lymphoma is a progressive disorder that is characterized by an enlarged spleen and lymph nodes.

2. True   False   The tonsils have no role in the immune system.

3. True   False   A reaction to poison ivy is an example of anaphylaxis.

4. True   False   SLE is an example of an autoimmune disease.

5. True   False   Hemolysis is a form of lymphatic cancer.

6. True   False   Splenomegaly is enlargement of the spleen.

7. True   False   An accumulation of lymph in the soft tissue is called lymphedema.

8. True   False   Drugs are or may be used to prevent or reduce the body's normal reactions to invasions of harmful organisms.

9. True   False   Peyer's patches are located in the back of the throat.

10. True   False   The axilla is one area where there is a concentration of lymph nodes.

CHAPTER 11

The Respiratory System

LEARNING OBJECTIVES

Upon completion of this chapter, you should be able to:

- Name the major parts of the respiratory system and describe the functions of each part.
- State the primary function of the respiratory system.
- Identify and use the word elements of the respiratory system.
- Build, spell, and pronounce medical terms that relate to the respiratory system.
- Describe symptoms, disorders, treatments, and surgical procedures relating to the respiratory system.
- Describe the major drug classifications used to treat respiratory system disorders.
- Identify and interpret selected abbreviations relating to the respiratory system.
- Analyze and define the new terms introduced in this chapter.

Word Elements • The Respiratory System

WORD ELEMENT	REFERS TO
bronch/o; bronchi/o	bronchus
laryng/o	larynx
nas/o, rhin/o	nose
-oxia	oxygen
pharyng/o	pharynx
-phonia	voice
phren/o	diaphragm
pleur/o	pleura
-pnea	breathing
pneum/o, pneumon/o	air; lung
pulmon/o	lung
sinus/o	sinus cavity
thorac/o-, thorac/i, thoracic/o-	thorax, chest
trache/o	trachea

An Overview of the Respiratory System

The respiratory system consists of the **nose (nasal cavity)**, **pharynx**, **larynx**, **bronchi**, **bronchioles**, **alveoli**, and **lungs** (Fig. 11-1). The primary purpose of the respiratory system is to furnish oxygen to the body's cells and to remove gaseous waste products (i.e., carbon dioxide). Figure 11-2 is a diagram that shows the process of gas exchange, which is accomplished through **external** and **internal respiration**.

External respiration is the process whereby air is brought into the lungs and oxygen and carbon dioxide (a waste product) are exchanged in the blood within the capillaries surrounding the alveoli. Internal respiration is the process whereby oxygen and carbon dioxide move between the blood and the body cells.

Structure and Function

As mentioned earlier, several structures make up the respiratory system. The following sections discuss each part and its role in respiratory function.

THE NOSE

Air enters the body through the nose, which is lined with small hairs called **cilia**, and passes into the **nasal cavity** where it is warmed and moistened. **Mucus** coats the lining of the nasal cavity to filter out particles too small to be blocked by the cilia.

THE PHARYNX

The **pharynx**, also known as the throat, has three divisions: the **nasopharynx** (nas/o means "nose"; pharynx means "throat"), **oropharynx** (or/o means "mouth" or "opening"; pharynx

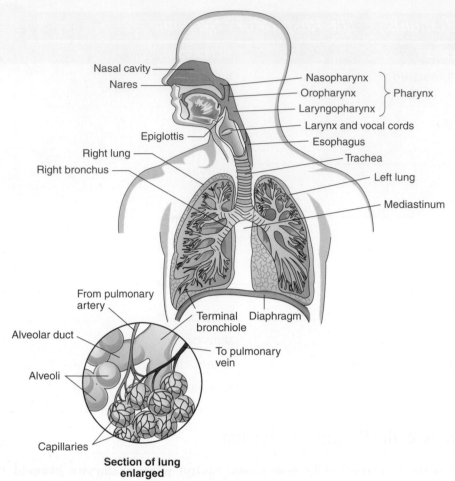

FIGURE 11-1   The respiratory system. An overview of the respiratory anatomical terms. The main structures include the nasal cavity, pharynx (three divisions), larynx, trachea, bronchi, bronchioles, and alveoli. Enlarged section of the terminal bronchiole showing the relationship between the alveoli and blood capillaries. External respiration occurs as oxygen moves from the alveoli into the blood and carbon dioxide moves from the blood out into the alveoli where it will be exhaled. Modified from Cohen BJ. Medical Terminology: An Illustrated Guide, 5th Ed. Philadelphia: Lippincott Williams & Wilkins, 2007.

means "throat"), and **laryngopharynx** (laryng/o means "larynx" or "voice box"; pharynx means "throat") (Fig. 11-1A). The nasopharynx is posterior to the nasal cavity; the oropharynx is the middle portion located behind the mouth; and the laryngopharynx is the lower portion behind the larynx. Associated with the pharynx are three pairs of lymphoid (lymph/o means "lymph tissue"; -oid means "resembling") tissue called tonsils (tonsils were introduced in Chapter 10). The adenoids, also known as pharyngeal tonsils, are located in the nasopharynx, the palatine tonsils are in the oropharynx, and the **lingual** (lingu means "tongue"; -al is an adjective suffix) tonsils are at the base of the posterior portion of the tongue (Fig. 11-3). As discussed in Chapter 10, the tonsils are accessory organs that aid in filtering bacteria.

THE LARYNX

The **larynx** (voice box) is a cartilaginous structure located between the pharynx and trachea (Fig. 11-4). The larynx is held open by a number of cartilages, the largest being the thyroid car-

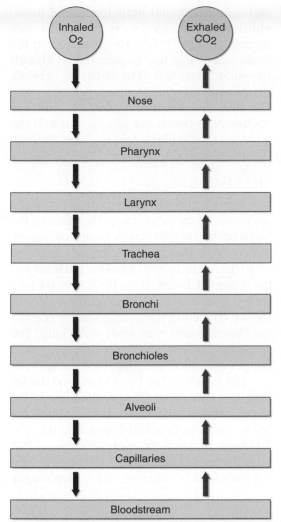

FIGURE 11-2   **Pathway of inhaled/exhaled air.** (Red arrows indicate oxygenated air; blue arrows represent deoxygenated air.) Oxygen (O_2) enters the respiratory system through the nose and travels down through the larynx and pharynx and into the lungs where a gas exchange takes place. Oxygen moves into the bloodstream where it is carried to the cells and is exchanged with carbon dioxide (CO_2). The carbon dioxide passes back up through the respiratory structures and is exhaled.

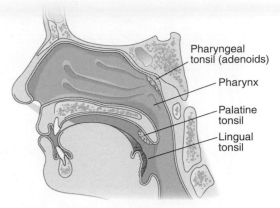

FIGURE 11-3   **The pharynx and tonsils.** The pharyngeal tonsil or adenoids are located in the nasopharyngeal region or upper portion of the throat. The palatine tonsils are located in the oropharynx or back of the mouth. The lingual tonsils are located at the base of the tongue. From Cohen BJ. Medical Terminology: An Illustrated Guide, 5th Ed. Philadelphia: Lippincott Williams & Wilkins, 2007.

tilage (Adam's apple). Also contained in the larynx are the **vocal cords** (Fig. 11-5). These folds of mucous membrane vibrate as air from the lungs flows over them to produce sound.

The space between the vocal cords is termed the **glottis** (comes from the Greek word *glottis* meaning "opening"). The glottis is closed during swallowing to keep food out of the respiratory tract (Fig. 11-5A). Note in Figure 11-5B that the glottis is widely opened when a person takes a forced breath to allow air down into the respiratory tract. The little leaf-shaped cartilage located above the glottis is called the **epiglottis** (epi- means "upon"; glottis means "opening in the vocal cords"). Along with the glottis in the closed position, this flap-like structure swings downward during swallowing to cover the larynx so food does not enter the trachea and the lungs.

THE TRACHEA

The **trachea** (windpipe) is a cartilaginous tube that extends from the pharynx to the main bronchi. It is composed of smooth muscle and is kept open with C-shaped rings of cartilage. The trachea is lined with cilia to help sweep foreign material out of the air passage. The purpose of the trachea is to provide an open airway to the lungs.

THE BRONCHI, BRONCHIOLES, AND ALVEOLI

The inferior portion of the trachea branches off into two major airways called the **right** and **left bronchus** (plural: bronchi). Air passes down through the bronchi, which subdivide into

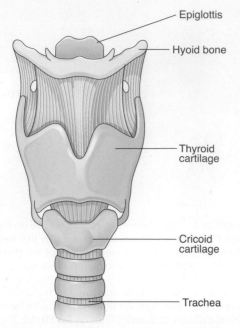

FIGURE 11-4   The larynx. The larynx (voice box) is a cartilaginous structure located between the pharynx and trachea. It is held open by a number of cartilages, the largest being the thyroid cartilage (Adam's apple). A little leaf-shaped cartilage located above the glottis is called the epiglottis (epi- means "upon"; glottis means "opening in the vocal cords"). This flap-like structure swings downward during swallowing to cover the larynx so food does not enter the trachea and the lungs. From Cohen BJ. Medical Terminology: An Illustrated Guide, 5th Ed. Philadelphia: Lippincott Williams & Wilkins, 2007.

increasingly smaller branches called **bronchioles** (bronch/o means "bronchi"; -iole means "smaller"). The air terminates in the bronchial tree in tiny air sacs called **alveoli** (singular: alveolus) (Fig. 11-1B). A network of thin-walled capillaries surrounds each alveolar sac. During respiration, the gas exchange between the alveolar air and the pulmonary capillary takes place through the alveolar walls.

THE LUNGS

The lungs lie on either side of the heart and are protected by the rib cage. They take up the major portion of the thoracic cavity and are enclosed in the **pleura**, a membrane composed of two principal layers, called the **parietal** and the **visceral** layers (Fig. 11-6). The parietal (outer) layer lines the thoracic cavity and forms the sac containing each lung. The visceral (inner) layer closely surrounds each lung. The space in between contains a lubricating fluid that prevents friction during respiration.

The right lung has three lobes, and the left lung has two lobes. The **mediastinum**, the space between the two lungs, contains the heart, aorta, trachea, esophagus, and bronchi. The **apex**, or superior part of each lung, is located at the level of the clavicle. The base, or inferior part of each lung, rests on the **diaphragm**,

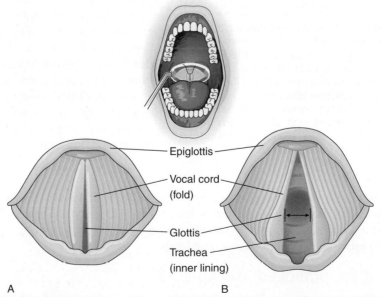

FIGURE 11-5   The vocal cords, a superior view. A. The glottis in a closed position. **B.** The glottis in an open position. From Cohen BJ. Medical Terminology: An Illustrated Guide, 5th Ed. Philadelphia: Lippincott Williams & Wilkins, 2007.

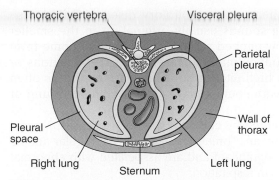

FIGURE 11-6   Pleura. A horizontal cross-sectional view of the lungs illustrating the pleural linings and pleural space. The parietal pleura is the outer lining, and the visceral pleura is the inner lining. The space in between the two linings is called the pleural space. Modified from Cohen BJ. Medical Terminology: An Illustrated Guide, 5th Ed. Philadelphia: Lippincott Williams & Wilkins, 2007.

which is the major muscle of respiration that separates the thoracic cavity from the abdomen. See Figure 11-1A for the location of the diaphragm.

The lungs and airways bring in fresh, oxygen-enriched air and get rid of waste carbon dioxide made by the cells in the body. They exchange these gases through external and internal respiration. As mentioned earlier, external respiration is the act of breathing (bringing air into and out of the lungs). Internal respiration occurs when oxygen passes from the bloodstream into the tissue cells. At the same time, carbon dioxide moves from the tissue cells into the bloodstream. This process of gas exchange between the tissue cells happens after air is inhaled into the alveoli. Oxygen from the air passes into the blood and is carried to the body's cells, while carbon dioxide passes back from the tissue cells into the blood and is eventually exhaled.

Practice and Practitioners

A number of health care professionals work within the specialty area of the respiratory system. A **pulmonologist** (pulmon/o means "lung"; -logy means "study of"; -ist means "one who specializes") is a physician who specializes in **pulmonology** (pulmon/o means "lung"; -logy means "study of"), the study of diagnosing and treating lung and respiratory disorders. An **otolaryngologist** (ot/o means "ear"; laryng/o means "larynx" or "voice box"; -logy means "study of"; -ist means "one who specializes") is also known as an **otorhinolaryngologist** (ot/o means "ear"; rhin/o means "nose"; laryng/o means "larynx" or "voice box"; -logy means "study of"; -ist means "one who specializes"). Both specialists refer to a physician who diagnoses and treats diseases and disorders of the ears, nose, and throat. **Respiratory therapists** are allied health care professionals who specialize in airway management, mechanical ventilation, and blood acid-base balance. They work closely with physicians and nurses.

Disorders and Treatments

The pathway through which air moves in and out of the lungs needs to remain **patent** (a common English word that when used as a medical term means "physically open") in order for proper oxygen and carbon dioxide exchange to take place. When this pathway becomes partially blocked, the body's normal response is a sneeze or cough. Sneezing is a reflex response to an irritant, inflammation, or foreign material in the nasal passages. Coughing may be associated with irritation from nasal discharge from the oropharynx or from foreign material in the lower respiratory tract. A persistent cough may be a symptom of a respiratory disorder or a chronic irritation.

A "productive" cough is one that occurs when **sputum** or other secretions accumulate in the lungs and need to be removed for optimal airway **patency** ("state of being open"; noun form of the adjective patent) and oxygen exchange. Sputum is a mucoid (muc/o means "mucus"; -oid means "resembling" or "like") discharge from the respiratory tract. Its characteristics are associated with several respiratory conditions. Normal secretions are relatively thin, colorless, and clear. Yellowish-green, cloudy, or thick mucus usually indicates a bacterial infection. Rusty or dark-colored sputum, such as **hemoptysis** (hem/o means "blood"; -ptysis means "spitting"), may be a sign of other respiratory disorders.

Abnormal breath sounds are another indication of respiratory disease. **Rales**, also known as crackles, are high-pitched popping sounds usually originating in the smaller airways. **Rhonchi** (singular: rhonchus) are low-pitched sonorous sounds that come from the larger airways. **Wheezing** or whistling sounds may indicate excessive secretions or partially obstructed airways, and **stridor** is a high-pitched squeaking sound that is often heard on inspiration. The absence of any breath sounds may signal a collapsed lung or non-aeration.

Breathing patterns and rates may also be altered by certain respiratory diseases. Normal breathing, **eupnea** (eu- means "normal"; -pnea means "breathing"), should be regular and effortless. Changes in rate, depth, and rhythm are significant and are associated with abnormal conditions. The following is a list of abnormalities in respiration:

- **Tachypnea** (tachy- means "rapid"; -pnea means "breathing"): Rapid rate of respiration (may be normal during exercise)
- **Bradypnea** (brachy- means "slow"; -pnea means "breathing"): Abnormal slowness of respiration
- **Apnea** (a- means "without"; -pnea means "breathing"): Cessation of respiration; short periods of apnea normally occur during sleep
- **Dyspnea** (dys- means "difficult or painful"; -pnea means "breathing"): Difficult or painful respiration
- **Orthopnea** (ortho- means "straight"; -pnea means "breathing"): Discomfort or difficulty in breathing while lying flat; difficulty is relieved by sitting up
- **Cheyne-Stokes:** A rhythmic respiratory pattern in which a variation in depth of respirations alternates with periods of apnea
- **Kussmaul breathing:** Rapid deep respirations characteristic of an acid-base imbalance (frequently seen in uncontrolled diabetes)

A number of disorders affect the respiratory system. Some of them are briefly discussed under the following broad categories: infectious disorders, obstructive lung diseases, and expansion disorders.

INFECTIOUS DISORDERS

The respiratory tract provides easy access for microorganisms to enter the body. The body's defense mechanisms increase mucus production to produce a runny nose to wash away organisms. A cough may ensue to clear the airways of mucoid discharge. Following are a few of the common infections that occur in the respiratory system.

Common Cold (Infectious Rhinitis)

As previously mentioned, the nose and upper respiratory tract have cilia and mucus that help ward off infectious agents. However, there are more than 100 viruses that are easily spread by contaminated items or respiratory droplets. Symptoms may include fever, swollen mucous membranes, watery discharge from the nose, a cough, and sometimes sneezing. Persistent coughing will cause throat irritation. Treatment usually is aimed at alleviating discomfort caused by such symptoms. Over-the-counter medications such as acetaminophen can help treat a fever and accompanying headaches, and **decongestants** (de- means "to undo or reduce") reduce edema and congestion in the respiratory airways.

Sinusitis

Sinusitis (sinus means "sinus" or "hollow space in the bone"; -itis means "inflammation"), a bacterial infection of the sinuses, is usually secondary to a cold or allergy. The sinus passageways become clogged, and drainage is obstructed. A buildup of mucus in the sinuses can cause considerable discomfort. Decongestants and analgesics are the most common types of treatment.

Croup

Croup, also called **laryngotracheobronchitis** (laryng/o means "larynx" or "voice box"; trache/o means "trachea" or "windpipe"; bronch/o means "bronchus" or "airway"; -itis means "inflammation"), usually affects children younger than 3 years. It is caused by a number of different infections that affect the upper respiratory tract. Laryngeal inflammation produces a characteristic barking cough, hoarse voice, and inspiratory stridor. The infection usually lasts a few days. Humidification and cool air often relieve the obstruction.

Epiglottitis

Epiglottitis (epi- means "upon"; glottis means "opening between the vocal cords"; -itis means "inflammation") is an acute infection of the larynx and epiglottis. The infection has a rapid onset and causes swelling of the laryngeal tissues. The patient frequently appears anxious, sits upright, and has a difficult time swallowing. Treatment usually consists of oxygen, antibiotics, and, in severe cases, a **tracheostomy** (trache/o means "trachea" or "windpipe"; -stomy means "create an opening").

Influenza (Flu)

Influenza is a viral infection that may affect both the upper and lower respiratory tracts. It is highly contagious, and some strains are particularly detrimental to the older population. Symptoms include fever, general aches and pains, tiredness, sore throat, **hemoptysis** (hem/o means "blood"; -ptysis means "spitting"), and nasal congestion. **Pneumonia** (pneumon/o means "lung"; -ia means "condition") is a frequent complication of the flu, especially in patients with chronic pulmonary and/or cardiovascular diseases. Pneumonia is an inflammation of the lungs accompanied by the pooling of fluids, which causes impaired air exchange in the alveoli. Flu vaccines are offered annually to match the predicted flu strains and are recommended for health care workers and people older than 65 years. Antiviral medications are available, but it is recommended that they be administered within 2 days of the onset of symptoms. Otherwise, treatment is symptomatic and supportive unless a bacterial infection results, in which case antibiotics might be administered.

Laryngitis

Laryngitis (laryng/o means "larynx"; -itis means "inflammation") is an inflammation of the larynx. **Dysphonia** (dys- means "difficult" or "painful"; phon/o means "voice"; -ia means "condition of"), or hoarseness, or weak voice or loss of voice is common with inflamed vocal cords.

Pertussis

Pertussis, also known as whooping cough, is a contagious bacterial infection of the upper respiratory tract. Previously known as a childhood disease, pertussis has in recent years occurred in adolescents and adults. Its primary symptom is a convulsive, spasmodic cough. Pertussis can be prevented with a vaccine.

Tuberculosis

Tuberculosis (TB) is an infectious disease caused by a bacterium. It usually attacks the lungs, although it may affect other parts of the body also. A person may have TB and not realize it, as the bacilli may be dormant. As the disease progresses, symptoms such as fever, night sweats, anorexia, general weakness, and weight loss may occur. A cough develops, producing a thick, blood-tinged sputum. Long-term treatment, including a combination of drugs, is usually needed. Patient compliance with the drug regimen is most important to eradicate the infection.

OBSTRUCTIVE LUNG DISEASES

Obstructive disease impairs airflow through the respiratory tree. The obstruction may be caused by an increased production of secretions or actual destruction of the lung tissues. Cystic fibrosis, emphysema, and asthma are a few of the diseases that fall into this category.

Cystic Fibrosis

Cystic fibrosis (CF) is a genetic disorder in which the lungs become clogged with excessive amounts of abnormally thick mucus. Although the respiratory system is the site of much of the damage, CF originates in the digestive system and is caused by abnormal exocrine secretions, which also block the pancreatic and bile ducts. In the respiratory system, the mucus obstructs the bronchioles and small bronchi, causing infections and other respiratory disorders. Recurrent infections may cause **bronchiectasis** (bronchi/o means "bronchus"; -ectasis means "dilation"), which impairs airflow and oxygen exchange. Bronchiectasis is a chronic expansion or dilation of the bronchi or bronchioles that may be caused by recurrent infections. Treatment includes a number of pharmacologic agents to help decrease the viscosity of the mucus and antibiotics to fight infections. Daily physical therapy known as chest physiotherapy (CPT) is implemented to facilitate the drainage of the mucus from the airways. CPT incorporates percussion and vibration techniques along with postural drainage, where the patient lies on his or her side, head downward, to help drain the lungs. The therapist strikes the chest wall with a cupped hand (percussion) and uses rapid massage (vibration) to loosen secretions.

Emphysema

In **emphysema**, the alveolar walls become chronically distended, leading to destruction and permanently inflated alveolar spaces (Fig. 11-7A). The alveolar walls become thin and are predisposed to rupture. There is a loss of surface area, thus affecting perfusion and oxygen exchange. Air becomes trapped in the alveoli, creating over-inflation of the lungs and a distended thoracic cage (Fig. 11-7B). Frequent infections occur as a result of the increased mucus production. The mucus in this case occurs as a result of chronic irritants such as smoking. Treatment includes elimination of irritants (e.g., smoking), good nutrition and hydration, and moderate exercise. Drug therapy includes antibiotics; **bronchodilators** (bronch/i/o means "bronchus"; dilator means "increase diameter" or "open up"), which promote better air flow; and oxygen therapy. Emphysema falls into the category of chronic obstructive pulmonary disease (COPD).

Asthma

Asthma is a bronchial obstructive disease resulting from hypersensitive airways. The bronchi and bronchioles respond excessively to irritants, and the smooth muscle of the airways contracts, a condition called **bronchoconstriction**, which causes an obstruction in the airway and interferes with the oxygen supply. Coughing, wheezing, chronic dyspnea, a tight feeling in the chest, and cyanosis (cyan/o means "blue"; -osis means "abnormal condition"), a condition exhibited by a dusky or bluish color of the skin, are common symptoms. Treatment consists of avoidance of the irritant (e.g., cats), good ventilation in the home, reduction of anxiety when attacks occur, and drugs to open the airways (bronchodilators).

EXPANSION DISORDERS

Adequate lung expansion is necessary for proper ventilation and gas exchange to take place. Some disease conditions place restrictions on the lung's capacity, thereby causing non-aeration of the lung tissues. **Atelectasis** and **pneumothorax** (pneum/o means "air" or "lung") are two of these conditions.

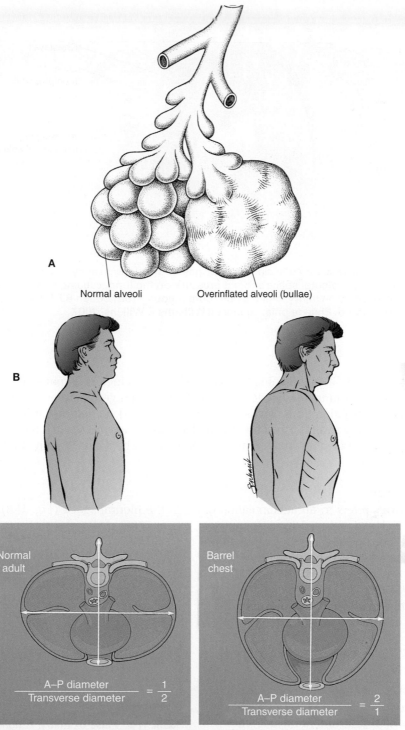

A

Normal alveoli   Overinflated alveoli (bullae)

B

Normal
adult

$$\frac{\text{A–P diameter}}{\text{Transverse diameter}} = \frac{1}{2}$$

Barrel
chest

$$\frac{\text{A–P diameter}}{\text{Transverse diameter}} = \frac{2}{1}$$

FIGURE 11-7 Emphysematous alveoli and barrel chest. A. Emphysematous alveoli. This illustration depicts a diseased alveolus (terminal end of the airway). In emphysema, the alveoli become chronically distended, impeding gas exchange. Air gets trapped inside the dilated alveoli, causing overinflation of the lungs. **B.** Barrel chest. Emphysema can ultimately lead to an enlarged thoracic cage, sometimes called a "barrel chest." The rib cage shape increases its anterior-posterior diameter due to trapped air in the lungs. Modified from Werner R, Benjamin BE. A massage therapist's guide to pathology, 2nd Ed. Baltimore: Lippincott Williams & Wilkins, and Smeltzer SC, Bare BG. Medical-Surgical Nursing, 9th Ed. Philadelphia: Lippincott Williams & Wilkins, 2000.

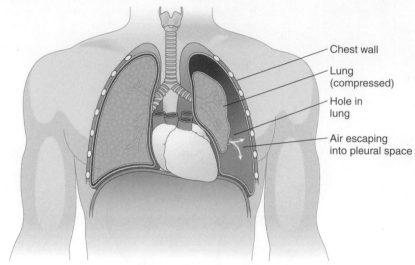

Chest wall

Lung (compressed)

Hole in lung

Air escaping into pleural space

FIGURE 11-8 **Pneumothorax.** A collection of air or gas in the pleural cavity. An injury to lung tissue allows air to leak into the pleural space and put pressure on the lung, causing it to collapse. A pneumothorax can be caused by an injury, or it may be spontaneous. From Cohen BJ. Medical Terminology: An Illustrated Guide, 5th Ed. Philadelphia: Lippincott Williams & Wilkins, 2007.

Atelectasis

Atelectasis (*ateles* is Greek meaning "incomplete"; -ectasis means "expansion") is the collapse of a lung or part of a lung, leading to decreased gas exchange. There are a variety of causes, including total obstruction from mucus, a tumor, or restricted ventilation caused by pain, as in a postoperative surgery setting. Small areas of atelectasis are asymptomatic, but larger areas may cause dyspnea, increased respiratory and heart rates, and chest pain. Treatment depends on the underlying cause.

Pneumothorax

Pneumothorax refers to an accumulation of air in the pleural space (Fig. 11-8). Pneumothorax may be closed (caused by a spontaneous collapse) or open (caused by a puncture wound). General signs of a pneumothorax are decreased breath sounds in the area of the collapse, dyspnea, and chest pain. Treatment consists of re-expansion of the lung as quickly as possible and supportive care.

DIAGNOSTIC PROCEDURES AND TREATMENTS

Both invasive and noninvasive procedures are used to diagnose respiratory disorders. The noninvasive procedures include chest X-rays, lung scans, **pulse oximetry** (ox means "oxygen"; -metry means "to measure") (Fig. 11-9), **arterial blood gases (ABGs)**, and computed tomography (CT) scans. Invasive procedures may include a thoracentesis (thorac/o means "thorax"; -centesis means "to puncture")

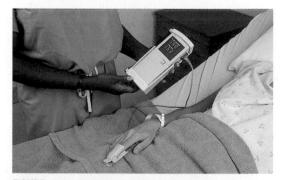

FIGURE 11-9 **Pulse oximetry.** A noninvasive test to indirectly measure the oxygen saturation of arterial blood. A monitor is placed over a translucent part of the body, usually a fingertip or earlobe. It is connected to a medical device that measures the oxygen saturation of the patient's blood. From Cohen BJ. Medical Terminology: An Illustrated Guide, 5th Ed. Philadelphia: Lippincott Williams & Wilkins, 2007.

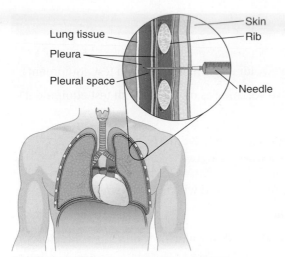

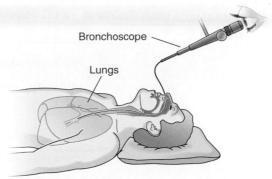

FIGURE 11-11 Bronchoscopy. Introduction of a bronchoscope through the nose that is then guided down into the bronchi. Visual examination (suffix -scopy means "visual examination") can be made of the bronchial tree; biopsies may be taken from the bronchi; and secretions may be removed for analysis or to reduce respiratory distress. From Cohen BJ. Medical Terminology, 4th Ed. Philadelphia: Lippincott Williams & Wilkins, 2003.

FIGURE 11-10 Thoracentesis. Excess fluid can accumulate inside the pleural space. A puncture (suffix -centesis means "to make a puncture") is made into the thorax, and a needle is inserted through the thoracic wall and into the pleural space. This procedure is done to withdraw fluid, or sometimes it is done to inject medicine. A thoracentesis is frequently done for therapeutic reasons such as to remove excess fluid, which will reduce respiratory distress. From Cohen BJ. Medical Terminology: An Illustrated Guide, 5th Ed. Philadelphia: Lippincott Williams & Wilkins, 2007.

(Fig. 11-10) and a **bronchoscopy** (bronch/o means "bronchus"; -scopy means "a lighted instrument for examination") (Fig. 11-11).

Respiratory therapists often perform **pulmonary function tests** on patients to assess breathing and ventilation. Lung volumes are measured with a **spirometer** (spir/o means "breath"; -meter means "measure") to assess progress and to monitor treatments.

Pharmacology

Sneezing, coughing, nasal congestion, fever, wheezing, and dyspnea are all symptoms of respiratory disorders that can be treated with pharmacologic agents. Following are some of the drug classifications used in treating respiratory conditions: **antipyretics** (anti- means "against"; pyret/o means "fever"; -ic is an adjective form); **bronchodilators** (bronchi/o means "bronchus"; dilator means "increase diameter" or "open up"); **mucolytics** (muc/o means "mucus"; -lytic means "digesting" or "dissolving"); **corticosteroids** (treat inflammatory and allergic conditions); **expectorants** (stimulate respiratory secretions to treat dry, irritating coughs); **decongestants** (reduce nasal congestion); **antibiotics** (anti- means "against"; biotic is an adjective form of bio or life); and **antihistaminics** (anti- means "against"; histaminic is an adjective form of histamine).

Abbreviation Table • *The Respiratory System*

ABBREVIATION	MEANING
ABG	arterial blood gas
CF	cystic fibrosis
CO_2	carbon dioxide
COPD	chronic obstructive pulmonary disease

(continued)

ABBREVIATION	MEANING
CXR	chest X-ray
ERV	expiratory reserve volume (as measured with test equipment)
IRV	inspiratory reserve volume (as measured with test equipment)
O$_2$	oxygen
PFT	pulmonary function test
R	respiratory rate
RV	residual volume (as measured with test equipment)
SOB	shortness of breath
T&A	tonsils and adenoids (also tonsillectomy and adenoidectomy)
TB	tuberculosis
TLC	total lung capacity (as measured with test equipment)
TV	tidal volume (as measured with test equipment)

Study Table • The Respiratory System

TERM AND PRONUNCIATION	ANALYSIS	MEANING
Structure and Function		
alveoli (al-VEE-oh-lee); singular: alveolus	diminutive of the Latin word *alveus* (cavity, hollow)	small cavities in which oxygen is removed from the air delivered by the bronchioles (note: alveoli are also found in other body systems)
apex (AY-pex)	a Latin word meaning summit, peak, tip	word used to describe the upper tip of each lung
base	common English word	word used to describe the bottom of each lung
bronchi (BRON-kee); singular: bronchus (BRON-kuss)	bronch/o-, bronch/i- (bronchus)	tubes (right and left) branching off from the trachea and into the lungs
bronchiole (BRON-kee-ole)	bronch/o-, bronch/i- (bronchus)	very small branches of bronchi that extend into the lungs
cilia (SIHL-ee-ah)	plural of the Latin word *cilium* (eyelash; eyelid)	small hairs in the upper respiratory tract that sweep foreign matter and mucus out of the respiratory tract
diaphragm (DY-uh-fram)	from the Greek word *diaphragma* (partition, barrier)	the major muscle of respiration located at the base of the thoracic cavity

TERM AND PRONUNCIATION	ANALYSIS	MEANING
epiglottis (ep-ih-GLOT-ihs)	*epi-* (upon) + the Greek *glottis* (tongue, mouth of the windpipe)	a mucous membrane-covered, leaf-shaped piece of cartilage at the root of the tongue
external respiration	common English words	process whereby air is brought into the lungs, and oxygen and carbon dioxide (waste product) are exchanged in the blood within the capillaries of the alveoli
glottis (GLOT-is)	a Greek word meaning tongue, mouth of the windpipe	vocal folds and apparatus of the larynx
internal respiration	common English words	process whereby the oxygen and carbon dioxide are exchanged at the cellular level
laryngopharynx (LAYR-in-je-o- FAYR-inx)	*laryng/o* (larynx); *-al* (adjective suffix); *pharyng/o* (pharynx)	lower portion of the pharynx
larynx (LAYR-inx)	*laryng/o* (larynx)	voice box, vocal cords
mediastinum (MEE-dee-ahs-TYN-um)	from the Latin word *mediastinus* (midway)	area between the lungs that houses the heart, aorta, trachea, esophagus, and bronchi
mucus (MYU-kus)	a Latin word meaning slime, mold	clear secretion produced in the respiratory tract
nasal (NAY-zuhl)	*nas/o* (nose); *-al* (adjective suffix)	adjective referring to the nose
nasopharynx (NAY-zoh-FAYR-inx)	*nas/o* (nose); *pharyng/o* (pharynx)	upper portion of the pharynx
oropharynx (O-roh-FAYR-inx)	from the Latin word *oris* (mouth); *pharyng/o* (pharynx)	middle portion of the pharynx
patency (PAY-tehn-see)	from the Latin word *patere* (lie open, be open)	the state of being open
patent (PA-tehnt; or PAY-tehnt)	from the Latin word *patere* (lie open, be open)	open; adjective form of patency
pharynx (FAYR-inx)	a Greek word meaning throat	passageway just below the nasal cavity and mouth
phrenic (FREN-ik)	from the Greek word *phren* (mind)	adjective referring to the diaphragm; synonymous with diaphragmatic
pleura (PLU-rah)	a Greek word meaning side of the body, rib	serous membrane that surrounds the lung; *parietal pleura* is the outer layer; *visceral pleura* is the inner layer

(continued)

TERM AND PRONUNCIATION	ANALYSIS	MEANING
pulmonary (PULL-muhn-ayr-ee)	*pulmon/o* (lung); *-ary* (adjective suffix)	adjective frequently used to modify another term in or associated with the lungs
sputum (SPYOU-tum)	from the Latin word *spuere* (to spit)	thick mucus ejected through the mouth
trachea (TRAY-kee-uh)	from the Greek word *trakheia* (windpipe)	windpipe
vocal cords	common English words	folds of mucus membranes that are used in speech production

Common Disorders

apnea (APP-nee-uh)	*a-* (without); *-pnea* (breathing)	absence of breathing
asthma (AZ-mah)	A Greek word meaning a panting	a lung disease characterized by reversible inflammation and constriction
atelectasis (at-eh-LEK-tah-sihs)	from the Greek word *ateles* (incomplete); *-ectasis* (expansion)	collapse of a lung or part of a lung, leading to decreased gas exchange
bradypnea (BRAH-dip-NEE-ah)	*brady-* (slow); *-pnea* (breathing)	abnormal slowness of respiration
bronchial pneumonia (BRAWN-kee-uhl nu-MO-nee-ah); also called *bronchopneumonia*	*bronchi/o* (bronchus); *-al* (adjective suffix); *pneumon/o* (air, lung)	inflammation of the smaller bronchial tubes
bronchiectasis (BRON-kee-EK-tay-sis)	*bronchi/o* (bronchus); *-ecstatis* (expansion)	chronic dilation of the bronchi
bronchiolitis (bron-kee-oh-LY-tihs)	*bronchi/o* (bronchus); *-itis* (inflammation)	inflammation of the bronchioles
bronchiostenosis (BRON-kee-oh-steh-NOH-sis)	*bronchi/o* (bronchus); *sten/o* (narrowing); *-osis* (abnormal condition of)	narrowing of the bronchial tubes
bronchitis (bron-KY-tihs)	*bronchi/o* (bronchus); *-itis* (inflammation)	inflammation of the mucous membrane of the bronchial tubes
bronchoconstriction (BRON-koh-kon-STRIK-shun)	*bronch/o* (bronchus) + constriction	the bronchi become narrowed or constricted
bronchodilation (BRON-ko-DYE-lay-shun)	*bronch/o* (bronchus) + dilation	the bronchi become more open or dilated
bronchopneumonia (BRON-koh-nu-MO-nee-uh); also called *bronchial pneumonia*	*bronch/o* (bronchus); *pneumon/o* (air, lung); *-ia* (condition)	inflammation of the smaller bronchial tubes

TERM AND PRONUNCIATION	ANALYSIS	MEANING
bronchospasm (BRON-ko-spaz-uhm)	*bronch/o* (bronchus) + spasm	abnormal contraction of bronchi
Cheyne-Stokes (SHAYN STOHKS)	named after John Cheyne, British physician, and William Stokes, Irish physician, who first described the disorder in the 19th century	a rhythmic respiratory pattern where there is a variation in depth of respirations alternating with periods of apnea
croup (krupe); laryngotracheobronchitis	obsolete English verb (to croak); *laryng/o* (larynx); *trache/o* (trachea); *bronchi/o* (bronchus)	a viral infection that causes swelling of the larynx and epiglottis; a barking noise is characteristic
cystic fibrosis (SIS-tik FYE-broh-sis)	from the Greek word *kystis* (bladder, pouch); from the Latin word *fibra* (fiber); *-osis* (abnormal condition)	genetic disorder in which the lungs become clogged with excessive amounts of abnormally thick mucus
dysphonia (DIS-fohn-ya)	*dys-* (difficult); *phon/o* (sound); *-ia* (condition)	difficult or painful speech
dyspnea (DISP-nee-uh)	*dys-* (difficult); *-pnea* (breathing)	difficult breathing
emphysema (ehm-fih-SEE-mah)	a Greek word meaning swelling	condition in which the alveoli are inefficient because of distension
hemoptysis (HEE-mop-ti-sis)	*hem/o* (blood); *-ptysis* (spitting)	blood-tinged frothy sputum
influenza (IN-flew-EN-zah); flu	an Italian word meaning influence (of planets or stars)	highly contagious viral infection of the upper respiratory tract that is spread by droplets
Kussmaul (KUHS-mowl)	named after 19th century German physician who first noted it among patients with advanced diabetes mellitus	rapid deep respirations that are characteristic of an acid-base imbalance (frequently seen in uncontrolled diabetes)
laryngitis (LAYR-ihn-jy-this)	*laryng/o* (larynx); *-itis* (inflammation)	inflammation of the larynx
laryngospasm (lah-RIHN-go-spaz-uhm)	*laryng/o* (larynx) + spasm	involuntary contraction of the larynx
laryngostenosis (lah-RIHN-go-steh-NO-sihs)	*laryng/o* (larynx); *sten/o* (narrowing); *-osis* (abnormal condition)	a narrowing of the larynx
orthopnea (or-THOP-NEE-ah)	*ortho-* (straight, correct); *-pnea* (breathing)	discomfort or difficulty in breathing while lying flat; difficulty is relieved by sitting up

(continued)

TERM AND PRONUNCIATION	ANALYSIS	MEANING
pertussis (per-TUSS-ihs)	from the Latin *per-* (through) + *tussis* (cough)	an acute infectious inflammation of the larynx, trachea, and bronchi caused by *Bordetella pertussis*
pharyngitis (fair-in-JY-tihs)	*pharyng/o* (pharynx); *-itis* (inflammation)	inflammation of the pharynx
pharyngospasm (fah-RIN-goh-spas-uhm)	*pharyng/o* (pharynx) + spasm	involuntary contraction of the pharynx
phrenoplegia (freh-no-PLEE-jee-ah)	*phren/o* (diaphragm); *-plegia* (paralysis)	paralysis of the diaphragm
pneumolith (NOO-mo-lith)	*pneum/o* (air, lung); from the Greek word *lithos* (stone)	calculus in a lung
pneumonia (noo-MONE-yah) (synonym for *pneumonitis*)	*pneumon/o* (air, lung); *-ia* (condition)	inflammation of a lung caused by infection, chemical inhalation, or trauma
pneumonitis (noo-mo-NY-tihs) (synonym for *pneumonia*)	*pneumon/o* (air, lung); *-itis* (inflammation)	inflammation of a lung caused by infection, chemical inhalation, or trauma
pneumothorax (NOO-moh-thoh-rax)	*pneumon/o* (air, lung); from the Greek word *thorakos* (breastplate, chest)	accumulation of air in the pleural space
rales (RAYLS)	from the French word *râler* (to make a rattling sound in the throat)	abnormal breath sound; crackles
rhinitis (ry-NY-tihs)	*rhin/o* (nose); *-itis* (inflammation)	inflammation of the inner lining of the nasal cavity
rhinopathy (ry-NAW-pah-thee)	*rhin/o* (nose); *-pathy* (disease)	any disease of the nose
rhinorrhea (ry-no-REE-ah)	*rhin/o* (nose); *-rrhea* (discharge)	discharge from the rhinal mucous membrane
rhonchi (RON-kye)	from the Greek *rhonchos* (snore)	abnormal breath sound; low-pitched sonorous sounds
sinusitis (sy-nuh-SY-tihs)	*sinus/o* (sinus); *-itis* (inflammation)	inflammation of the respiratory sinuses
stridor (STRY-dohr)	a Latin word meaning harsh, high pitched	high-pitched squeaking sound frequently associated with croup
tachypnea (TAK-ip-NE-ah)	*tachy-* (rapid); *-pnea* (breathing)	abnormal rapid respiration
tracheitis (tray-kee-EYE-tihs)	*trache/o* (trachea); *-itis* (inflammation)	inflammation of the trachea

TERM AND PRONUNCIATION	ANALYSIS	MEANING
tracheostenosis (TRAY-kee-oh-steh-NO-sihs)	*trache/o* (trachea); *sten/o* (narrowing); *-sis* (condition)	abnormal narrowing of the trachea
tuberculosis (tu-BURK-yu-loh-sihs)	from the Latin word- *tuberculum* (small swelling, pimple); *-osis* (abnormal condition)	disease caused by presence of *Mycobacterium tuberculosis*, most commonly affecting the lungs
wheezing (WEE-zing)	common English word	abnormal breath sounds; whistling sounds heard with upper airway obstruction

Diagnosis and Treatment

TERM AND PRONUNCIATION	ANALYSIS	MEANING
antihistaminic (anti-HISS-tah-MIN-ik)	*anti-* (against); from the Greek word *histos* (tissue); from the Latin *amine* (ammonia, compound); *-ic* (adjective suffix)	drug used to treat acute allergic reactions
antipyretic (anti-PYE-reh-tik)	*anti-* (against); from the Greek *pyretos* (fever); *-ic* (adjective suffix)	drug used to reduce fever
arterial blood gas	*arteri/o* (artery) + blood + gas, common English words	measures the partial pressures of oxygen and carbon dioxide in the arterial blood
bronchodilator (bron-ko-DYE-lay-tor)	*bronch/o* (bronchus); from the Latin word *dilatare* (to spread wide)	drug used to expand the bronchi
bronchoscope (BRON-ko-skope)	*bronch/o* (bronchus); *-scope* (instrument for viewing)	a device for visually inspecting the interior of a bronchus
bronchoscopy (bron-KOSS-ko-pee)	*bronch/o* (bronchus); *-scopy* (use of instrument for viewing)	inspection using a bronchoscope
decongestant (DEE-kon-jes-tant)	*de-* (away from, cessation); from the Latin word *congerere* (to bring together)	drug used to reduce edema and congestion
laryngoscope (lah-RIHN-go-skope)	*laryng/o* (larynx); *-scope* (instrument for viewing)	instrument with a light at the tip to aid in visual inspection of the larynx
laryngoscopy (LAYR-ihn-GOSS-koh-pee)	*laryng/o* (larynx); *-scopy* (use of instrument for viewing)	visual inspection of the larynx with the aid of a laryngoscope

(continued)

TERM AND PRONUNCIATION	ANALYSIS	MEANING
pharyngoscope (fah-RIN-goh-skope)	*pharyng/o* (pharynx); *-scope* (instrument for viewing)	instrument with a light at the tip to aid in the visual inspection of the pharynx
pharyngoscopy (FAH-rihn-GAW-skoh-pee)	*pharyng/o* (pharynx); *-scopy* (use of instrument for viewing)	visual inspection of the pharynx with aid of a pharyngoscope
postural drainage (PAHS-chu-ral)	common English words	a physical therapy technique where the patient lies on his or her side on a decline to help drain the lungs
pulmonary function tests	*pulmon/o* (lung); *-ary* (adjective suffix) + function + tests, common English words	measurement of lung volumes to assess breathing and ventilation; instrument used is a spirometer
pulse oximeter (ahk-SIM-eh-tuhr)	from the Latin word *pellere* (to push, drive); from the Greek words *oxys* (sharp) and *metron* (measure)	a device that measures the oxygen saturation of arterial blood by reference to light wave lengths
pulse oximetry (ahk-SIM-eh-tree)	from the Latin word *pellere* (to push, drive); from the Greek words *oxys* (sharp) and *metron* (measure)	a small instrument is placed on a finger or thin body part that measures the oxygen saturation of arterial blood
rhinoscope (RY-noh-skope)	*rhin/o* (nose); *-scope* (instrument for viewing)	a small mirror with a thin handle; used in rhinoscopy
rhinoscopy (ry-NAW-skoh-pee)	*rhin/o* (nose); *-scopy* (use of instrument for viewing)	visual inspection of the nasal areas
Surgical Procedures		
bronchoplasty (BRAWN-koh-plass-tee)	*bronch/o* (bronchus); *-plasty* (surgical repair)	surgical repair of a bronchus
laryngectomy (LAYR-ehn-JEK-toh-mee)	*laryng/o* (larynx); *-ectomy* (excision)	excision of the larynx
laryngoplasty (lah-RIHN-go-plass-tee)	*laryng/o* (larynx); *-plasty* (surgical repair)	surgical repair of the larynx
laryngotomy (layr-ihn-GOT-oh-mee)	*laryng/o* (larynx); *-tomy* (cutting operation)	incision into the larynx
pharyngoplasty (fah-RIHN-go-plass-tee)	*pharyng/o* (pharynx); *-plasty* (surgical repair)	surgical repair of the pharynx

TERM AND PRONUNCIATION	ANALYSIS	MEANING
pharyngotomy (FAYR-ihn-GOT-oh-mee)	*pharyng/o* (pharynx); *-tomy* (cutting operation)	surgical incision into the pharynx
pneumonectomy (NOO-mo-NEK-toh-mee)	*pneumon/o* (air, lung); *-ectomy* (excision)	removal of pulmonary lobes from a lung
pneumonorrhaphy (noo-mo-NOR-ah-fee)	*pneumon/o* (air, lung); *-rrhaphy* (surgical suturing)	suturing of a lung
pneumonotomy (noo-mo-NOT-ah-mee)	*pneumon/o* (air, lung); *-tomy* (cutting operation)	incision into a lung
rhinoplasty (RY-no-plass-tee)	*rhin/o* (nose); *-plasty* (surgical repair)	surgery performed on the nose
rhinotomy (ry-NAW-toh-mee)	*rhin/o* (nose); *-tomy* (cutting operation)	surgical incision into the nose
sinusotomy (sy-nuh-SOT-oh-mee)	*sinus/o* (sinus); *-tomy* (cutting operation)	incision into a sinus
spirometer (spy-ROM-eh-tehr)	from the Latin word *spirare* (breath, blow, live); from the Greek word *metron* (measure)	a device used to measure respiratory gases
thoracentesis (THOH-rah-sen-TEE-sihs)	*thorac/o* (thorax); *-centesis* (surgical puncture)	insertion of a needle into the pleural cavity to withdraw fluid for diagnostic purposes, to drain excess fluid, or to re-expand a collapsed lung
tracheoplasty (TRAY-kee-oh-plass-tee)	*trache/o* (trachea); *-plasty* (surgical repair)	surgical repair of the trachea
tracheostomy (tray-kee-OS-toh-mee)	*trache/o* (trachea); from the Greek *stoma* (mouth)	surgical creation of an opening into the trachea to form an airway or to prepare for the insertion of a tube for ventilation
tracheotomy (tray-kee-AH-toh-mee)	*trache/o* (trachea); *-tomy* (cutting operation)	incision into the trachea for purpose of restoring airflow to the lungs

Practice and Practitioners

otolaryngologist (oh-to-LAYR-ihn-GAW-loh-jist)	*ot/o* (ear); *laryng/o* (larynx); *-logist* (one who specializes)	physician who specializes in diagnosis and treatment of ear, nose, and throat diseases
otolaryngology (oh-to-LAYR-ihn-GAW-loh-jee)	*ot/o* (ear); *laryng/o* (larynx); *-logy* (study of)	branch of medical study concerned with the ear, nose, and throat and diagnosis and treatment of its diseases

(continued)

TERM AND PRONUNCIATION	ANALYSIS	MEANING
pulmonologist (PULL-muhn-AW-loh-jist)	*pulmon/o* (lung); *-logist* (one who specializes)	physician who specializes in diagnosing and treating respiratory disorders
pulmonology (PULL-muhn-AW-loh-jee)	*pulmon/o* (lung); *-logy* (study of)	medical specialty of diagnosing and treating respiratory disorders
respiratory therapist	from the Latin word *respirare* (breathe, blow back, blow again) + therapist	allied health care professional who specializes in airway management, mechanical ventilation, and blood acid-base balance

EXERCISES

EXERCISE 11-1   Figure Labeling: The Respiratory System

capillaries	nasal cavity	alveoli	esophagus
diaphragm	mediastinum	nares	alveolar duct
left lung	terminal bronchiole	trachea	right lung
right bronchus	nasopharynx	laryngopharynx	larynx (vocal cords)
epiglottis	pharynx	oropharynx	

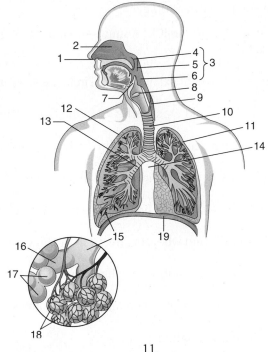

1. _____   11. _____

2. _____   12. _____

3. _____   13. _____

4. _____   14. _____

5. _____   15. _____

6. _____   16. _____

7. _____   17. _____

8. _____   18. _____

9. _____   19. _____

10. _____

EXERCISE 11-2   Case Study

MEDICAL RECORD

Analyze the following medical record and answer the questions below.

HISTORY: A 30-year-old female who c/o a nonproductive cough, dyspnea, and a fever of 3 days; patient has a negative history for smoking and has otherwise been in good health.

PHYSICAL EXAM: T 102°F, BP 104/65, R 26, P 108
    Tachypnea is accompanied by mild cyanosis, and inspiratory rales are noted during a stethoscope exam. WBC is elevated, CXR shows diffuse infiltrates at the bases of both lungs. An ABG taken while the patient was breathing room air was abnormal and showed the patient had low oxygen content in the blood. A sputum specimen contained WBCs.

DIAGNOSIS: Pneumonia of unknown etiology.

TREATMENT PLAN: Admit patient to the ICU. Administer antibiotics and oxygen by face mask and monitor patient's status.

1. What are the findings on physical examination? Circle the answer.

   A. Fast breathing, blue skin, and crackles heard in the lungs as the patient inhales

   B. Slow breathing, blue skin, and rales heard in the lungs as the patient holds her breath

   C. Slow breathing, blue skin, and rhonchi heard in the lungs as the patient exhales

   D. Fast heart rate, blue skin, and rales heard in the lungs as the patient inhales

   E. Fast breathing, blue skin, and wheezing heard in the lungs as the patient inhales

2. What is the patient's chief complaint? Circle the answer.

   A. Cannot breathe, fever, and coughing up material from lungs

   B. Dry cough and difficulty breathing

   C. Fever, coughing up sputum, and breathing fast

   D. Hoarse throat, dry cough, and fever

   E. Fever with a dry cough and difficulty breathing

EXERCISE 11-3   Matching

Match the term in Column A with the correct definition in Column B.

COLUMN A

1. _____ alveoli

2. _____ diaphragm

3. _____ pulmonary

4. _____ trachea

5. _____ epiglottis

6. _____ pneumonia, pneumonitis

7. _____ larynx

8. _____ bronchioles

9. _____ asthma

10. _____ pharynx

11. _____ emphysema

12. _____ bronchitis

13. _____ dyspnea

14. _____ tracheotomy

COLUMN B

A. the lid or flap that helps prevent food and drink from entering the trachea

B. the "voice box"

C. indicating something in or associated with the lungs

D. the major muscle of the respiratory system

E. tiny "sacs" in the lungs that receive oxygen from the bronchioles and transfer it to the capillaries

F. the "windpipe"; air flows through it to the bronchi

G. inflammation of a lung, caused by infection, chemical inhalation, or trauma

H. incision into the trachea

I. inner lining of the lung

J. the smallest extensions of the bronchi, which pass air directly to the alveoli

K. a lung disease characterized by reversible inflammation and constriction

L. throat

M. narrowing of a bronchial tube

N. inflammation of the mucous membrane of the bronchial tubes

15. _____ bronchiostenosis

O. difficult breathing

16. _____ apnea

P. inspection using a bronchoscope

17. _____ visceral pleura

Q. absence of breathing

18. _____ bronchoscopy

R. condition in which the alveoli are inefficient due to distension

EXERCISE 11-4   Definitions

Write the medical term for each definition.

1. the process of breathing in

_____

2. spitting up of blood

_____

3. any disease of the chest

_____

4. inflammation of sinus

_____

5. difficulty in speaking

_____

6. air in the pleural cavity

_____

7. incision into the pleura

_____

8. pain in the pleural region

_____

9. herniation of lung tissue or pleura

_____

EXERCISE 11-5   Word Building

Use bronch/o or bronchi/o to build the following terms:

1. inflammation of the bronchi

_____

2. drug used to open bronchi

_____

3. drug used to constrict bronchi

_____

4. chronic dilation of the bronchioles

_____

Use the suffix -itis to build the following terms:

5. inflammation of the larynx _____

6. inflammation of the bronchi _____

7. inflammation of a sinus _____

8. inflammation of the epiglottis _____

Use the suffix -pnea to build the following terms:

9. rapid breathing _____

10. slow breathing _____

11. painful or difficult breathing _____

12. difficulty breathing while lying down _____

EXERCISE 11-6   Case Study

An 88-year-old female is seen in the physician's office complaining of SOB, dizziness, orthopnea, elevated temperature, and productive cough. She was referred to the hospital for evaluation. Bubbling rales are heard upon inspiration over the R bronchi. RUL congestion is seen on X-ray exam. Vital signs are as follows: temperature 102, pulse 100 and rapid, respirations 24 and labored. She was placed on antibiotic treatment, postural drainage, and IPPB or intermittent positive pressure breathing. She was released to her family with medications after 3 days of hospitalization.

1. Define:

    A. Bubbling rales _____

    B. Orthopnea _____

    C. SOB _____

2. What is postural drainage? _____

    _____

EXERCISE 11-7 Crossword Puzzle: Respiratory System

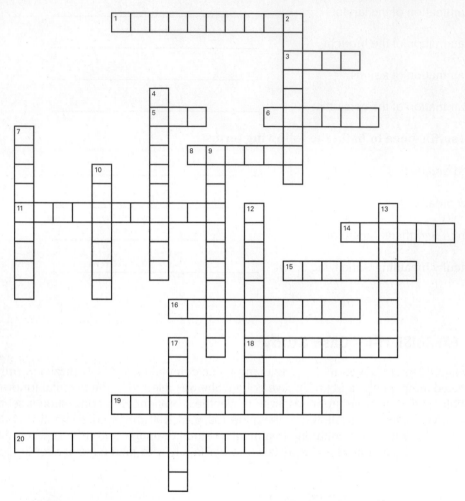

ACROSS

1. small bronchi
3. suffix meaning breathing
5. abbreviation for arterial blood gas
6. disease characterized by wheezing and inflammation of the bronchi
8. mucus expectorated from the mouth
11. area between lungs
14. vocal cords are found here
15. throat
16. inflammation of the bronchi
18. terminal end of the bronchial tree
19. instrument used to visualize inside the bronchi
20. needle inserted into the pleural space

DOWN

2. type of COPD with overexpansion of alveoli
4. inflammation of the voicebox
7. same as pneumonitis
9. study of the lungs
10. windpipe
12. collapsed lung
13. singular form for bronchi
17. inflammation of the nose

CHAPTER 11 QUIZ

Multiple Choice

1. Pertussis is the medical term for:
   a. strep throat
   b. diphtheria
   c. whooping cough
   d. Lyme disease

2. Expectoration of blood is called:
   a. hematemesis
   b. hemoptysis
   c. anosmia
   d. dysphonia

3. What is the uppermost part of the pharynx?
   a. oropharynx
   b. laryngopharynx
   c. nasopharynx
   d. hypopharynx

4. What is the serous membrane that lines the walls of the pulmonary cavity?
   a. visceral pleura
   b. parietal pleura
   c. visceral peritoneum
   d. parietal peritoneum

5. What is the term for slow breathing?
   a. bradyphasia
   b. tachypnea
   c. bradypnea
   d. tachyphasia

6. Which procedure involves making an opening in the trachea to facilitate breathing?
   a. intubation
   b. tracheocentesis
   c. tracheoplasty
   d. tracheostomy

7. Which of the following would probably cause dysphonia?
   a. rhinitis
   b. laryngitis
   c. otitis
   d. ophthalmodynia

8. What is surgical puncture of the lungs?
   a. pneumoconiosis
   b. pneumocentesis
   c. pneumomelanosis
   d. pneumogenesis

9. What is pleurisy (pleuritis)?
   a. effusion of fluid into the air/tissue of the lungs
   b. softening of the lungs
   c. engorgement of the pulmonary vessels with fluid
   d. inflammation of the membrane that surrounds the lungs and lines the walls of the chest cavity

10. Which of the following is the same as pharyngodynia?
    a. sore throat
    b. inflammation of the pharynx
    c. examination of the throat
    d. a fungal condition of the pharynx

11. What is the membrane that surrounds the lungs?
    a. pharynx
    c. pleura
    b. palate
    d. polyp

12. What is the term for difficult breathing in all positions except an upright position?
    a. dysphonia
    c. dyspnea
    b. hyperpnea
    d. orthopnea

13. Which term means the drawing of air into the lungs?
    a. respiration
    c. inspiration
    b. orthopnea
    d. hypoxia

14. What is another term for *pneumonia?*
    a. pleuropneumonia
    c. pulmonary edema
    b. pneumonitis
    d. pulmonary insufficiency

15. What is chronic dilation of the bronchi?
    a. bronchiectasis
    c. bronchiolitis
    b. bronchopathy
    d. bronchoscopy

16. What is a collapse of part of a lung or alveoli called?
    a. asthma
    c. SIDS
    b. atelectasis
    d. cystic fibrosis

17. A thin watery discharge from the nose is known as?
    a. hemoptysis
    c. rhinorrhea
    b. rhinitis
    d. rhinolithiasis

18. What is a lobectomy?
    a. incision of the lung
    c. excision of a lobe of an organ
    b. excision of a lung
    d. bilateral incision of the skull

19. What condition describes alternating periods of apnea and dyspnea?
    a. Kussmaul breathing
    c. atelectasis
    b. Cheyne-Stokes respirations
    d. rales

20. What type of drug is used to decrease the viscosity of mucus?
    a. antipyretic
    c. mucolytic
    b. antibiotic
    d. diuretic

CHAPTER 12

The Digestive System

LEARNING OBJECTIVES

Upon completion of this chapter, you should be able to:

- Name and briefly describe the functions of the digestive system and its accessory organs.
- Identify and use the word elements of the digestive system.
- Briefly describe symptoms and treatments in response to disorders of the digestive system.
- Name the major drug classifications used to treat digestive system disorders.
- Identify and interpret selected abbreviations relating to the digestive system.
- Analyze and define the new terms introduced in this chapter.
- Label a diagram of the digestive system.

Word Elements • The Digestive System

WORD ELEMENT	REFERS TO
abdomin/o	abdomen
bucc/o	cheek
cheil/o	lip
chol/e, chol/o	bile, gall
cholangi/o	bile duct
cholecyst/o	gallbladder
choledoch/o	common bile duct
col/o, colon/o	colon
dent/i, dent/o	teeth
duoden/o	duodenum
-emesis	vomit
enter/o	intestine
esophag/o	esophagus
gastr/o	stomach
gingiv/o	gums
gloss/o	tongue
hepat/o	liver
ile/o	ileum
jejun/o	jejunum
lapar/o	abdomen
-lith	stone
pancreat/o	pancreas
-pepsia	digestion
phag/o	eating; swallowing
-phagia	eat or swallow
proct/o	anus and rectum
pylor/o	pylorus
rect/o	rectum
-scope	device for visual examination
-scopy	visual examination
sial/o	salivary glands
sigmoid/o	sigmoid colon
stomat/o	mouth

An Overview of the Digestive System

The digestive system is composed of a continuous tract beginning with the oral cavity and ending at the anus (Fig. 12-1). This tract, called the **alimentary canal** or the **gastrointestinal (GI) tract** (gastr/o means "stomach"), is complemented by accessory organs that convert food and fluids into a form that permits the body to absorb nutrients. The GI tract is divided into two sections: the *upper GI tract*, which consists of the oral cavity, esophagus, and stomach, and the *lower GI tract*, which consists of the intestines. The three main functions of the digestive system are *digestion*, *absorption*, and *elimination*. The GI tract and accessory organ terms are introduced in this chapter.

The specialists concerned with most aspects of the digestive system are **gastroenterologists** (gastr/o means "stomach"; enter/o means "intestine") and **proctologists** (from the Greek word *proktos* meaning "rectum" and the suffix -logy meaning "study of"). The specialties are gastroenterology and proctology, respectively.

Structure and Function

The body requires food and nutrients to sustain life. However, the food we eat needs to be converted into a form our bodies can use, and that conversion is the job performed by the digestive tract and associated organs.

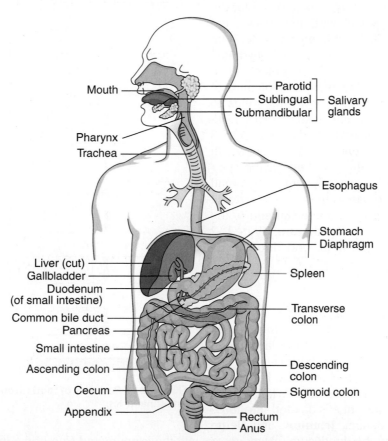

FIGURE 12-1   Digestive system. Some of the divisions of the large and small intestines are shown. The accessory organs are the salivary glands, liver, gallbladder, and pancreas. From Cohen BJ. Medical Terminology: An Illustrated Guide, 5th Ed. Philadelphia: Lippincott Williams & Wilkins, 2007.

THE UPPER GI TRACT

Digestion begins in the oral cavity where food is broken apart by **mastication** (comes from the Latin word meaning "to chew"). Saliva produced by the salivary glands moistens the food, which helps form a bolus (small mass of masticated food) that is then pushed back and downward with the tongue. Next, the bolus enters the **pharynx** (introduced in Chapter 11 as part of the respiratory tract) and from there into the **esophagus**. The esophagus, a collapsible tube, lubricates the food with mucus and moves it into the stomach by **peristalsis** (wave-like muscular contractions). The **cardiac sphincter** ("cardiac" because of its proximity to the heart) is also called the lower esophageal sphincter (LES). It is a ring-like muscle that controls food flow from the esophagus into the stomach.

The stomach is the center of the system, both physically and functionally. Its first job is to act as a temporary storage place for the food we eat, which allows time for its second job—secreting acid and enzymes to help break down proteins, fats, and carbohydrates. Digestion thus includes not only mechanical changes, such as the reduction of particle size and liquefaction (converting solids to liquids), but also the chemical changes needed to produce fuel for the body's cells. After 3 or 4 hours, the content of the stomach, which by this stage is a liquid called chyme (pronounced kyme), begins to enter the small intestine. Chyme passes through the **pyloric sphincter**, a muscle at the distal end of the stomach, and into the **duodenum**. Figure 12-2 illustrates the pathway of food through the GI tract.

THE LOWER GI TRACT

The lower GI tract begins with the small intestine, which extends from the pyloric sphincter to the first part of the large intestine. Although it is about 20 feet in length, it is known as the small intestine because it is smaller in diameter than the large intestine. The small intestine is divided into three parts: the duodenum, **jejunum**, and **ileum**

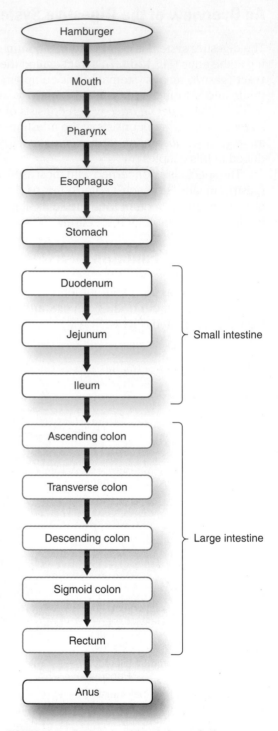

FIGURE 12-2 Pathway of food through the gastrointestinal tract.

(Fig. 12-3). From the duodenum, chyme moves into the jejunum and from there into the ileum. The **ileocecal sphincter** (ile/o means "ileum"; cecal is the adjective form of cecum) controls the flow from the ileum into the **cecum**, the first part of the large intestine.

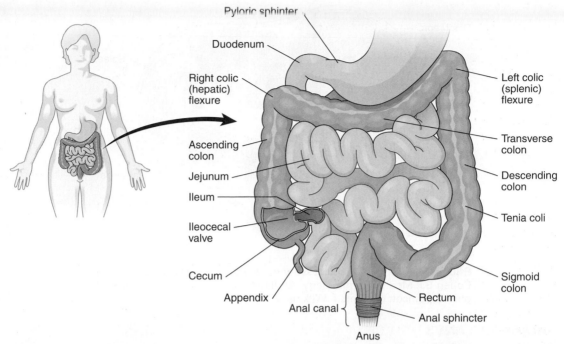

FIGURE 12-3   The small and large intestines The small intestine, illustrated in light pink, is made up of the duodenum, jejunum, and ileum. The large intestine, illustrated in darker pink, can be divided into the ascending colon, transverse colon, and the descending colon. The intestinal tract terminates at the anus. From Cohen BJ, Wood DL. Memmler's The Human Body in Health and Disease, 10th Ed. Baltimore: Lippincott Williams & Wilkins, 2004.

> *The word* ileum *might sound familiar to you. In Chapter 5, you learned that* ilium *is the name of one of the three bones making up the hip. Ilium and ileum are pronounced the same even though they have different roots. A convenient way to remember which word is which is to associate ilium with hip, which also has an* i *in it, and ileum with enter/o, the root for intestine.*

The large intestine extends from the distal portion of the ileum to the anus. It is divided into three parts: the **cecum**, **colon**, and **rectum**. The cecum is the beginning part of the large intestine. Attached to the cecum is a blind tube called the **vermiform appendix**. Vermiform, which means worm-like, is usually omitted; the single word *appendix* is the preferred term. The appendix consists of lymphatic tissue and is, functionally speaking, part of the immune system.

The colon is subdivided into four parts: the **ascending colon**, **transverse colon**, **descending colon**, and **sigmoid colon** (see Fig. 12-3). The last part, the sigmoid colon, continues from the descending colon and connects to the rectum. The rectum takes up approximately the last 6 inches of the large intestine and terminates at the anus, through which waste products are eliminated.

Accessory Organs

The **salivary glands**, **liver**, **gallbladder**, and **pancreas**, although not part of the alimentary canal, play a key role in the digestive process and are referred to as **accessory organs** of the digestive system (Fig. 12-4).

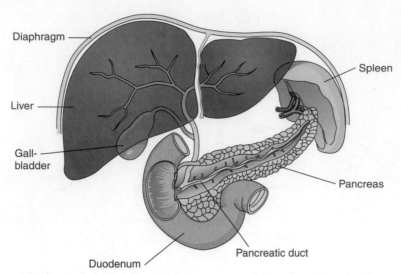

FIGURE 12-4 Some of the accessory organs of digestion. Modified from Cohen BJ. Medical Terminology: An Illustrated Guide, 5th Ed. Philadelphia: Lippincott Williams & Wilkins, 2007.

SALIVARY GLANDS

The senses of taste and smell stimulate the salivary glands to secrete saliva (sial/o means "saliva"), a watery liquid that contains enzymes that begin the digestive process. Saliva also helps eliminate bacteria in the mouth and keeps the teeth (dent/i means "tooth") and tongue (gloss/o means "tongue") clean. Figure 12-1 shows the location of the salivary glands.

LIVER

The liver (hepat/o means "liver"), located in the upper right quadrant of the abdomen under the dome of the diaphragm, plays many important roles in digestion, metabolism, and detoxification of harmful substances. One of its main digestive functions is the manufacture and secretion of bile. Our bodies need bile to process fats before they are released into the bloodstream. Once bile is produced in the liver, it travels down the **common bile duct** to the gallbladder for storage.

A few other functions of the liver include:
- Stores glucose in the form of glycogen.
- Manufactures blood proteins and blood clotting factors.
- Destroys old red blood cells.
- Stores some vitamins and iron.

As you can see, the liver is a most important organ whose functions are integrated into many of the body's systems.

GALLBLADDER

Although the liver produces and recycles bile, the gallbladder, which is located in a depression under the liver, stores, condenses, and delivers the bile to the small intestine. The gallbladder is also sometimes referred to as the cholecystis or cholecyst, from the word root *cholecyst/o* (see Fig. 12-4).

PANCREAS

The pancreas (pancr/o and pancreat/o mean "pancreas") is an elongated feather-shaped organ that lies posterior to the stomach. It has both digestive and endocrine functions. It produces digestive enzymes that aid in processing carbohydrates and fats in foods, as well as secreting hormones directly into the bloodstream (discussed in Chapter 8).

A summary of the digestive organs and their functions is provided in Table 12-1.

Table 12-1   Summary of the Digestive System Organs and Functions

Organ	Functions
Oral cavity	breaks food apart by mastication (chewing); food bolus formed
Salivary glands	secretes saliva to moisten food
Pharynx	common passageway for both food and air
Esophagus	peristalsis moves food bolus downward to stomach
Stomach	converts food to semi-liquid state and imparts chemical changes
Small intestine	where most digestion and absorption takes place
Large intestine	where water is removed from the feces and elimination occurs
Liver	stores glycogen; manufactures and secretes bile; manufactures blood proteins; destroys old red blood cells; detoxifies harmful substances
Gallbladder	stores and delivers bile
Pancreas	secretes juices and enzymes into small intestine; secretes insulin

Disorders and Treatments

Several digestive system conditions necessitate a "team approach" to assist with their many facets. A condition may require an adjustment of dietary intake, such as a reduction or elimination of caffeine and alcohol, to promote the healing of ulcers or possibly stress-reduction techniques to prevent inflammatory bowel conditions. Various drugs are used to treat gastrointestinal disorders, and various surgeries are used to remove diseased components. Several invasive and noninvasive tests are used to diagnose conditions of the GI tract and accessory organs. These and some of the clinical manifestations of the digestive system are discussed in the following sections.

DISORDERS OF THE UPPER GI TRACT

Disorders of the upper GI tract may involve infections, cancer, or structural problems. Infections such as **stomatitis** (stomat/o means "mouth") and **gingivitis** (gingiv/i means "gums") occur in the oral cavity. **Parotiditis** (also known as parotitis), is an inflammation of the parotid gland that is characterized by a swelling of the gland, usually bilateral. (See Fig. 12-1 for location of the parotid gland.) Other abnormal conditions such as **dental caries** or cavities and **bruxism** (an involuntary clenching or grinding of teeth) can occur in the mouth.

A few common disorders of the upper digestive tract include the following:

- **Dysphagia** is difficulty in swallowing and may be caused by stenosis (narrowing) of the esophagus, strictures, ulcers, chronic inflammation, paralysis, or **esophagitis** (esophag/o means "esophagus"; -itis means "inflammation of"). Diagnostic tests may include a **barium swallow upper GI series** (X-ray of the upper GI tract using a contrast medium) or **gastroscopy** (examination of the esophagus and stomach using a **gastroscope**, a special lighted instrument. Depending on the cause, treatment may involve surgical intervention, esophageal dilations, or drug therapy.
- A **hiatal hernia** is a condition in which part of the stomach protrudes through the opening (hiatus) in the diaphragm into the thoracic cavity. This type of hernia often causes heartburn or **epigastric** (epi- means "above"; gastr/o means "stomach"; -ic is an adjective suffix) pain and is usually diagnosed by means of a barium swallow upper GI test or **endoscopy** (end/o means "within"; -scopy means "an instrument used to view"). Drug therapy may relieve heartburn discomfort, and surgical intervention may be necessary in severe cases (Fig. 12-5).
- **GERD (gastroesophageal reflux disease)** is the upward flow of stomach acid into the esophagus. This condition creates pain in the *epigastric* (above the stomach or just below the breast bone) region. Drug therapy usually relieves the discomfort.

Hiatal Hernia

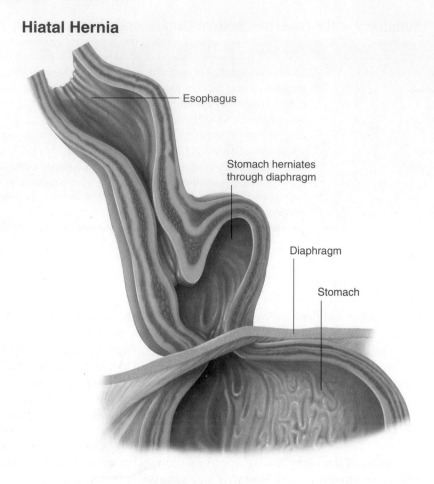

Esophagus

Stomach herniates
through diaphragm

Diaphragm

Stomach

FIGURE 12-5   Hiatal hernia.

- **Gastritis**, which occurs when the gastric mucosa is inflamed, may progress to ulceration if left untreated. Causes include repeated infections, allergies to food, ingestion of spicy foods, medications such as nonsteroidal anti-inflammatory drugs (NSAIDs), or corrosive agents. Treatment consists of elimination of the causative agent and may also include drug therapy.

DISORDERS OF THE LOWER GI TRACT

Disorders of the lower GI tract include obstructions, inflammation, or structural abnormalities. Some of these conditions are described below.

- **Crohn disease** is an inflammation in the mucosal lining of the intestine (usually small intestine) and may result in ulcers and destruction of the intestinal lining or total obstruction. Symptoms may include cramping, diarrhea, **melena** (bloody stools), anorexia, weight loss, and fatigue. In severe cases, sections of the GI tract are removed, and a **stoma** (an opening) is created on the surface of the abdomen to accommodate waste elimination.
- **Appendicitis** is a common acute inflammatory disease. It can become abscessed and may rupture, causing **peritonitis** (an inflammation of the peritoneum, which is the sac that lines the abdominal cavity).
- **Diverticula** are abnormal pouches in the intestinal wall that form as increased pressure pushes the wall of the colon outward at certain weakened points. Sometimes if there is not

enough fiber or bulk in the diet, the colon has to work harder to push the food through, and this may cause increased pressure in the colon. The condition **diverticulosis** occurs when these pouches develop in the colon. They do not always cause problems or create symptoms. When bacteria or fecal material collect in the pouches, inflammation can result, and this is termed **diverticulitis**, or an inflammation of the diverticula. These conditions can be diagnosed by tests such as a colonoscopy (an examination of the colon with a lighted instrument) or a barium enema X-ray. They are treated with diet modifications and drug therapy.

- **Intestinal obstruction** refers to a lack of movement of the intestinal contents through the intestine. The condition occurs more frequently in the small intestine because of its small diameter. Functional obstructions result from neurologic impairments such as a spinal cord injury, whereas mechanical obstructions result from tumors or physical obstructions. **Intussusception**, one type of mechanical obstruction, is a telescoping of a section of bowel inside an adjacent section. Another condition, a **volvulus**, is a twisting of the bowel. Either of these last two disorders can be fatal if not treated quickly.

- **Inguinal hernia** is the protrusion of a small loop of intestine through a weak spot in the lower abdominal wall or groin. Surgical repair is the most frequent type of treatment.

- **Cancer** of the GI tract frequently affects the colon and rectum. The cancer may develop from a **polyp**, a growth protruding from a stalk. Polyps may be removed by means of an instrument called a **colonoscope** during a **colonoscopy** (the diagnostic procedure).

DISORDERS OF THE ACCESSORY ORGANS OF THE DIGESTIVE SYSTEM

Many of the conditions that affect the digestive system accessory organs are obstructions caused by stones, tumors, or inflammatory processes. A few of these are described below.

- **Cholelithiasis** (chol/e means "gall"; lith/o means "stone"; -iasis means "condition"), or gallstones, describes a condition in which calculi or stones reside in the gallbladder or bile ducts. These can cause **cholecystitis**, an inflammation of the gallbladder. **Cholangiolitis** usually refers to an inflammation of the smallest bile duct, and **choledocholithiasis** (chol/e means "gall"; doch/o means "duct") refers to an obstruction of the biliary tract by gallstones. Symptoms of cholelithiasis may include nausea and vomiting, pain in the upper right quadrant, and sometimes **jaundice** (yellowish color of the skin). The normal course of treatment is surgical removal of the gallbladder.

- **Hepatitis** is an inflammation of the liver. **Jaundice**, or **icterus**, is a symptom of hepatitis. The whites of the eyes and mucous membranes take on a yellow appearance caused by the presence of **bilirubin** in the blood. There is no treatment to destroy the viruses in the body, but supportive care is most useful. Vaccines are available now for hepatitis A and hepatitis B.

- **Cirrhosis** (cirrh means "yellow") of the liver is a chronic liver disease; the liver becomes firm and nodular, and the disease can progress to necrosis and liver failure. It is characterized by jaundice, fatigue, and **ascites** (fluid in the peritoneal cavity), and in the early stages of the disease, **hepatomegaly** (hepat/o means "liver"; -megaly means "enlarged") may be present.

A few additional conditions, symptoms, or disorders of the digestive system include **anorexia** (loss of appetite), **bulimia** (binge eating followed by self-induced vomiting and misuse of laxatives), **eructation** (belching or burping gas), **hyperemesis** (hyper- means "excessive"; -emesis means "vomit"), **dyspepsia** (impairment of digestion or *indigestion*), and **hemorrhoids** (enlarged veins in or near the anus). **Diarrhea** (Greek meaning "to flow") may be a symptom characterized by frequently "loose" or watery stools. It may be seen with food poisoning, intestinal infections, intestinal worms, or increased activity in the colon. The opposite condition, **constipation**, is a decrease in the frequency of bowel movements, difficulty in passing stools, and/or hard dry stools. Constipation can be classified as acute or chronic. In acute conditions, there may be an intestinal obstruction, such as a tumor, or an inflammation, such as diverticulitis. In chronic conditions, sometimes the muscles in the wall of the colon become weak and are unable to push and expel the stool.

Pharmacology

Medications can be prescribed to relieve symptoms, or they may be obtained over the counter. Some of the common drug classifications for the digestive system are as follows:

- **Antacids** neutralize acid production.
- **Antidiarrheals** are drugs that relieve diarrhea by absorbing the excess fluid or by decreasing intestinal motility.
- **Antiemetics** are taken to relieve vomiting.
- **Antiflatulence** drugs are taken to reduce gas (**flatus**).
- **Emetics** stimulate or induce vomiting.
- **H2 blockers** are drugs used to treat ulcers and conditions such as GERD. They act by blocking the release of acid.
- **Protein pump inhibitors** are medications prescribed to reduce the production of acid by blocking an enzyme that is necessary for acid production. The reduction of acid prevents ulcers and allows any ulcers that exist in the esophagus, stomach, and duodenum to heal.
- **Protective agents** are taken for ulcers. They provide a topical protective layer over the ulcer, allowing it to heal.

For some digestive disorders, nutrition, vitamins and medications must be given intravenously (IV). These patients are considered **NPO** (can take "nothing by mouth"). **Total parenteral nutrition (TPN)** is a type of complete nutrition that is given through an IV while the patient is closely monitored. (Parenteral means that the medication is being given in a means other than through the digestive tract; *para* is Greek for "apart from"; enteral is the adjective form of enter/o, referring to the intestine). TPN is administered through a special IV called a central line. This type of IV catheter is placed "centrally" (i.e., with the tip in a central large vein). For patients who are required to eat nothing for extended periods of time, TPN may be administered.

Abbreviation Table • The Digestive System

ABBREVIATION	MEANING
BE	barium enema
BM	bowel movement
EGD	esophagogastroduodenoscopy
GB	gallbladder
GBS	gallbladder X-ray series
GERD	gastroesophageal reflux disease
GI	gastrointestinal
HCl	hydrochloric acid
IBS	irritable bowel syndrome
LES	lower esophageal sphincter
NGT	nasogastric tube
NPO	nothing by mouth
PO	per os, or by mouth
TPN	total parenteral nutrition
UGI	upper gastrointestinal

Study Table • The Digestive System

TERM AND PRONUNCIATION	ANALYSIS	MEANING
Structure and Function		
alimentary canal (al-ih-MEN-tah-ree)	from the Latin word *alimentarius* (pertaining to food) + canal	the digestive tract, the gastrointestinal (GI) tract
antibody (AN-tih-body)	*anti-* (against) + body	antibodies contained in saliva that act as antibacterial agents
bilirubin (BIHL-ee-ROO-bin)	from the Latin *bilus* (bile) and *ruber* (red)	waste produced by worn out RBCs breaking down
cardiac sphincter (KAR-dee-ak sfink-ter)	*cardi/o* (heart); *-ac* (adjective suffix); from the Greek word *sphingein* (to bind tight)	the ring-like muscle between the esophagus and stomach that controls food flow
colon (KOH-luhn); also called the *large intestine*	from the Greek word *kolon* (large intestine)	the large intestine, divisible into the ascending, transverse, descending, and sigmoid colons
common bile duct	common English words	tube that transports bile from the liver to the gallbladder
deglutition (dee-glu-TISH-uhn)	from the Latin word *deglutire* (to swallow, overwhelm, abolish)	swallowing
duodenal (doo-oh-DEE-nuhl)	from the Greek word *dodekadaktylon* (literally "12 fingers long"; named by Greek physician Herophilus) + *-al* (adjective suffix)	adjective form of duodenum used in the terms naming some digestive system disorders
duodenum (doo-oh-DEE-num)	from the Greek *dodekadaktylon* (12 fingers long)	segment of the small intestine connecting with the stomach
esophagus (ee-SOF-ah-guhs)	from the Greek *oisophagos* (gullet, literally "what carries and eats")	the part of the digestive tract between the pharynx and stomach
fundus (FUN-duhs)	a Latin word meaning bottom	the part of the stomach lying above the cardia notch
gallbladder	from Old English *galla* (to shine, yellow); from Old English *bledre* (to blast, blow up, swell up)	small pear-shaped organ that stores bile

(continued)

TERM AND PRONUNCIATION	ANALYSIS	MEANING
gastric (GAS-trik)	*gastr/o* (stomach); *-ic* (adjective suffix)	adjective form of stomach
gastrointestinal tract (GAS-troh-in-TES-tin-ahl)	*gastr/o* (stomach); from Latin *intestina*, plural of *intestinus* (internal, inward, intestine) + tract	the alimentary canal; also, simply, the GI tract
ileocecal sphincter (EEL-ee-oh-see-kal)	*ile/o* (ileum); from the Latin *caecum*, (blind); *-al* (adjective suffix); sphincter (from the Greek word *sphingein*: to bind tight)	muscular ring that separates the distal portion of the ileum and the beginning of the cecum (large intestine)
ileum (ILL-ee-uhm)	a Latin word meaning flank, groin	the longest segment of the small intestine, which leads into the large intestine
intestine (ihn-TESS-tin); the term includes the small intestine and the large intestine, also called the *colon*	from Latin *intestina*, plural of *intestinus* (internal, inward, intestine)	the small intestine is divisible into the duodenum, jejunum, and ileum; the large intestine comprises the cecum, colon, rectum, and anus
jejunum (jeh-JOO-nuhm)	from the Latin word *jejunus* (empty, fasting, abstinent, hungry)	eight-foot-long segment of the small intestine between the duodenum and the ileum
pancreas (PAN-kree-as)	from the Greek words *pan* (all) and *kreas* (flesh, meat)	organ of the digestive system that has both exocrine and endocrine functions; secretes enzymes that aid in digestion
pancreatic (pan-kree-AT-ik)	*pancreat/o* (pancreas); *-ic* (adjective suffix)	adjective for pancreas
peristalsis (pear-ih-STAL-sis)	from the Greek word *peristaltiko* (clasping and compressing)	wave-like muscular contractions that move food along in the digestive tract
pharynx (FAYR-inx)	from the Greek word *pharunx* (throat)	passageway just below the nasal cavity and mouth
pyloric sphincter (pye-LOHR-ik sfink-ter)	*pylor/o* (pylorus); *-ic* (adjective suffix); sphincter (from the Greek word *sphingein*: to bind tight)	ring muscle between the stomach and duodenum
salivary glands (SAL-ih-vahr-ee)	from the Latin word *salivarius* (slimy, clammy) + gland from the Latin word *glans* (acorn)	collectively, the parotid, sublingual, and submandibular salivary glands
stoma (STOH-mah)	a Greek word meaning mouth, opening	an artificial opening

TERM AND PRONUNCIATION	ANALYSIS	MEANING
stomach (STUM-uhk)	from the Greek word *stoma* (mouth, opening)	digestive organ composed of four parts: the fundus, the cardia, the body, and the antrum

Common Disorders

anorexia (an-orh-ECKS-ee-ah)	from the Greek *an* (without) + *orexis* (appetite, desire)	loss of appetite
appendicitis (ay-PEN-dih-SY-tis)	from the Latin word *appendix* (something attached); *-itis* (inflammation)	inflammation of the appendix
ascites (ay-SYTE-ees)	from the Greek word *askos* (bag)	abnormal accumulation of fluid in the peritoneal cavity
bruxism (BRUKS-ism)	from the Greek word *ebryxa*, root of *brykein* (to gnash the teeth) + *-ism* (condition)	involuntary grinding of the teeth that usually occurs during sleep
bulimia (bull-EE-mee-ah)	from the Greek word *boulemia* (hunger)	eating disorder characterized by episodes of binge eating followed by self-induced vomiting and misuse of laxatives
cholangiolitis (KOH-lan-GY-oh-LY-tis)	*cholangi/o* (bile, duct); *-itis* (inflammation)	inflammation of the bile ducts
cholecystitis (KOH-lee-siss-TY-tiss) cholecyst (KOH-leh-sihst)	*cholecyst/o* (gallbladder); *-itis* (inflammation)	inflammation of the gallbladder
cholecystopathy (KOH-lee-siss-TOP-ah-thee)	*cholecyst/o* (gallbladder); *-pathy* (disease)	any disease of the gallbladder
choledocholithiasis (KOH-le-DOKO-lith-EYE-ah-sis)	*choledoch/o* (common bile duct); *-lithiasis* (condition of having stones)	inflammation of the bile duct caused by gall stones
cholelithiasis (KOH-lee-lih-THYE-ah-sis)	*chol/e* (bile, gall); *-lithiasis* (condition of having stones)	formation or presence of stones in the gallbladder or common bile duct
cirrhosis (sir-OH-sis)	from the Greek word *kirrhos* (tawny), named for the orange-yellow appearance of a diseased liver	chronic disease of the liver
colitis (ko-LY-tihs)	*col/o* (colon); *-itis* (inflammation)	inflammation of the colon
constipation (kon-stih-PAY-shun)	from the Latin word *constipare* (to press or crowd together)	decrease in the frequency of bowel movements, difficulty in passing stools, and/or hard dry stools

(continued)

TERM AND PRONUNCIATION	ANALYSIS	MEANING
Crohn disease	named after American B.B. Crohn (1884–1983), one of the team that described it in 1932	chronic inflammation of part(s) of the intestinal tract
dental caries (kayr-eez)	*dent/i* (tooth); *-al* (adjective suffix) + *caries*, a Latin word meaning rot, rottenness, corruption	tooth decay
diverticulitis (dye-ver-tik-yoo-LYE-tis)	from the Latin word *diverticulum* (a side road); *-itis* (inflammation)	inflammation of a diverticulum or sac in the intestinal tract
duodenitis (doo-odd-eh-NY-tihs)	*duoden/o* (duodenum); *-itis* (inflammation)	inflammation of the duodenum
dyspepsia (dis-PEP-see-ah)	from the Greek word *dyspeptos* (hard to digest); *-ia* (condition of)	impairment of digestion
dysphagia (dis-FA-jee-ah)	*dys-* (difficulty); *phag/o* (eating, swallowing); *-ia* (condition of)	difficulty swallowing
enteritis (ehn-teh-RY-tihs)	*enter/o* (intestine); *-itis* (inflammation)	inflammation of the intestine
enterohepatitis (EN-teh-roh- hep-ah-TI-tihs)	*enter/o* (intestine); *hepat/o* (liver); *-itis* (inflammation)	inflammation of the intestine and liver
enteropathy (en-tehr-OP-ah-thee)	*enter/o* (intestine); *-pathy* (disease)	any intestinal disease
eructation (ee-RUK-tay-shun)	from the Latin word *erucationis* (a belching forth)	act of belching or burping gas up from the stomach
gastric ulcers (GAS-trik)	*gastr/o* (stomach); *-ic* (adjective suffix) + ulcer, from the Latin *ulcus*, related to the Greek word *helkos* (wound, sore)	erosion of the gastric mucosa
gastritis (gas-TRY-tihs)	*gastr/o* (stomach); *-itis* (inflammation)	inflammation of the stomach
gastrocele (GAS-troh-seel)	*gastr/o* (stomach); *-cele* (hernia)	hernia of the stomach
gastroduodenitis (GAS-troh-doo-oh-deh-NY-tihs)	*gastr/o* (stomach); *duoden/o* (duodenum); *-itis* (inflammation)	inflammation of the stomach and duodenum
gastroenteritis (GAS-troh-en-teh-RY-tihs)	*gastr/o* (stomach); *enter/o* (intestine); *-itis* (inflammation)	inflammation of the stomach and intestine

TERM AND PRONUNCIATION	ANALYSIS	MEANING
gastroesophageal reflux disease (GERD) (GAS-troh-ee-sof-a-JEE-al)	*gastr/o* (stomach); *esophag/o* (esophagus); *-al* (adjective suffix); + reflux disease	upward flow of stomach acid into the esophagus
gingivitis (JIN-jeh-vye-tis)	*gingiv/o* (gums); *-itis* (inflammation)	inflammation of the gums
hemorrhoids (hem-ROYDs)	from the Greek word *haimorrhoides* derived from *haima* (blood); and *rhoos* (a flowing)	enlarged veins in or near the anus that may cause pain or bleeding
hepatitis (hep-ah-TY-tihs)	*hepat/o* (liver); *-itis* (inflammation)	inflammation of the liver
hepatogenic (heh-pah-toh-JEN-ik)	*hepat/o* (liver); *-genic* (originating)	originating in the liver
hepatomegaly (heh-PAH-to-MEG-ah-lee)	*hepat/o* (liver); *-megaly* (enlargement)	enlarged liver
hiatal hernia (HYE-ay-tahl HER-nee-ah)	from the Latin word *hiatus* (gaping, opening); *-al* (adjective suffix) + the Latin word *hernia* (rupture)	protrusion of the stomach through the diaphragm into the thoracic cavity
hyperemesis (hy-per-EM-ih-sis)	*hyper-* (excessive); *-emesis* (vomit)	excessive vomiting
inguinal hernia (ING-gwi-nahl HER-nee-ah)	from the Latin word *inguinalis* (of the groin) + the Latin word *hernia* (rupture)	out-pouching of intestines into the inguinal or groin region
intussusception (in-tuh-suh-SEP-shun)	from the Latin word *intus* (within); from the Latin word *suscipere* (undertake; support, accept)	one part of the intestine slipping or telescoping over another
jaundice (JAWN-dis) or icterus (IK-tehr-us)	from Middle French word *jaunisse* (yellow)	yellowish cast to the skin, sclera (white part of the eye), and mucous membranes caused by bile deposits
jejunitis (jeh-joo-NY-tihs)	*jejun/o* (jejunum); *-itis* (inflammation)	inflammation of the jejunum
melena (MEL-in-nah)	from the Greek word *melas* (black)	blood in the stool
pancreatitis (PAN-kree-ah-TY-tihs)	*pancreat/o* (pancreas); *-itis* (inflammation)	inflammation of the pancreas
pancreatopathy (PAN-kree-ah-TOP-ah-thee)	*pancreat/o* (pancreas); *-pathy* (disease)	any disease of the pancreas

(continued)

TERM AND PRONUNCIATION	ANALYSIS	MEANING
parotiditis (pah-RAH-ti-DYE-tis)	parotid from the Greek words *para-* (beside) and *otos* (ear); *-itis* (inflammation)	inflammation of the parotid salivary glands
peritonitis (PAYR-ih-toh-NYE-tis)	from the Greek words *peri-* (around) and *teinein* (to stretch); *-itis* (inflammation)	inflammation of the peritoneal cavity
polyp (PAHL-ip)	from the Latin word *polypus* (cuttlefish)	growth protruding from a stalk in the digestive tract
sialoadenitis (SY-ah-loh-ah-deh-NY-tihs)	*sial/o* (saliva, salivary gland); *aden/o* (gland); *-itis* (inflammation)	inflammation of a salivary gland
sialoangiitis (SY-ah-loh-an-jee-EYE-tihs)	*sial/o* (saliva, salivary gland); *angi/o* (vessel); *-itis* (inflammation)	inflammation of a salivary duct
sialorrhea (SY-ah-loh-REE-ah)	*sial/o* (saliva, salivary gland); *-rrhea* (discharge)	excessive production of saliva
sialostenosis (SY-ah-loh-steh-NO-sihs)	*sial/o* (saliva, salivary gland); *-stenosis* (narrowed, blocked)	narrowing of a salivary duct
stomatitis (STOH-mah-tye-tis)	*stomat/o* (mouth); *-itis* (inflammation)	inflammation of the mouth

Diagnosis and Treatment

antacids (ant-AS-ids)	from *anti-* (against) + acids	medications used to neutralize acid production
antidiarrheal (an-ty-DYE-ah-REE-al)	*anti-* (against); from the Greek *dia-* (through) + *-rrhea* (discharge); *-al* (adjective suffix)	drugs that relieve diarrhea by absorbing the excess fluid or by decreasing intestinal motility
antiemetic (an-ty-EE-meh-tik)	*anti-* (against); *-emesis* (vomit); *-ic* (adjective suffix)	drugs used to relieve vomiting
antiflatulence (an-ty-FLAT-yoo-lens)	*anti-* (against); from the Latin word *flatus* (a blowing; a breaking wind)	drugs taken to relive gas or flatus
colonoscope (ko-LAWN-uh-skope)	*colon/o* (colon); *-scope* (instrument for viewing)	device used in colonoscopy
colonoscopy (ko-luh-NAW-skuh-pee)	*colon/o* (colon); *-scopy* (viewing)	visual examination of the colon with a colonoscope
duodenoscopy (doo-oh-deh-NOS-kuh-pee)	*duoden/o* (duodenum); *-scopy* (viewing)	visual examination of the duodenum with the aid of an endoscope
emetic (ee-MET-ik)	*emesis* (vomit); *-ic* (adjective suffix)	drugs that stimulate or induce vomiting; frequently used in poisoning cases

TERM AND PRONUNCIATION	ANALYSIS	MEANING
enteroscope (en-TEHR-oh-skope)	*enter/o* (intestine); *-scope* (instrument for viewing)	lighted instrument for visually examining the intestines
enteroscopy (en-tehr-OS-koh-pee)	*enter/o* (intestine); *-scopy* (viewing)	visual examination of the intestines
gastroscope (gas-TROH-skope)	*gastr/o* (stomach); *-scope* (instrument for viewing)	lighted instrument for visually examining the stomach
gastroscopy (gas-TRAH-scoh-pee)	*gastr/o* (stomach); *-scopy* (viewing)	visual examination of the stomach with a lighted instrument
H2 blockers or H2-receptor antagonists	H2 (or histamine2), a common chemical in the body, signals the stomach to make acid; H2 blockers oppose histamine's action and reduce the amount of acid the stomach produces; + blocker, a common English word	drugs that block the release of gastric acid; used to treat GERD
hepatoscopy (he-pah-TOSS-kuh-pee)	*hepat/o* (liver); *-scopy* (viewing)	visual examination of the liver
sialography (sy-ah-LOG-rah-fee)	*sial/o* (saliva, salivary gland); *-graphy* (the process of recording)	radiography of salivary glands and ducts
Practice and Practitioners		
gastroenterologist (GAS-troh-en-tehr-OL-oh-jist)	*gastr/o* (stomach); *enter/o* (intestine); *-logist* (one who studies a certain field)	a specialist in the diagnosis and treatment of digestive system disorders
gastroenterology (GAS-troh-en-tehr-OL-oh-jee)	*gastr/o* (stomach); *enter/o* (intestine); *-logy* (the study of)	the specialty concerned with the digestive system
internal medicine	two common English words	specialty in the diagnosis and nonsurgical treatment of serious and/or chronic illnesses; the phrase is quite commonly used in North America (but not necessarily elsewhere); it also covers subspecialties in specific organs, such as the liver, kidneys, etc.
internist (IN-tur-nist)	internal (English adjective meaning inside) + *-ist* (practitioner)	a specialist in internal medicine
proctologist (prok-TAH-lo-jist)	*proct/o* (anus and rectum); *-logist* (one who studies a certain field)	a specialist in the diagnosis and treatment of rectal and anal disorders

(continued)

TERM AND PRONUNCIATION	ANALYSIS	MEANING
proctology	*proct/o* (anus and rectum); *-logy* (study of)	study of the rectum and anus

Surgical Procedures

TERM AND PRONUNCIATION	ANALYSIS	MEANING
anastomosis (ah-NAS-tah-MOH-sis)	from the Greek word *anastomoein* (to bring to a mouth)	creation of an opening between two hollow organs
cholecystectomy (KOH-lee-siss-TEK-toh-mee)	*cholecyst/o* (gallbladder); *-ectomy* (surgical removal)	excision of the gallbladder
cholecystotomy (KOH-lee-siss-TOT-oh-mee)	*cholecyst/o* (gallbladder); *-tomy* (incision)	incision into the gallbladder
colectomy (ko-LEK-toh-mee)	*col/o* (colon); *-ectomy* (surgical removal)	excision of all or part of the colon
colopexy (KOH-loh-pehk-see)	*col/o* (colon); *-pexy* (surgical fixation)	fixation of the colon
colostomy (koh-LOSS-tuh-mee)	*col/o* (colon); *-stomy* (permanent opening)	surgical establishment of an opening into the colon
colotomy (ko-LOT-uh-mee)	*col/o* (colon); *-tomy* (incision)	incision into the colon
duodenectomy (doo-oh-deh-NEK-toh-mee)	*duoden/o* (duodenum); *-ectomy* (surgical removal)	excision of the duodenum
duodenostomy (doo-oh-deh-NOS-toh-mee)	*duoden/o* (duodenum); *-stomy* (permanent opening)	surgical establishment of an opening in the duodenum
gastrectomy (gas-TREK-toh-mee)	*gastr/o* (stomach); *-ectomy* (surgical removal)	excision of part of the stomach
hepatopexy (HEH-pah-to-pek-see)	*hepat/o* (liver); *-pexy* (surgical fixation)	fixation of the liver
jejunectomy (jeh-joo-NEK-toh-mee)	*jejun/o* (jejunum); *-ectomy* (surgical removal)	excision of all or part of the jejunum
jejunoplasty (jeh-JOON-oh-plass-tee)	*jejun/o* (jejunum); *-plasty* (surgical repair)	surgical repair of the jejunum
jejunotomy (jeh-joo-NOT-oh-mee)	*jejun/o* (jejunum); *-tomy* (incision)	incision into the jejunum
pancreatotomy (PAN-kree-ah-TOT-ah-mee)	*pancreat/o* (pancreas); *-tomy* (incision)	incision into the pancreas
sialoadenectomy (SY-al-oh-ah-deh-NEK-tah-mee)	*sial/o* (saliva, salivary gland); *aden/o* (gland); *-ectomy* (surgical removal)	excision of a salivary gland
sialoadenotomy (SY-al-oh-ah-deh-NOT-ah-mee)	*sial/o* (saliva, salivary gland); *aden/o* (gland); *-tomy* (incision)	incision of a salivary gland

EXERCISES

EXERCISE 12-1   Figure Labeling: The Digestive System

anus	mouth	submandibular glands
gallbladder	small intestine	esophagus
rectum	descending colon	pharynx
ascending colon	pancreas	transverse colon
liver	stomach	sublingual gland
sigmoid colon	duodenum	
cecum	parotid gland	

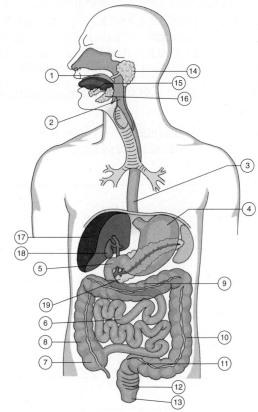

1. _____
2. _____
3. _____
4. _____
5. _____
6. _____
7. _____
8. _____
9. _____
10. _____

11. _____
12. _____
13. _____
14. _____
15. _____
16. _____
17. _____
18. _____
19. _____

EXERCISE 12-2   Chart Note

The chart note contains 12 phrases that can be reworded with a medical term that was learned in this unit. Each phrase is identified with an underline. Write the medical term on the line provided.

CURRENT COMPLAINT: Patient is a 72-year-old female seen by a (1) <u>physician who specializes in the treatment of the gastrointestinal tract</u> with complaints of severe lower abdominal pain and extreme (2) <u>difficulty with having a bowel movement</u>.

PAST HISTORY: Patient has a history of the (3) <u>presence of gallstones</u> requiring a (4) <u>surgical removal of the gallbladder</u> 10 years ago and chronic (5) <u>acid backing up from the stomach into the esophagus</u>.

SIGNS AND SYMPTOMS: The patient's abdomen is distended with (6) <u>fluid collecting in the abdominal cavity</u>. (7) <u>X-ray of the colon after inserting barium dye with an enema</u> revealed (8) <u>the presence of multiple small tumors growing on a stalk</u> throughout the colon. (9) <u>Visual examination of the colon by a fiberscope inserted through the rectum</u> was performed, and biopsies were taken of a tumor located by microscopic examination.

DIAGNOSIS: Carcinoma of the (10) <u>section of colon between the descending colon and the rectum</u>.

TREATMENT: (11) <u>Surgical removal of the colon</u> between the descending colon and the rectum with a colostomy (<u>surgical creation of an opening of the colon through the abdominal wall</u>).

1. _____

2. _____

3. _____

4. _____

5. _____

6. _____

7. _____

8. _____

9. _____

10. _____

11. _____

EXERCISE 12-3   Word Building

To build the term, use the combining form that is provided and add an appropriate suffix.

COMBINING FORM	BODY PART	CREATE A TERM
1. or/o	mouth	adjective form for oral cavity
2. stomat/o	mouth	inflammation of mouth
3. bucc/o	cheek	adjective form for cheek
4. cheil/o	lip	condition of the lip
5. gingiv/o	gum	removal of gum tissue (mouth)
6. gloss/o	tongue	incision into the tongue
7. lingu/o	tongue	adjective form for tongue
8. gastr/o	stomach	stomach pain
9. pharyng/o	throat	adjective form for pharynx
10. enter/o	intestine	inflammation of the small intestine
11. duoden/o	duodenum	adjective form for duodenum
12. jejun/o	jejunum	an adjective form of jejunum
13. ile/o	ileum	inflammation of the ileum
14. col/o	colon	removal of the colon

15. rect/o	rectum	a herniation of the rectum
		_____
16. an/o	anus	adjective form for anus
		_____
17. proct/o	anus/rectum	one whose medical specialty is the anus and rectum
		_____
18. hepat/o	liver	an enlarged liver
		_____
19. bil/i	bile	a bile pigment that is formed from the destruction of RBCs _____
20. cholecyst/o	gallbladder	removal of the gallbladder
		_____

EXERCISE 12-4   Abbreviations and Acronyms

Write the expansion for each abbreviation or acronym.

1. BE   _____

2. BM   _____

3. GI   _____

4. IBS   _____

5. GERD _____

EXERCISE 12-5   Crossword Puzzle: Digestive System

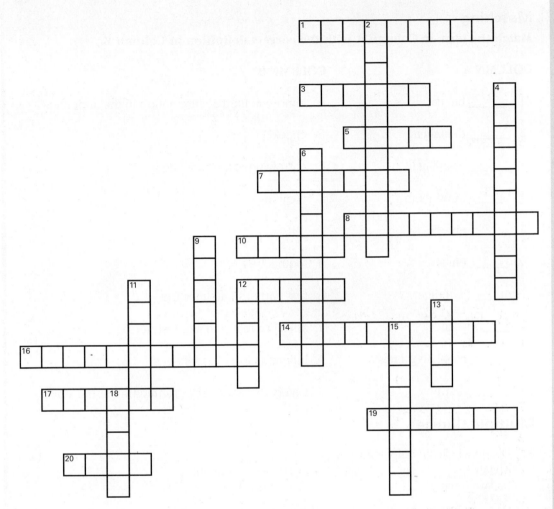

ACROSS
1. difficulty swallowing
3. liquid secreted from salivary gland
5. growth from a stalk found in intestines
7. binge eating
8. chronic liver disease
10. erosion of intestinal mucosa
12. root for stomach
14. burping
16. excessive vomiting
17. pertaining to the cheek
19. second portion of small intestine
20. distal end of the GI tract

DOWN
2. inflammation of the peritoneum
4. inflammation of the mouth
6. gastrointestinal tract
9. gas
11. blood in the stool
12. root for tongue
13. root for salivary gland
15. loss of appetite
18. first part of large intestine

CHAPTER 12 QUIZ

Matching

Match the term in Column A with the correct definition in Column B.

COLUMN A

1. _____ buccal

2. _____ dentalgia

3. _____ esophagitis

4. _____ duodenum

5. _____ enteric

6. _____ emesis

7. _____ jaundice

8. _____ ascites

9. _____ esophagostenosis

10. _____ diarrhea

COLUMN B

A. abnormal fluid accumulation in the abdomen

B. cheek

C. narrowing of the esophagus

D. vomiting

E. yellow

F. toothache

G. first part of small intestine

H. adjective referring to intestine(s)

I. inflammation of esophagus

J. watery discharge from the rectum; liquid stools

Multiple Choice

11. Dysphagia is difficulty with:
    a. talking
    b. swallowing
    c. elimination
    d. digestion

12. Anorexia is:
    a. difficulty in digestion
    b. hyperemesis
    c. loss of appetite
    d. a small ulcer

13. Gas in the stomach or intestines is:
    a. gavage
    b. icterus
    c. flatus
    d. dysentery

14. Diverticulitis is an inflammation of:
    a. small pouches in the intestine
    b. the vermiform appendix
    c. the hypopharynx
    d. descending colon

15. Movement of the bowels by which their contents are propelled toward the rectum is:
    a. pyloroplasty
    b. volvulus
    c. peristalsis
    d. gastroenteric

16. The buccal mucosa is in the:
    a. nostril
    b. stomach and intestines
    c. mouth, inside the cheek
    d. greater curvature of the stomach

17. Belching is called:
    a. volvulus
    b. eructation
    c. gastroenteric
    d. halitosis

18. Vomiting blood is called:
    a. hematitis
    b. indigestion
    c. mastication
    d. hematemesis

19. Telescoping of the intestines into themselves is called:
    a. gastrojejunostomy
    b. intussusception
    c. volvulus
    d. sphincter

20. A colonoscopy is:
    a. an endoscopic study of the colon
    b. an upper endoscopy with biopsy
    c. a type of barium enema
    d. an endoscopic study of the small intestine

CHAPTER 13

The Urinary System

LEARNING OBJECTIVES

Upon completion of this chapter, you should be able to:

- List the major organs of the urinary system and their functions.
- Build urinary medical terms from the word elements.
- Describe disorders, treatments, and procedures relative to the urinary system.
- Describe the major drug classifications used to treat urinary disorders.
- Interpret abbreviations associated with the urinary system.
- Analyze and define the new terms introduced in this chapter.

Word Elements • The Urinary System

WORD ELEMENT	MEANING	EXAMPLE
cyst/o	bladder	cystitis
glomerul/o	glomerulus	glomerulonephritis
-iasis	suffix meaning "condition" or "state"	nephrolithiasis
lith/o	stone	nephrolithotomy
nephr/o, ren/o	kidney	nephritis, renal
noct/o	night	nocturia
olig/o	little, few	oliguria
poly-	prefix meaning "much" or "many"	polyuria
py/o	pus	pyuria
pyel/o	pelvis	pyelonephritis
ur/o, urin/o	urine	urography
ureter/o	ureter	ureterolith
urethr/o	urethra	urethralgia

An Overview of the Urinary System

The urinary system is composed of the **kidneys**, **ureters**, **urinary bladder**, and **urethra**. Figure 13-1 illustrates the location of each of these structures. The primary function of the urinary system is to remove wastes and toxins from the body. The process starts with the kidneys, which remove certain wastes from the bloodstream. The kidneys then convert the waste to urine (water that contains other substances in solution) and transport it to the bladder via the ureters. The urine is then eliminated through the urethra. This process regulates the amount of water in the body and maintains the proper balance of acids and electrolytes, such as salts, and is a necessary function for human survival. The flow chart illustrates this fundamental process.

The physician who specializes in the diagnosis and treatment of urinary disorders is called a **urologist** (ur/o is the combining form meaning "urine"; -logist means "one who studies"), and the specialty practice is **urology** (ur/o means "urine"; -logy means "study of"). The physician who treats the kidney and kidney disorders is called a **nephrologist** (nephr/o means "kidney"; -logist means "one who studies"). The area of specialty is named **nephrology** (nephr/o means "kidney"; -logy means "study of").

> ✳ *The root* cyst/o *is used to form terms having to do with the urinary bladder. Those same terms, however, are often used in reference to the gallbladder. Therefore,* cystalgia, cystectomy, *and* cystopexy *can mean, respectively, pain in, excision of, and surgical fixation of either the urinary bladder or the gallbladder. The term* cystectomy *can also mean excision of a cyst, a word that refers to an abnormal sac that has nothing to do with either the urinary bladder or the gallbladder. All of these usages come from the Greek word* kystis, *which means bladder, and careful users who wish to refer specifically to the gallbladder couple the Greek word* chole *(which means bile) with* cyst/o. *This distinction yields the terms* cholecystalgia, cholecystectomy, cholecystopexy, *and so on.*

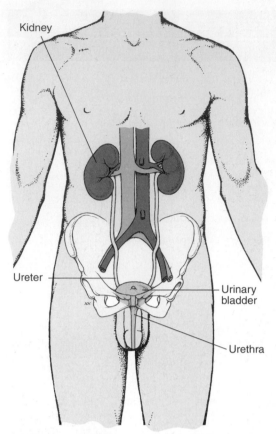

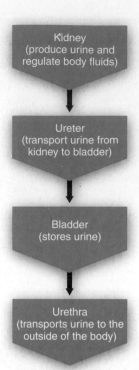

FIGURE 13-1 Primary structures of the urinary system. Anterior view of the kidneys, ureters, bladder, and urethra (male). From Stedman's Medical Dictionary, 27th Ed. Baltimore: Lippincott Williams & Wilkins, 2000.

Flow chart illustrating the process of urine formation and excretion. The process of urine formation begins in the kidneys. The kidneys filter waste products from the blood and convert them to urine. The urine is transported from the kidneys by the ureters to the bladder, where it is stored until it is expelled through the urethra via the process of urination.

Structure and Function

The kidneys are bean-shaped organs (hence the name, kidney bean) and are about the size of a fist; they lie at the back of the abdominopelvic cavity, along each side of the spinal column. Each kidney is covered by a thin membrane called the renal capsule. A thicker layer of fatty tissue, called the **perirenal** (peri- means "around"; ren/o means "kidney"; -al creates the adjective form) **fat**, provides protection to this vital organ and surrounds the renal capsule. Finally, a thin layer of connective tissue, called the **renal fascia**, forms each kidney's outer covering. The **hilum** is the indented, or narrowest, part of the kidney, where blood vessels and nerves enter. Figure 13-2 shows the structure of the kidneys.

The kidneys remove two natural products of metabolism while producing urine: **urea** and **uric acid**, along with other waste products from the blood. The kidneys also filter, reabsorb, and secrete nonwaste products back into the system.

Filtration and the urine production process begin in the **nephron**, the functional unit of the kidney. Each kidney has approximately 1 million nephrons. Each nephron contains a tiny filtration unit called the **glomerulus**, which consists of a cluster of capillaries. As blood travels through the capillaries, a continuous exchange of substances occurs between the glomerulus and the nephron. The walls of the capillaries permit waste products, water, and electrolytes to pass through and collect in the kidney tubules. The end product, **urine**, is transported out of the nephron into the renal pelvis and enters the **ureter**, where it is carried to and stored in the **urinary bladder**.

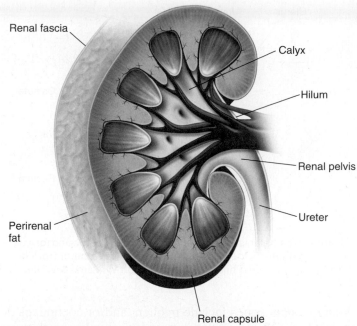

Renal fascia

Calyx

Hilum

Renal pelvis

Ureter

Perirenal fat

Renal capsule

FIGURE 13-2   Kidney. Sagittal view of the kidney and internal structures. (From *A Short Course in Medical Terminology, First Edition*, C. Edward Collins: p. 210, Figure 14-2.**)**

The bladder collects the urine until the volume reaches a certain level, which triggers the urge to **urinate** or **void** (expel the urine) called the **micturition** reflex (comes from Latin word *micturio*, which means "to urinate"). Urine is expelled through the **urethra**, a tube that measures approximately 1.5 inches long in the female and 8 inches long in the male. The female urethra carries only urine, whereas the male urethra conveys both urine and semen.

Urination or voiding is regulated by two **sphincters**, which are circular muscles that surround the urethra. They are the internal urethral sphincter, which is located at the entrance to the urethra and is involuntarily controlled, and the external urethral sphincter, which is located at the distal end of the urethra and is under conscious control.

Disorders and Treatment

Disorders of the urinary system can encompass any or all of the urinary structures. These conditions can range from an irritating leakage of urine when you sneeze to chronic renal failure. Some of the more common disorders are discussed in the following sections.

INCONTINENCE AND RETENTION

Incontinence, the loss of urinary control, has many causes, some of which are listed below:
- Spinal cord damage
- Brain damage
- Prostate surgery
- Pregnancy
- Aging

Stress incontinence is the inability to control urine under physical stress such as laughing, coughing, running, or sneezing.

Retention is the inability to empty the bladder. This may occur for a variety of reasons, such as the result of anesthesia or prostate enlargement. Sometimes with a spinal cord injury, retention occurs when the micturition reflex is blocked. There may be overflow incontinence as a result.

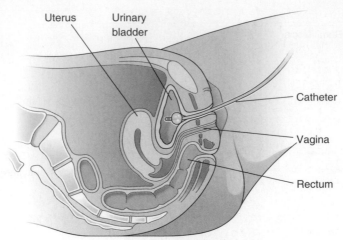

Uterus   Urinary bladder

Catheter

Vagina

Rectum

FIGURE 13-3 **Catheterization.** A catheter is inserted into the urinary meatus and forwarded into the bladder. The balloon on the tip of the catheter is then inflated to prevent the catheter from being dislodged. From Cohen BJ. Medical Terminology, 4th Ed. Philadelphia: Lippincott Williams & Wilkins, 2003.

Symptoms of urinary incontinence include frequent and/or continuous dribbling and loss of urine. Treatment may be as simple as wearing protective pads or may require the use of an indwelling **catheter**. An indwelling urinary catheter is a tube that is placed through the urethra into the urinary bladder. It drains the urine into a bag outside of the body (Fig. 13-3).

URINARY TRACT INFECTIONS

Urinary tract infections (UTIs) are extremely common. Bacteria that infect the urinary tract can ascend the urethra into the bladder. Left untreated, organisms can travel further into the urinary system. **Cystitis** (cyst/o means "bladder"; -itis means "inflammation") and **urethritis** (urethr/o means "urethra"; -itis means "inflammation") are infections of the lower urinary tract, generally referred to as bladder infections, whereas **pyelonephritis** (pyel/o means "pelvis"; nephr/o means "kidney"; -itis means "inflammation") and **nephritis** (nephr/o means "kidney"; -itis means "inflammation") are infections of the upper urinary tract, generally referred to as kidney infections. Women are more prone to bladder infections due to the shortness of the urethra, the proximity of the urethra to the anus, susceptibility to poor toilet habits, and frequent irritation through the use of tampons, bubble baths, and so on. Older males with prostate hypertrophy (enlargement) can retain urine. This may encourage bacterial growth and infection. Obstructions of the urinary tract can also promote retention of urine, leading to an infection.

Glomerulonephritis (glomerul/o means "glomerulus"; nephr/o means "kidney"; -itis means "inflammation") can involve one or both kidneys. This infection extends from the ureter into the renal pelvis of the kidney. It can result from infections from other body systems or can be a response from the body's immune system. Left untreated, it can cause **renal failure** in which the kidneys fail to produce urine.

Pain in the lower abdomen is a frequent symptom of a **UTI**, along with **dysuria** (dys- means "painful" or "difficult"; ur/o means "urine"; -ia creates the adjective form), frequency, and urgency. Systemic signs include fever, general malaise, and leukocytosis (abnormal white blood cell counts).

Treatment of UTIs includes taking a prescribed antibiotic along with increasing fluid intake. If the infection recurs, then assessment of a predisposing factor might be necessary.

RENAL FAILURE

The kidneys can suddenly fail for many different reasons. Exposure to toxins, shock, infections such as glomerulonephritis, and other renal disorders can damage the nephrons. Symptoms in-

Hemodialysis

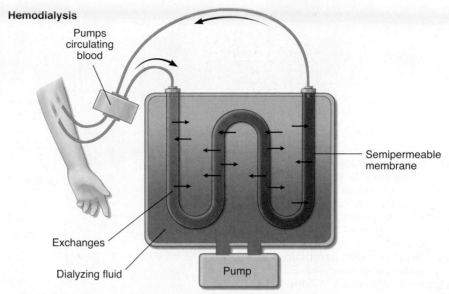

FIGURE 13-4   **Dialysis.** During hemodialysis, blood from an artery is pumped into a filter, which acts as the semipermeable membrane. The solution, which has the same chemical composition as the blood except for waste products, flows in and around the filter. The waste products in the blood diffuse through the semipermeable membrane into the solution. From Premkumar K. The Massage Connection Anatomy and Physiology. Baltimore: Lippincott Williams & Wilkins, 2004.

clude **oliguria** (olig/o means "scanty" or "few"; ur/o means "urine"; -ia creates the adjective form) progressing to **anuria** (an- means "none" or "without"; ur/o means "urine"; -ia creates the adjective form), with an increase in the patient's blood urea nitrogen (BUN) or a decrease in the glomerular filtration rate (GFR). **BUN** is a blood test that detects waste products in the blood, and **GFR** refers to the volume of water that is filtered through the glomerulus. The failure may be reversible if the primary problem is treated. In acute renal failure, **dialysis** (a method of artificial kidney function) and drug therapy with the use of **diuretics** (dia- means "through"; ur/o means "urine"; from the Greek *dia* meaning "through" and *ourein* meaning "urine") can help a patient through the acute stages while the nephrons recover. In chronic renal failure (CRF), there is permanent damage to the kidneys. Some symptoms of CRF include anuria, **azotemia** or **uremia** (ur/o means "urine"; -emia means "blood"; presence of urea or nitrogenous wastes in the blood), and electrolyte imbalances. CRF affects all body symptoms. **Hemodialysis** (hemo- means "blood"; *dialyo* comes from the Greek word meaning "to separate"), **perito-neal** (comes from the Greek word *peritonaion* meaning "to stretch over") **dialysis**, or a kidney transplant is necessary to sustain life in patients with CRF (Figs. 13-4, 13-5, and 13-6).

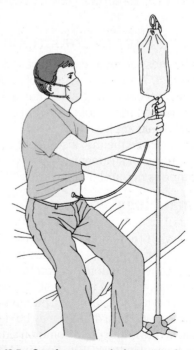

FIGURE 13-5   **Continuous ambulatory peritoneal dialysis (CAPD).** After applying a mask, a bag of solution is attached to the tube entering the patient's abdominal area so that the fluid flows into the peritoneal cavity. Modified from Nursing Procedures, 4th Ed. Ambler: Lippincott Williams & Wilkins, 2004.

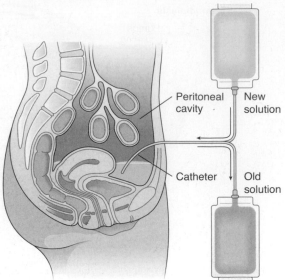

FIGURE 13-6 Peritoneal dialysis. In peritoneal dialysis, a semipermeable membrane richly supplied with blood vessels lines the peritoneal cavity. The new solution drains into the peritoneal cavity and remains for a period of time. The waste products diffuse from the network of blood vessels into the solution and are drained out. Reprinted with permission from Cohen BJ. Medical Terminology, 4th Ed. Philadelphia: Lippincott Williams & Wilkins, 2004.

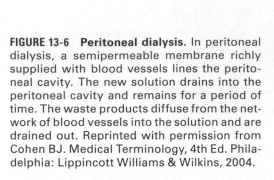

The roots nephr/o *and* ren/o *are both used to refer to the kidneys.* Nephr/o *is used in the names of most kidney disorders and treatments, but* ren/o *is an option in some. Applying standard suffixes yields* nephritis, nephralgia, nephrectomy, nephrorrhaphy, nephrotomy, nephromegaly *(or* renomegaly*), and* nephropathy *(or* renopathy*). In other uses, the term* nephrology *is more common than* renology, *but the adjective* renal *is far more common than its counterpart,* nephric.

URINARY TRACT OBSTRUCTIONS

Kidney stones, or renal calculi, are a common problem and can develop anywhere along the urinary tract. They can cause an obstruction in urinary flow, which can further lead to urinary stasis and infection. With renal calculi, the patient frequently experiences intense pain in the flank region or renal colic. Treatment consists of removing the stone(s) or obstruction. This can be done using less noninvasive techniques such as through a **cystoscope** (cyst/o means "bladder"; -scope means "instrument used to view"), a **ureteroscope** (ureter/o means "ureter"; -scope means "instrument used to view"), extracorporeal shock wave lithotripsy (ESWL), or percutaneous nephrolithotomy (Fig. 13-7).

Pharmacology

Drugs used in treating diseases of the urinary system include diuretics, antibiotics, antibacterials, and other drugs that influence the strength of contraction of the urinary bladder. Diuretics promote urine excretion and can be divided into categories according to their action. The physician orders the type of diuretic depending on the condition being treated. Congestive heart failure, hypertension, cirrhosis, pulmonary edema, and increased intracranial pressure are some conditions in which a diuretic may be ordered. Fluid and electrolyte imbalance, especially hypokalemia, is one of the more common side effects of taking a diuretic. Some examples of diuretics include Lasix, HydroDIURIL, Esidrix, Aldactazide, Dyazide, and mannitol.

Antibiotics or antibacterials are used to treat urinary tract infections. These can be bacteriostatic or bactericidal in action. Bacteriostatic medications inhibit the growth of bacteria, whereas bactericidal medications kill the bacteria (-cidal is a suffix meaning "to kill"). It is very important that patients take the full course of antibiotics to eradicate the infecting organisms. Patients

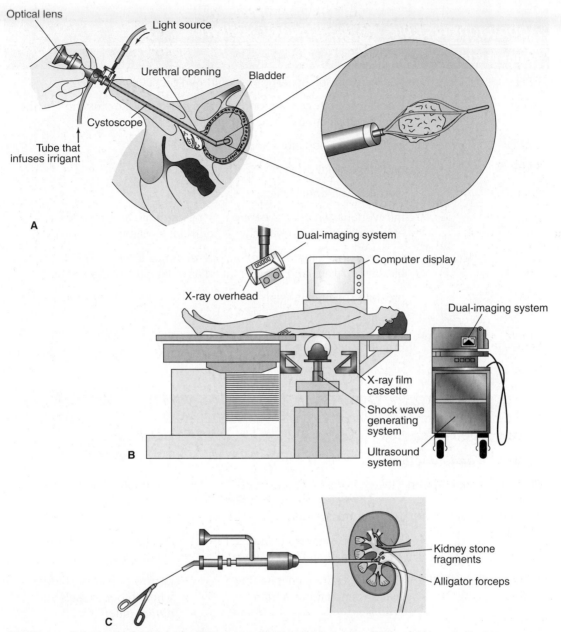

FIGURE 13-7   Renal calculi. There are different methods to treat renal calculi or stones. **A.** During a cystoscopy, the stone is visualized, captured, fragmented, and removed. **B.** Extracorporeal shock wave lithotripsy (ESWL) is used for most symptomatic nonpassable upper urinary tract stones. The shock waves fragment the stone. **C.** Percutaneous nephrolithotomy is used to treat larger stones. A percutaneous tract is formed, and a nephroscope is inserted through it. Then the stone is extracted or pulverized. From Smeltzer SC, Bare BG. Textbook of Medical-Surgical Nursing, 9th Ed. Philadelphia: Lippincott Williams & Wilkins, 2000.

should be encouraged to increase their fluid intake when they have a urinary tract infection. Some examples of urinary antibiotics include Septra, Bactrim, Macrodantin, and Furadantin.

Antispasmodics are used in patients who experience frequency and incontinence. These drugs help to reduce the strength and contraction of the bladder muscle. Some examples of antispasmodic agents include Vesicare, Detrol, and Ditropan.

Cholinergic drugs are used to treat postoperative or postpartum urinary retention. They increase the contraction of the urinary bladder. An example of a cholinergic drug is Urecholine.

Abbreviation Table • The Urinary System

ABBREVIATION	MEANING
BPH	benign prostatic hypertrophy; enlarged prostate
BUN	blood urea nitrogen; a blood test to measure kidney function by the level of nitrogenous waste and urea that is in the blood
CAPD	continuous ambulatory peritoneal dialysis
ESRD	end-stage renal disease
GFR	glomerular filtration rate
IVP	intravenous pyelogram; contrast is injected into a vein and is excreted by the kidney to show the urinary system
KUB	kidneys, ureter, and bladder; also a reference to an X-ray of the kidneys, ureters, and bladder taken as a flat plate of the abdomen
PSA	prostate-specific antigen
UA	urinalysis
UTI	urinary tract infection

Study Table • The Urinary System

TERM AND PRONUNCIATION	ANALYSIS	MEANING
Structure and Function		
electrolyte (ee-LEK-troh-lyte)	from the Greek words *electron* (electron); and *lytos* (soluble)	electricity-conducting compound in solution
glomerulus (gloh-MER-yu-luhs)	a Latin word meaning small ball, round knot	capillary network found inside each nephron
hilum (HY-luhm)	a Latin word meaning a small thing, a trifle	narrow part of the kidney where blood vessels and nerves enter
kidney (KID-nee)	originally *kidenere*, perhaps a compound of Old English *cwið* "womb" + *ey* "egg," in reference to the shape of the organ	organ that excretes urine
nephron (NEFF-ron)	from the Greek word *nephros* (kidney)	tiny structure within the kidney in which the urine-production process begins
perirenal fat (PERH-ih-REE-nahl)	*peri-* (around); *ren/o* (kidney) *-al* (adjective suffix)	fatty tissue surrounding the renal capsule

TERM AND PRONUNCIATION	ANALYSIS	MEANING
renal fascia (REE-nahlFASH-ee-ah)	*ren/o* (kidney); *-al* (adjective suffix) + *fascia*, a Latin word meaning band, sash	protective outer covering of the kidney
retroperitoneal (reh-troh-pehr-ih-toh-NEE-al)	*retro-* (backwards, behind); from the Greek word *peritonaion* (to stretch over)	space between the parietal peritoneum and the muscles and bones of the peritoneum
sphincters (SFINK-tehrs)	from the Greek word *sphincter* (band, anything that binds tight)	circular muscle that surrounds a tube such as the urethra and constricts the tube when it contracts
urea (yu-REE-ah)	from the French word *urée* (urine)	natural waste product of metabolism that is excreted in urine
ureters (yu-REE-tehrs; also YUR-eh-tehrs)	from the Greek word *oureter*, from *ourein* (to urinate)	two tubes that transfer urine from the kidneys to the urinary bladder
urethra (yu-REE-thrah)	from the Greek word *ourethra*, from *ourein* (to urinate)	tube that conducts urine away from the bladder for expulsion
uric acid (YUR-ik)	*ur/o* (urine); *-ic* (adjective suffix) + acid, common English Word	natural waste product of metabolism that is excreted in urine
urinary bladder (YUR-ihn-ayr-ee BLAD-dehr)	from the Greek word *ouron* (urine) + Anglo-Saxon, *blaedre* (bladder)	temporary storage receptacle for urine
urinate (YUR-ihn-ayt)	*urin/o* (urine) + *-ate* (verb suffix)	passing of urine
urine (YUR-ihn)	from the Greek word *ouron* (urine)	water and soluble substances excreted by the kidneys
void (voy-d)	from Old French *voide* (empty, hollow, waste)	to urinate

Common Disorders and Symptoms

albuminuria (al-byu-mihn-YUR-ee-ah)	from the vulgar Latin *albumen* (egg white) + *ur/o* (urine); *-ia* (condition)	presence of protein in urine
anuria (an-YUR-ee-ah)	*an-* (without); *ur/o* (urine); *-ia* (condition)	absence of urine formation
calculus (KAL-kyu-luhs); plural: calculi (KAL-kyu-lye)	a Latin word meaning stone	a kidney stone (in the context of this body system)

(continued)

TERM AND PRONUNCIATION	ANALYSIS	MEANING
cystalgia (sihs-TAL-jee-ah)	*cyst/o* (bladder); *-algia* (pain)	pain in a bladder, most often used to signify the urinary bladder
cystitis (sihs-TY-tihs)	*cyst/o* (bladder); *-itis* (inflammation)	inflammation of the bladder
cystocele (SIHS-toh-seel)	*cyst/o* (bladder); *-cele* (hernia)	hernia of the bladder
cystolith (SIS-toh-lith)	*cyst/o* (bladder); *-lith* (stone)	bladder stone
diuretic (dy-yu-REHT-ik)	from the Greek *dia-* (through) + *ourein* (urine)	drug that promotes the excretion of urine
dysuria (dihs-YUR-ee-ah)	*dys-* (difficult); *ur/o* (urine); *-ia* (condition)	difficult or painful urination
enuresis (ahn-your-REE-sis)	from Greek *enourein* (to urinate in)	bedwetting
glomerulonephritis (glom-MER-yu-lo-neh-FRY-tihs)	*glomerul/o* (glomerulus); *nephr/o* (kidney); *-itis* (inflammation)	renal disease characterized by inflammation of glomeruli (not the result of kidney infection)
glycosuria (gly-kohs-YUR-ee-ah)	*glycos-* (sugar); *ur/o* (urine); *-ia* (condition)	urinary excretion of carbohydrates
hematuria (he-mat-YUR-ee-ah)	*hemat/o* (blood); *ur/o* (urine); *-ia* (adjective suffix)	urinary excretion of blood
incontinence (in-KON-tih-nents)	from the Latin word *incontinentia* (inability to retain)	inability to control urine
nephralgia (neh-FRAL-jee-ah)	*nephr/o* (kidney); *-algia* (pain)	pain in the kidneys
nephritis (neh-FRY-tihs)	*nephr/o* (kidney); *-itis* (inflammation)	inflammation of the kidney
nephrolithiasis (NEFF-ro-lih-THY-ah-sihs)	*nephr/o* (kidney); *lith/o* (stone); *-iasis* (condition)	the presence of renal calculi
nephromegaly (neh-fro-MEG-ah-lee)	*nephr/o* (kidney); *-megaly* (enlargement)	enlargement of one or both kidneys; renomegaly
nephropathy (neh-FROP-ah-thee)	*nephr/o* (kidney); *-pathy* (disease)	any disease of the kidney
nephroptosis (neh-FROP-hot-sis)	*nephr/o* (kidney); *-ptosis* (falling downward, prolapse)	prolapse of the kidney
nocturia (noc-TUR-ee-ah)	*noct/o* (night); *ur/o* (urine); *-ia* (condition)	excessive urination at night
oliguria (oh-lih-GUR-ee-ah)	*olig/o* (few); *ur/o* (urine); *-ia* (condition)	diminished urine production

TERM AND PRONUNCIATION	ANALYSIS	MEANING
polyuria (pol-ee-YUR-ee-ah)	*poly-* (much, many); *ur/o* (urine); *-ia* (condition)	excessive urine production
pyelonephritis (PY-loh-NEH-FRY-tihs)	*pyel/o* (pelvis); *nephr/o* (kidney); *-itis* (inflammation)	inflammation of the renal or kidney pelvis due to local bacteria infection
pyuria (pu-YOUR-ee-ah)	*py/o* (pus); *ur/o* (urine); *-ia* (condition)	pus in the urine
renal calculus (REE-nahl KAL-ku-luhs)	*ren/o* (kidney); *calculus*, a Latin word meaning stone	a kidney stone
renal failure (REE-nahl)	*ren/o* (kidney); *-al* (adjective suffix) + failure, common English word	impairment of renal function, either acute or chronic, with retention of urea, creatinine, and other waste products
renal hypoplasia (REE-nahl HY-poh-PLAYZ-ee-ah)	*ren/o* (kidney); *hypo-* (below normal); *-plasia* (formation, development)	an underdeveloped kidney
retention (ree-TEN-shun)	from the Latin word *retentionem* (a retaining, a holding back)	the inability to empty the bladder
uremia (yu-REE-mee-ah) or azotemia (ays-oh-TEAM-ee-ah)	*ur/o* (urine); *-emia* (blood condition)	an excess of urea in the blood
ureteritis (yu-ree-teh-RY-tihs)	*ureter/o* (ureter); *-itis* (inflammation)	inflammation of a ureter
urethralgia (yu-ree-THRAL-jee-ah)	*urethr/o* (urethra); *-algia* (pain)	pain in the urethra (sometimes also called *urethrodynia*)
urethritis (yu-ree-THRY-tihs)	*urethr/o* (urethra); *-itis* (inflammation)	inflammation of the urethra
urethrostenosis (yu-REE-throh-steh-NO-sihs)	*urethr/o* (urethra); *sten/o* (narrow); *-sis* (condition)	narrowing of the urethra
urinary tract infection (yur-ihn-ARY)	*urin/o* (urine); *-ary* (adjective suffix); + tract + infection	microbial infection of any part of the urinary tract

Practice and Practitioners

nephrologist (neh-FROL-oh-jist)	*nephr/o* (kidney); *-logist* (one who studies a special field)	a medical specialist who diagnoses and treats disorders of the kidney
nephrology (neh-FROL-oh-jee)	*nephr/o* (kidney); *-logy* (study of)	medical specialty dealing with the kidneys
urologist (yu-ROL-oh-jist)	*ur/o* (urine); *-logist* (one who studies a special field)	a medical specialist who diagnoses and treats disorders of the urinary system

(continued)

TERM AND PRONUNCIATION	ANALYSIS	MEANING
urology (yu-ROL-oh-jee)	*ur/o* (urine); *-logy* (study of)	the medical specialty dealing with the urinary system

Diagnosis, Treatment, and Procedures

catheter (CATH-eh-tehr)	from the Greek word *kathienai* (to let down, thrust in)	a flexible tube that enables passage of fluid from or into a body cavity
cystectomy (sihs-TEK-toh-mee)	*cyst/o* (bladder); *-ectomy* (excision)	excision of the urinary bladder
cystopexy (SIHS-toh-pek-see)	*cyst/o* (bladder); *-pexy* (fixation)	surgical fixation of the urinary bladder
cystoscopy (sihs-TOS-ko-pee)	*cyst/o* (bladder); *-scopy* (use of an instrument for viewing)	visual inspection of the bladder by means of an instrument called a cystoscope
dialysis (dy-AL-ih-sihs)	a Greek word meaning dissolution, separation	filtration to remove colloidal particles from a fluid; a method of artificial kidney function
diuretic (dy-yu-REHT-ik)	from the Greek *dia-* (through) + *ourein* (urine)	a drug that promotes the excretion of urine
hemodialysis (HEE-mo-dy-AL-ih-sihs)	*hemo-* (blood) + *dialysis*, a Greek word meaning dissolution, separation	removal of unwanted substances from the blood by passage through a semipermeable membrane
lithotripsy (LITH-oh-trip-see)	*lith/o* (stone); *-tripsy* (crushing)	treatment in which a stone in the kidney, urethra, or bladder is broken up into small particles
nephrectomy (neh-FREK-toh-mee)	*nephr/o* (kidney); *-ectomy* (removal)	removal of a kidney
nephrolithotomy (NEH-froh-lih-THOT-oh-mee)	*nephr/o* (kidney); *lith/o* (stone); *-tomy* (incision into)	incision into the kidney to remove a calculus (kidney stone)
ureteroplasty (yu-REE-tehr-oh-plass-tee)	*ureter/o* (ureter); *-plasty* (surgical repair)	surgical repair of a ureter
ureterorrhaphy (yu-REE-tehr-OR-rah-fee)	*ureter/o* (ureter); *-rrhaphy* (surgical suturing)	suture of a ureter
ureteroscope (yu-REE-tehr-oh-skohp)	*ureter/o* (ureter); *-scope* (instrument for viewing)	instrument used to visually examine the ureter
urinalysis (yur-ih-NAL-ih-sihs)	*urin/o* (urine); *-alysis* from the English word analysis	analysis of urine

EXERCISES

EXERCISE 13-1   Figure Labeling: The Urinary System

Left kidney	Right kidney	Urethra
Left ureter	Right ureter	Urinary bladder

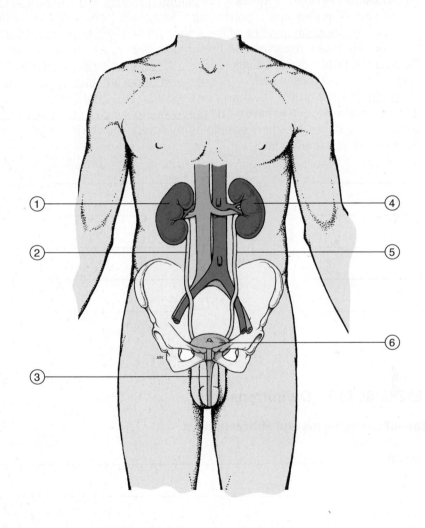

1. _____   4. _____

2. _____   5. _____

3. _____   6. _____

EXERCISE 13-2   Case Study

CASE STUDY

Read the following case study. There are 11 phrases that can be reworded with a medical term that was introduced in this chapter. Determine what the term is and write your answers in the space provided.

Heather is a 40-year-old female who saw (1) <u>a specialist who treats disorders of the urinary system</u> for complaints of urinary frequency, (2) <u>painful urination</u>, (3) <u>blood in her urine</u>, and low abdominal pain. She also was experiencing a low-grade fever and general fatigue. The doctor ordered a (4) <u>laboratory reading of her urine</u> and an (5) <u>X-ray of her kidneys, ureters, and bladder</u>. The laboratory results showed red blood cells in the urine, and the urine was cloudy with an odor. Tests indicated multiple (6) <u>small round calcified objects</u> in the (7) <u>urine reservoir</u>. Heather was diagnosed with a (8) <u>condition of having bacteria in the urinary tract</u> and also (9) <u>stones</u> in her bladder. The doctor ordered a(n) (10) <u>drug used to kill bacteria</u>, and he told Heather that she needed to have a (11) <u>procedure in which a scope is inserted into the bladder</u> to remove the stones. Heather's symptoms improved, and she returned to have the procedure. Her recovery was uneventful.

1. _____   7. _____

2. _____   8. _____

3. _____   9. _____

4. _____   10. _____

5. _____   11. _____

6. _____

EXERCISE 13-3   Definitions

Define the following terms and abbreviations:

1. nephrotomy   _____

2. nephrolithiasis   _____

3. dialysis   _____

4. CAPD   _____

5. pyuria   _____

6. ureteroplasty　_____

7. UTI　_____

8. ureterorrhaphy　_____

9. periurethral　_____

10. nephromegaly　_____

EXERCISE 13-4　Matching Terms with Definitions

Match the terms in Column 1 with the correct definitions in Column 2.

TERM

1. _____ nephron

2. _____ urethra

3. _____ renal calculus

4. _____ glomerulus

5. _____ micturition

6. _____ uric acid

7. _____ ureters

8. _____ hilum

9. _____ electrolyte

10. _____ UA

11. _____ nephralgia

12. _____ nephritis

DEFINITION

A. capillary network found inside each nephron

B. urination

C. pain in the bladder

D. tube that conducts urine away from the bladder for excretion

E. electricity-producing compound in solution

F. narrow part of the kidney where blood vessels and nerves enter

G. functional unit of the kidney

H. two tubes that transfer urine from the kidneys to the urinary bladder

I. X-ray of the ureter

J. natural waste product of metabolism excreted in the urine

K. a kidney stone

L. excision of a kidney, ureter, and at least part of the urinary bladder

13. _____ urethrostenosis

14. _____ nephrolithotomy

15. _____ nephroureterocystectomy

16. _____ ureterography

17. _____ cystalgia

18. _____ nephropathy

M. inflammation of the kidney

N. narrowing of the urethra

O. any disease of the kidney

P. pain in the kidneys

Q. incision into the kidney to remove a calculus (kidney stone)

R. urinalysis

EXERCISE 13-5   Word Building

Use the combining form *nephr/o* to build the following terms:

1. inflammation of the kidney   _____

2. inflammation of the kidney and the renal pelvis   _____

3. condition of having stones in the kidney   _____

4. incision into the kidney   _____

Use the root *ur* or *urin* to build the following terms:

5. a urinary stone   _____

6. urinary waste products in the blood   _____

7. examination of a urine sample   _____

8. excessive urination   _____

9. blood in the urine   _____

10. no urine production from the kidney   _____

EXERCISE 13-6   True or False

Put an X in the True or False column next to each statement. If False, write the correct answer in the Correction column for any statements you identify as false.

STATEMENT	TRUE	FALSE	CORRECTION, IF FALSE
1. Diuretics are medications that promote urination.	_____	_____	_____
2. Renal fascia is the fatty tissue surrounding the renal capsule.	_____	_____	_____
3. The two tubes that transfer urine from the kidneys to the urinary bladder are the urethritis.	_____	_____	_____
4. A natural waste product of metabolism that is excreted in urine is called urea.	_____	_____	_____
5. The urinary bladder serves as a temporary storage receptacle for urine.	_____	_____	_____
6. Narrowing of the urethra is referred to as urethrostenosis.	_____	_____	_____
7. The word element *-logist* in urologist means "study."	_____	_____	_____
8. An incision into the kidney to remove a kidney stone is called a nephrectomy.	_____	_____	_____
9. An incision into the ureter is called a ureteroplasty.	_____	_____	_____
10. Inflammation of the bladder is called cystodynia.	_____	_____	_____

EXERCISE 13-7   Crossword Puzzle: Urinary System

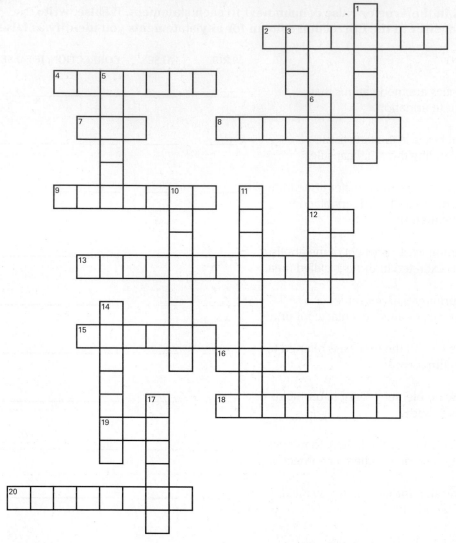

ACROSS

2. artificial kidney function
4. functional unit of the kidney
7. abbreviation for blood, urea, nitrogen
8. drug that promotes urination
9. urine reservoir
12. abbreviation for urinalysis
13. drooping kidney
15. urea in the blood
16. urinate
18. inflammation of the bladder
19. root for kidney
20. urinating at night

DOWN

1. painful urination
3. intravenous pyelogram
5. pus in the urine
6. blood in the urine
10. bedwetting
11. removal of the bladder
14. tube from the kidney to bladder
17. no urine production

CHAPTER 13 QUIZ

Using the knowledge gained from previous chapters and the terms introduced in this chapter and in the study table, place the proper term in the sentences below.

cystoscopy   dysuria   IVP   nephrolithiasis nephropexy
nephropyelitis   pyelolithotomy renal transplant ureterectomy

1. Tom suffered from chronic renal failure. His sister donated one of her normal kidneys to him and he had a(n) _____.

2. Cindy had a floating kidney that required surgical fixation. Her urologist performed a surgical procedure known as a (n) _____.

3. The surgeons operated on Robert to remove a calculus from his renal pelvis. The name of this surgery is _____.

4. Judy had to have one of her ureters removed due to a stricture. This procedure is called _____.

5. The physician had to examine Joshua's bladder for blood. They used a special instrument. This procedure is called a(n) _____.

Define the following terms

6. antibiotic _____

7. antispasmodic _____

8. BUN _____

9. enuresis _____

10. renal hyperplasia _____

Multiple Choice

11. The _____ carry the urine from the kidney pelvis down to the urinary bladder.
    a. urethra   c. cortex
    b. meatus   d. ureters

12. Which of the following is a *noninflammatory* condition of the kidney?
    a. pyuria   c. nephritis
    b. nephrosis   d. uremia

13. The inability to hold urine is called:
    a. polyuria   c. hematuria
    b. incontinence   d. enuresis

14. The abbreviation for an X-ray of the urinary system where a contrast material is injected intravenously is:
    a. BUN
    b. IVP
    c. KUB
    d. GFR

15. Excretion of urine from the bladder is properly termed as:
    a. voiding
    b. micturition
    c. urination
    d. all of the above

16. The functioning unit of the kidney is the:
    a. nephron
    b. cortex of the kidney
    c. glomeruli
    d. pelvis of the kidney

17. A pharmacologic agent that encourages urine excretion is classified as a(n):
    a. cholinergic
    b. antibiotic
    c. diuretic
    d. antispasmodic

18. What are glomeruli?
    a. complete functioning units of the kidney
    b. cavities in the kidney that collect urine from many ducts
    c. long, twisted structures where reabsorption occurs
    d. clusters of capillaries

19. What does anuria mean?
    a. no urine in the bladder
    b. no urine from the kidney
    c. painful urination
    d. pus in the urine

20. What term means destruction of kidney tissue?
    a. nephrolithiasis
    b. neurolysis
    c. nephrolysis
    d. resection

CHAPTER 14

The Reproductive System

LEARNING OBJECTIVES

Upon completion of this chapter, you should be able to:

- List the major organs of the male and female reproductive systems and describe their functions.
- Identify and use the word elements of the male and female reproductive systems.
- Briefly describe symptoms and treatments in response to disorders of the reproductive system.
- Describe the major drug classifications used to treat reproductive system disorders.
- Identify and interpret selected abbreviations relating to the reproductive system.
- Label diagrams of the male and female reproductive systems.
- Analyze and define the new terms introduced in this chapter.

Word Elements • The Reproductive System

ROOT	MEANING
amni/o	amnion; innermost of the extraembryonic membranes enveloping the embryo in utero and containing the amniotic fluid
balan/o	glans penis
cervic/o	cervix
circum/o	around
colp/o; vagin/o	vagina
gonad/o	gonads; sex glands
gynec/o	woman; female
lact/o	milk
mast/o; mamm/o	breast
men/o	menses; menstruation
nat/o	birth
oophor/o; oo	ovary; egg
orch/o; orchi/o; orchid/o; test/o	testes
ovari/o	ovary
prostat/o	prostate gland
salping/o	tube; fallopian tube
spermat/o; sperm/o	sperm
uter/o; hyster/o; metr/o	uterus
vas/o	vessel; vas deferens
vulv/o	vulva

An Overview of the Reproductive System

The primary function of the reproductive system is to perpetuate life. The reproductive process begins with **fertilization**, which occurs when a male **gamete** (also called a **sperm** or **spermatozoon**; plural: **spermatozoa**) fertilizes a female gamete (also called an **ovum**; plural: **ova**). The collective name for any female or male organ that produces a gamete is **gonad**.

The single cell formed at fertilization is called a **zygote**, which contains more than a trillion molecules, despite its diameter measuring only 0.1 mm. These trillions of molecules all communicate and work together in the **gestation** process. The period of gestation is the time lapse between the formation of the zygote and birth.

Obstetricians (from *obstetrix*, the Latin word for midwife) are the specialists who provide medical care to pregnant women and deliver babies. **Gynecologists** (gyn/o, gynec/o means "woman") diagnose and treat disorders of the female reproductive system, and **urologists** diagnose and treat disorders of the urinary and male reproductive systems. Two additional specialists are the **neonatologist**, who specializes in newborns (neo- means "new"; nat/o means "born"), and the **pediatrician**, who specializes in children (ped/o means "child").

Structure and Function

The reproductive systems in both the male and female may be divided into two groups: the organs of reproduction and the external genitalia. Both reproductive systems have similarities in that they produce special cells to replicate the species, yet they differ in their physical structure and function.

THE MALE REPRODUCTIVE SYSTEM

The male reproductive system is a combination of reproduction and urinary systems. It consists of the **testes** (singular: **testis**), various ducts, the urethra, and the following accessory glands: **seminal vesicles**, **prostate**, and the **bulbourethral** (bulb/o means "bulb-like"; urethr/o means "urethra"; -al is an adjective form) **glands**. The supporting structure and accessory organs are the **scrotum** and **penis**, which are considered the external organs of reproduction (Fig. 14-1).

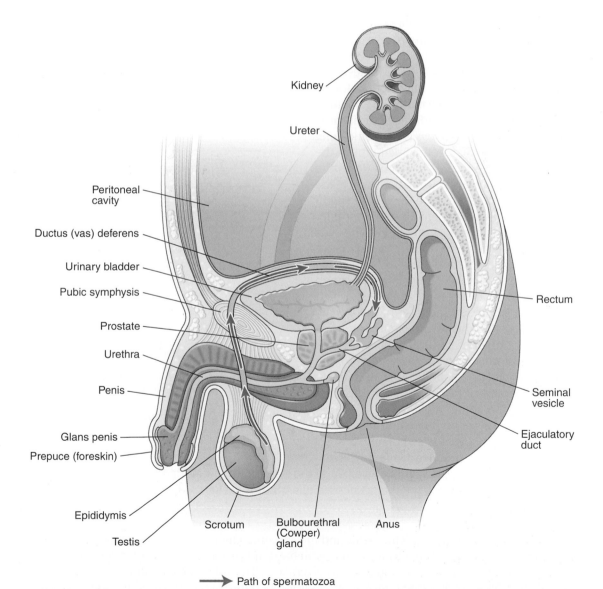

Kidney

Ureter

Peritoneal cavity

Ductus (vas) deferens

Urinary bladder

Pubic symphysis

Prostate

Urethra

Penis

Glans penis

Prepuce (foreskin)

Epididymis

Scrotum

Testis

Bulbourethral (Cowper) gland

Anus

Rectum

Seminal vesicle

Ejaculatory duct

⟶ Path of spermatozoa

FIGURE 14-1   Male reproductive system. A sagittal view of the male reproductive system. The blue arrows illustrate the pathway of sperm. Parts of the urinary and digestive systems are also shown. From Cohen BJ. Medical Terminology: An Illustrated Guide, 5th Ed. Philadelphia: Lippincott Williams & Wilkins, 2007.

The primary function of the male reproductive system is to produce sperm. The process, called **spermatogenesis** (spermat/o means "sperm"; genesis means "origin" or "beginning process"), involves cell division known as **meiosis**. Meiosis is a process that halves the number of chromosomes in a cell from 46 to 23.

Organs of Reproduction

As indicated earlier, the organs of reproduction in the male reproductive system include the testes, various ducts, and the urethra, along with their supporting structures. Spermatogenesis begins in the **testes** and is initiated by the secretion of **androgens** (andr/o means "masculine"; androgen means "male hormone"). The most significant of these hormones is **testosterone**. After spermatogenesis is complete, the **spermatozoa** (singular: **spermatozoon**) travel to the **epididymis** (epi- means "upon"; *didymis* is Greek meaning "twin" and "testes"), a coil-shaped tube at the upper part of the testicle that runs down the side and turns upward into the body where the sperm are stored to mature. Once the sperm mature, they leave the epididymis and enter the **ductus deferens**, also called the **vas deferens** (vas means "vessel"; deferen means "to carry away"), which leads to the ejaculatory duct in the prostate. From here, the sperm travel through the seminal vesicles, which are glands located at the base of the urinary bladder that join the vas deferens. The seminal vesicle produces a fluid that nourishes the sperm and forms much of the volume of the semen; the prostate gland located just below the urinary bladder secretes a thick alkaline fluid that assists sperm motility.

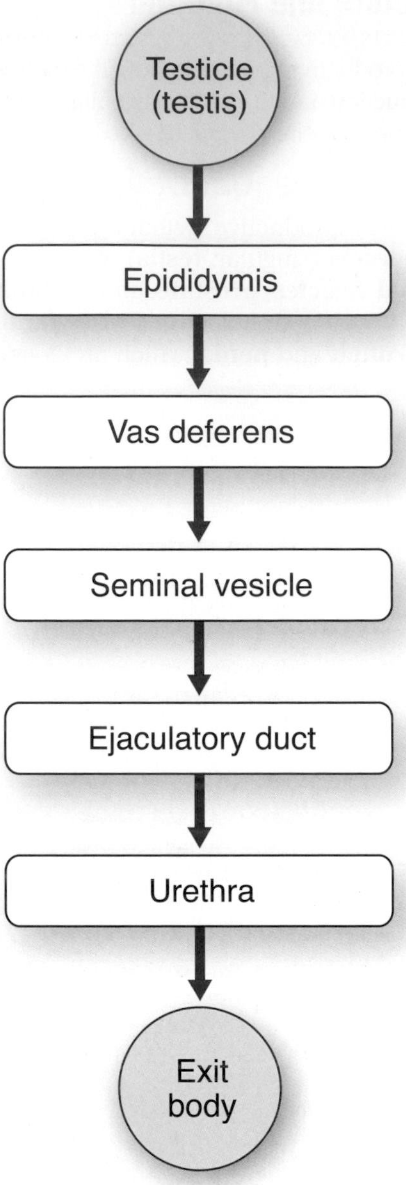

The Cowper's or bulbourethral glands are small pea-sized glands located on either side of the urethra. They produce a mucus-type secretion that joins the semen to become part of the ejaculated fluid during sexual intercourse. See the pathway of sperm from spermatogenesis to **ejaculation** in Figure 14-2.

FIGURE 14-2   Pathway of sperm.

External Genitalia

The external genitalia include the penis and the scrotum. Once the sperm is propelled through the reproductive ducts, it enters the urethra, which extends from the urinary bladder to the external opening on the end of the penis, and is ejaculated. The role of the scrotum is to house and protect the testes. The testes require a lower body temperature in order to produce sperm and are located outside of the body, suspended in the scrotal sac.

THE FEMALE REPRODUCTIVE SYSTEM

Similar to the male reproductive system, the female reproductive system has both internal and external organs. The internal organs of reproduction are the **uterus**, two **ovaries**, two **fallopian tubes**, **vagina**, and the **hymen** (Fig. 14-3). The external genitalia are collectively called the **vulva** and consist of the **labia majora**, **labia minora**, **clitoris**, **vaginal opening**, and **urinary meatus**. (Fig. 14-4). The **Bartholin's glands**, two small organs located on either side of the vagina, open into the area between the labia minora.

Organs of Reproduction

The **uterus** is a pear-shaped organ that has an upper rounded portion called the **fundus** and a lower narrow portion referred to as the **cervix**, which extends into the vagina. The uterus is composed of three layers of tissues: the **perimetrium** (peri- means "surrounding"; metr/o means "uterus"; -um is a singular noun ending), which is the outer surrounding layer; **myometrium** (my/o means "muscle"; metr/o means "uterus"; -um is a singular noun ending), which is the middle muscular layer; and the **endometrium** (endo- means within; metr/o means "uterus"; um is a singular noun ending), which is the inner layer that has a rich blood supply. The endometrium reacts to hormonal changes every month that result in **menstruation** (*mensis* is Latin for "month"), a shedding of the endometrial lining.

Two **ovaries** (singular: **ovary**) lie on either side of the uterus in the pelvic cavity. At birth, the ovaries of the female contain the immature **ova** (ova is plural for **ovum**, or egg). The maturation of the ova takes place in these almond-shaped organs, along with the production of hormones.

The **fallopian tubes**, or uterine tubes, extend out from the upper portion of the uterus. They end with finger-like projections, fimbriae (fimbria is singular), near the ovaries, and their primary

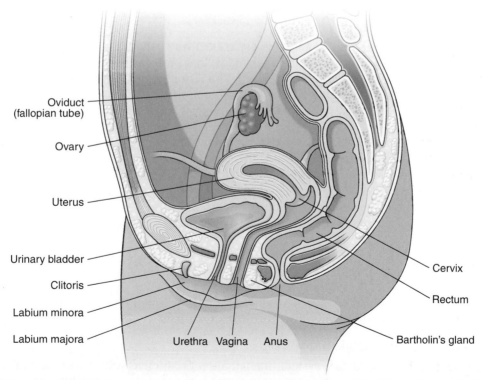

FIGURE 14-3 The female reproductive system and adjacent structures, sagittal view. The internal organs of reproduction are the uterus, two ovaries, two fallopian tubes, vagina, and hymen. From Cohen BJ. Medical Terminology: An Illustrated Guide, 5th Ed. Philadelphia: Lippincott Williams & Wilkins, 2007.

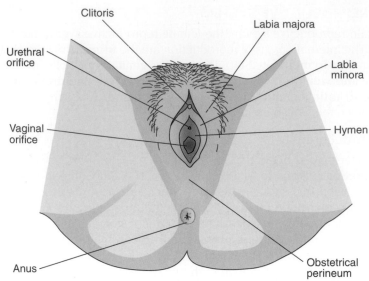

FIGURE 14-4 **The external genitalia of the female reproductive system.** Collectively, the parts of the female external genitalia are termed the "vulva" and consist of the labia majora, labia minora, clitoris, vaginal opening, urinary meatus, and Bartholin's glands. Modified from Cohen BJ. Medical Terminology: An Illustrated Guide, 5th Ed. Philadelphia: Lippincott Williams & Wilkins, 2007.

function is to catch the ovum as it leaves the ovary and propel it toward the uterus for implantation. Fertilization occurs in the fallopian tube.

External Genitalia

As mentioned earlier, the external genitalia are collectively called the **vulva** (Fig. 14-4). The **labia majora** and **labia minora** are the vaginal lips that protect the vaginal opening and the urinary meatus (labi/o and cheil/o mean "lips"). The **clitoris** is an organ of sensitive, erectile tissue located in front of the vaginal opening. The **Bartholin's glands** are two small rounded glands on either side of the vaginal opening. They produce a mucus secretion to lubricate the vagina.

The **vagina** is a muscular tube that extends from the **cervix** to the outside of the body. The vagina has the following functions:
- Allows for the passage of the monthly **menstrual** flow of blood and tissue.
- Receptacle for semen during sexual intercourse.
- Serves as the birth canal during a normal vaginal birth.

The **hymen** is a membranous fold of tissue that partially or completely covers the vaginal opening.

The **mammary** (mamm/o means "breast") **glands**, or breasts, are an important part of the female reproductive system since they nourish the newborn. These are milk-producing glands that develop during puberty. **Lactation** (lact/o means "milk"), the production of milk, causes the breasts to become enlarged and is relieved by a nursing infant. The **areola** is the dark-pigmented area that surrounds the nipple.

Menstrual Cycle and Fertilization

Similar to the male reproductive system, the female reproductive system also provides gametes for fertilization but goes a step further in that it also provides a nourishing environment suitable for a fertilized egg and the development of the zygote. This process of preparation is the **menstrual cycle**, a recurrent periodic change in the ovaries and uterus that occurs

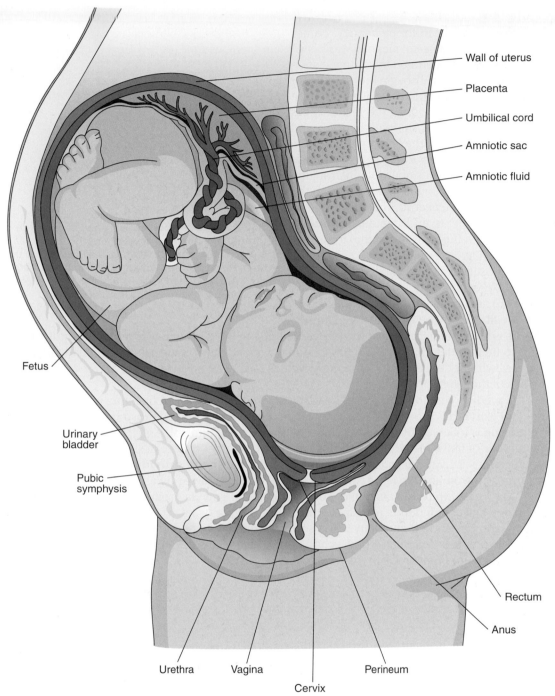

FIGURE 14-5   A pregnant uterus with intact fetus. From Cohen BJ. Medical Terminology: An Illustrated Guide, 5th Ed. Philadelphia: Lippincott Williams & Wilkins, 2007.

approximately every 28 days. Hormonal activity controls the menstrual cycle, which has three phases: **secretory** (secretion of hormones), **proliferative** (preparation of the endometrial lining for implantation if fertilization occurs), and **menses** (the end of one cycle and the beginning of another). If male spermatozoa are present during **ovulation**, the possibility of fertilization exists.

Pregnancy

Gestation, a synonym for pregnancy, comes from the Latin verb *gesto*, meaning "to bear." When the egg is penetrated by the male spermatozoon, it travels through the oviduct or fallopian tube and implants into the uterus; it is called an **embryo** during the first 8 weeks of gestation. Between the eighth week and birth, which under normal circumstances occurs between weeks 38 to 40, the term **fetus** is used. The fetus receives nourishment from the **placenta**, a spongy organ that attaches to the fetus by the umbilical cord. The **amniotic sac** surrounds the fetus and contains **amniotic fluid**, in which the fetus floats until it is ready to be born (Fig. 14-5).

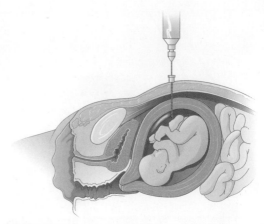

FIGURE 14-6 Amniocentesis. A needle is inserted through the abdominal wall, into the uterus, and a sample of amniotic fluid is removed from the amniotic sac. From Cohen BJ. Medical Terminology: An Illustrated Guide, 5th Ed. Philadelphia: Lippincott Williams & Wilkins, 2007.

Diagnostic tests and procedures associated with pregnancy include **amniocentesis** (Fig. 14-6), which involves the extraction of amniotic fluid from the **amniotic sac**. Amniocentesis is most commonly used to discover or rule out the presence of a genetic disorder, but it can also help in determining fetal lung maturity, which bears on the safety of an early delivery, indicates whether the mother's immune system is having an adverse effect, and reveals the age and sex of the fetus.

The medical term used in reference to a woman pregnant for the first time is **primigravida**. The term **gravida** is used in discussing a woman pregnant for the second and subsequent times, and gravida is followed by a number (most often a Roman numeral, e.g., I, II, etc.) that indicates the number of times the woman has been pregnant. Another way of designating the number of the pregnancy is by using Latin prefixes: **primigravida**, **secundigravida**, and so on. The medical term for a woman who has delivered a baby is **para**, followed by a number. Thus, a woman who has given birth to her first child would be called a gravida I, para I. A woman whose first pregnancy has concluded in a multiple birth, for example twins, would be gravida I, para II. A woman who has carried and delivered a second child would be known as a gravida II, para II. Another example is a woman who has had three pregnancies with only one carried to viability; this woman would be gravida III, para I.

Gravida comes from the Latin adjective gravis, *which medical dictionaries list as meaning "heavy." However, other meanings of* gravis *include "profound" and "important." Para comes from the Latin verb* pario, *which means "to bring forth, produce, or create."*

Disorders and Treatments

Disorders of the male and female reproductive systems sometimes vary. Disorders common to both the male and female reproductive systems are briefly described under the following headings: sexually transmitted diseases, other infections, structural abnormalities, and tumors. Additional conditions are included at the end of this section.

SEXUALLY TRANSMITTED DISEASES

Sexually transmitted diseases (STDs) occur through sexual intercourse or sexual contact. They include the following. **Human immunodeficiency virus (HIV)** attacks the immune system. It is transmitted through blood and infected body fluids during sexual intercourse with an infected partner. **Gonorrhea**, caused by bacteria, is highly contagious and is also transmitted through sexual contact. Signs and symptoms include painful urination and an abnormal discharge. This disease may also be transmitted to a child during birth. Silver nitrate eye drops or erythromycin ointment is given to all newborns immediately after birth to prevent gonorrhea as a preventive measure. **Chlamydia** is also an infection that is spread through sexual contact. Frequently, there are no noticeable symptoms at the onset, and if left untreated, the infection may spread to the reproductive organs in women. Antibiotics for the infected partner(s) are usually the recommended treatment. Repeated infections or spread of the infection in women can cause **pelvic inflammatory disease (PID)**. This is an infection of the uterus, ovaries, and fallopian tubes. The long-term effects of PID can cause scarring of the fallopian tubes (oviducts), which can block the tubes and prevent fertilization or pregnancy. If a woman has PID and an egg becomes fertilized, the egg may implant outside the uterus, which is known as an **ectopic** pregnancy (*ektopos* is Greek for "out of place"). An ectopic pregnancy can be life-threatening. **Syphilis** is another highly contagious disease and is also caused by bacteria. It is spread by sexual contact. Treatment consists of a course of antibiotics for the infected partners.

Lastly, infections are seen with the human papillomavirus (papilla is a small nipple-like process; -oma means "tumor"), also known as **HPV**. This is a contagious sexually transmitted virus that is spread through contact with infected genital skin, body fluids, and oral sex. There are many types of HPV. The virus may clear up on its own, but if it persists, it can lead to cervical cancer and genital warts. A vaccine is available that offers protection to a few of the types of HPV and may prevent cancers of the vagina and vulva.

OTHER INFECTIONS

Infections of the female reproductive system may result from exposure to bacteria, fungi, or viruses. Many of the conditions are marked by inflammation, the terms for which are indicated by the suffix -itis, which you learned in early chapters. They include the following: **mastitis** (mast/o means "breast"), **oophoritis** (oophor/o means "ovary") and **salpingitis** (salping/o means "fallopian tube"). Salpingitis is a condition that can lead to a closing off of the fallopian tubes and can result in infertility.

Male reproductive system infections include **epididymitis** (epi- means "upon"; *didymos* comes from Greek meaning "twin"), inflammation of the epididymis; and **prostatitis** (prostat/o means "prostate"; -itis means "inflammation"), inflammation of the prostate. **Balanitis** (balan/o means "glans penis") is inflammation of the head of the penis and usually occurs in uncircumcised male infants. Symptoms include redness and swelling and a foul-smelling discharge. Treatment usually consists of antibiotic therapy.

STRUCTURAL ABNORMALITIES

Structural abnormalities are found in both the male and female reproductive system. The differences will be presented first with the male reproductive system and then the female reproductive system.

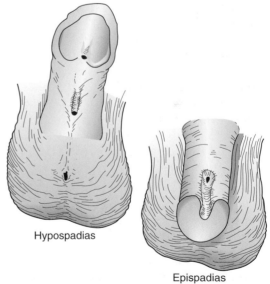

Hypospadias

Epispadias

FIGURE 14-7   Abnormal penile openings. Hypospadias is the term used when the urethral opening is located on the underside of the penis. Epispadias is the term for when the urethral opening is located on the topside of the penis. From Porth CM. Pathophysiology Concepts of Altered Health States, 7th Ed. Philadelphia: Lippincott Williams & Wilkins, 2005.

A birth defect in males where the urethral opening develops abnormally on the underside of the penis is called **hypospadias** (hypo- means "below" or "under"; spao is Greek for "tear"); when the opening develops abnormally on the topside of the penis, it is called **epispadias** (epi- means "on top" or "over") (Fig. 14-7). Surgical repair is usually performed in the first year of life to correct the placement of the abnormal opening.

One other structural condition of the male reproductive system involves the testes or male gonads. The testes develop in the abdominal cavity, and shortly before birth, they normally descend through a canal into the scrotum. When they do not descend or they remain "hidden" in the abdominal cavity, it is called **cryptorchidism** (crypt- means "hidden"; orchidism means "a condition of the testes").

In the female, the uterus may be out of position or actually may have a bend in the body of the organ. The following terms describe the variant conditions: **anteversion** (Fig. 14-8A) is an abnormal tipping forward of the entire uterus (ante- means "forward"; -version means "to turn"); **anteflexion** (Fig. 14-8B) is an exaggerated forward bend of the uterus; **retroversion** (Fig. 14-8C) is an abnormal tipping of the entire uterus backward (retro- means "backward"); and **retroflexion** (Fig. 14-8D) is an abnormal tipping with the body of the uterus bent back on itself. A **prolapsed uterus** involves the descent of the uterus or cervix into the vagina canal. Two other conditions involving structural abnormalities of the female reproductive system are a **cystocele** (cyst/o means "bladder"; -cele is a herniation or protrusion), which is a protrusion of the bladder into the anterior wall of the vagina (Fig. 14-9A), and a **rectocele**

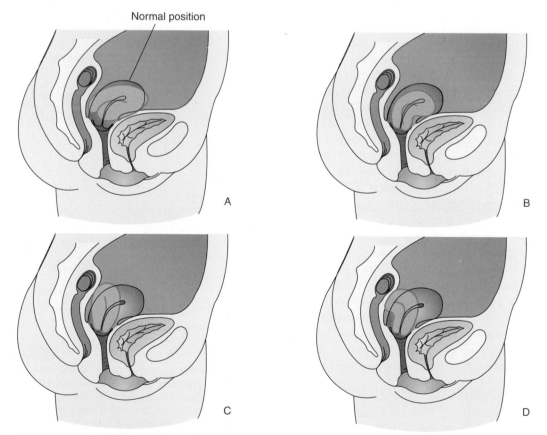

FIGURE 14-8   Uterine flexion and version. The blue-shaded figure represents the abnormal positioning of the uterus. **A.** Anteversion. **B.** Anteflexion. **C.** Retroversion. **D.** Retroflexion. From Pillitteri A. Maternal and Child Nursing, 4th Ed. Philadelphia: Lippincott Williams & Wilkins, 2003.

(rect/o means "rectum"), which is a protrusion of the rectum into the posterior wall of the vagina (Fig. 14-9B).

TUMORS

Tumors can affect any part of the male or female reproductive systems. Prostate cancer is one of the most common cancers in men. Genetics and age may play a role in its development. Another less common type of cancer in males is testicular (testicul means "testicle" or "testis") cancer. Although not nearly as common as prostate cancer, among males in the age group of 20 to 34 years, it is one of the most common types of male cancer.

Benign tumors in the female reproductive system are sometimes called **fibroids**. Cysts, which may also be considered a benign tumor, are usually caused by hormonal disturbances. They frequently occur in the ovaries and are characterized by enlarged ovaries. Infertility and menstrual abnormalities may be a result of polycystic ovary disease.

Cancer of the endometrium is the most common type of cancer in the female reproductive system. A biopsy may be used to detect the cancer, and a **hysterectomy** (hyster/o means "uterus"; -ectomy means "removal of") is a common type of treatment in which the uterus is removed.

Endometriosis (endo- means "within"; metr/o means "uterus"; -osis is an adjective suffix) is a condition many women have during their child-bearing years when estrogen levels are high. It occurs when the endometrial tissue that lines the uterus happens to grow outside the uterus. The tissue may grow on the intestines, on the outside of the uterus or ovaries, or on other organs in the abdomen (Fig. 14-10). This tissue becomes irritated dur-

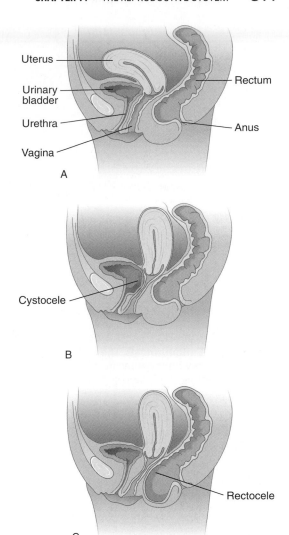

FIGURE 14-9 Herniation into the vagina. A. Normal positioning of the uterus. **B.** Cystocele: The bladder protrudes into the anterior wall of the vagina **C.** Rectocele: The rectum protrudes into the posterior wall of the vagina. From Cohen BJ. Medical Terminology: An Illustrated Guide, 5th Ed. Philadelphia: Lippincott Williams & Wilkins, 2007.

ing the menstrual cycle and may result in fluid-filled cysts that can be painful and result in scar tissue. Imaging tests such as computed tomography (CT) scans, magnetic resonance imaging (MRI), or ultrasounds are done to diagnose cysts or tissue growth outside of the uterus. A laparoscopy (lapar/o means "abdomen"; -scopy means "visualization with an instrument") is a surgical procedure where a viewing scope is introduced through the abdominal wall and allows visual inspection inside the abdominal cavity.

DIAGNOSTIC AND SURGICAL PROCEDURES

A variety of diagnostic tests and surgical procedures are performed on both men and women to detect and treat disorders of the reproductive system. Tests and procedures for the male will be discussed first, followed by those pertaining to the female.

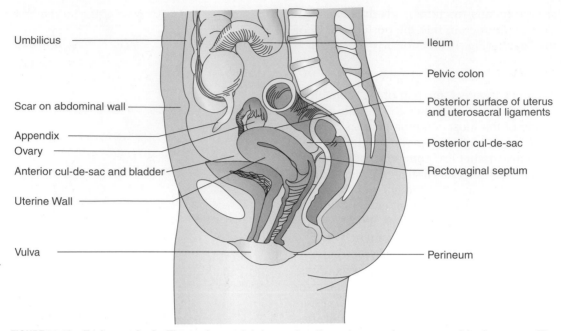

Umbilicus

Scar on abdominal wall

Appendix
Ovary

Anterior cul-de-sac and bladder

Uterine Wall

Vulva

Ileum

Pelvic colon

Posterior surface of uterus
and uterosacral ligaments

Posterior cul-de-sac

Rectovaginal septum

Perineum

FIGURE 14-10 **Endometriosis.** The endometrial tissue that lines the uterus grows outside the uterus. The tissue may grow on the intestines, ovaries, or other organs in the abdomen. From LifeART Nursing 1, CD-ROM. Baltimore: Lippincott Williams & Wilkins.

An enlarged prostate gland or cancerous gland may sometimes be detected by a digital (digit means "finger") exam, where the examiner palpates the prostate gland. Ultrasounds, CT scans, and MRIs are also performed on the prostate to detect abnormalities or cancer.

One surgical procedure that is performed for treatment of an enlarged prostate is called a transurethral resection of the prostate (TURP). Figures 14-11A and 14-11B illustrate the introduction of a cystoscope (cyst/o means "bladder"; -scope means "instrument for viewing") into the urethra and the resection of the enlarged prostate. In some cases, removal of the entire prostate

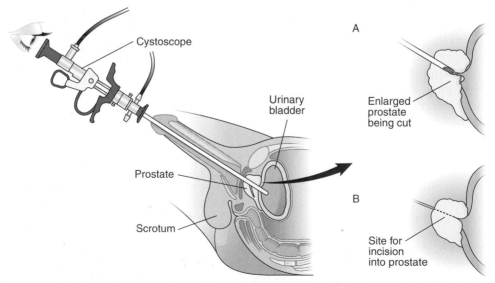

Cystoscope

Urinary
bladder

Prostate

Scrotum

A

Enlarged
prostate
being cut

B

Site for
incision
into prostate

FIGURE 14-11 **Prostate surgery procedure using a cystoscope.** From Cohen BJ. Medical Terminology: An Illustrated Guide, 5th Ed. Philadelphia: Lippincott Williams & Wilkins, 2007.

gland may be necessary. The medical term for this procedure is **prostatectomy** (prostat/o means "prostate"; -ectomy means "removal of").

Another common surgical procedure, a **vasectomy** (vas/o means "vessel" or "vas deferens" in this case; -ectomy "means removal of"), may be done on the male reproductive system for contraceptive (to prevent pregnancy) measures. A portion of the vas deferens, bilaterally, is removed to produce sterility (Fig. 14-12).

Some of the more common diagnostic and surgical treatments/procedures of the female reproductive system include the following:

- **Amniocentesis** (amni/o means "amnion"; -centesis means "surgical puncture"): As mentioned earlier, this is a procedure in which a sample of amniotic fluid is tested for fetal abnormalities (see Fig. 14-6).
- **Colposcopy** (colp/o means "vagina"; -scopy means "a visual examination with an instrument"): Visual examination of the tissues of the cervix and vagina using a **colposcope**.
- **Papanicolaou test**, or **Pap Smear** (named after Dr. Papanicolaou): Exfoliative biopsy or a scraping of the cervical tissues to diagnose cervical cancer and other conditions of the cervix and surrounding tissues.
- **Dilation and curettage (D&C):** Dilation of the cervix and curettage (removal) or scraping of the lining of the uterus.
- **Cone biopsy:** Surgical removal of a cone-shaped section of the cervix (Fig. 14-13).
- **Laparoscopy** (lapar/o means "abdomen"; -scopy means "a visual examination with an instrument"): Visual examination of the interior of the abdomen by means of a laparoscope.
- **Oophorectomy** (oophor/o means "ovary"): Removal of one ovary; **bilateral oophorectomy:** removal of both ovaries.

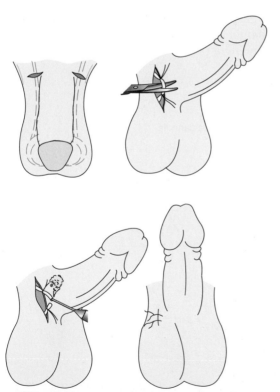

FIGURE 14-12   Vasectomy. External view of male genitalia showing vasectomy. A portion of the vas deferens, bilaterally, is removed to produce sterility. LifeART image copyright 2009. Lippincott Williams & Wilkins. All rights reserved.

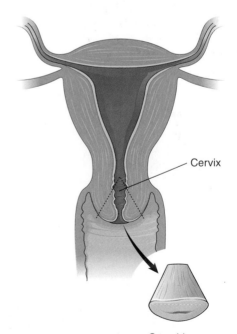

Cervix

Cone biopsy

FIGURE 14-13   Cone biopsy. The surgical removal of a cone-shaped section of the cervix. From Cohen BJ. Medical Terminology: An Illustrated Guide, 5th Ed. Philadelphia: Lippincott Williams & Wilkins, 2007.

- **Bilateral salpingo-oophorectomy** (salping/o means "fallopian tube" or "oviduct"; oophor/o means "ovary"): Removal of both ovaries and fallopian tubes.
- **Hysterosalpingograph (HSG)** (hyster/o means "uterus"; salping/o means "fallopian tube" or "oviduct"; -graph means "a recording"): A radiographic examination of the uterus and fallopian tubes after an injection of radiopaque material.
- **Hysterectomy** (hyster/o means "uterus"; -ectomy means "removal of"): The surgical removal of the uterus.
- **Mammography** (mamm/o means "breast"; -graphy means "process of recording"): A radiographic examination of the breast.
- **Mastectomy** (mast/o means "breast"; -ectomy means "to remove"): Removal of a breast.
- **Tubal ligation** (tubal is an adjective form of tube meaning a fallopian tube; ligation is to tie off or bind; ligo is Latin meaning "to bind"): A procedure that interrupts the continuity of the uterine or fallopian tubes by cutting the tubes to sterilize a female (Fig. 14-14).

Pharmacology

Pharmacologic treatment varies for the many conditions and disorders that affect the male and female reproductive systems. These may include antibiotics used in the infectious processes of the reproductive system; vaccines for certain sexually transmitted viruses; hormone therapy for conditions such as endometriosis, hormone-deficient conditions, and gender-specific cancers to name a few; nonsteroidal anti-inflammatory drugs (NSAIDs) for inflammatory conditions; and certain muscle relaxants and hormone inhibitors for treatment of benign prostatic hypertrophy (BPH) or an enlarged prostate.

As mentioned earlier, there are numerous drug classifications used for the reproductive system. To discuss the many individual drug names is larger than the scope of this text. For specific drug therapy nomenclature, we recommend referencing a pharmacology textbook or internet website specific to the reproductive condition.

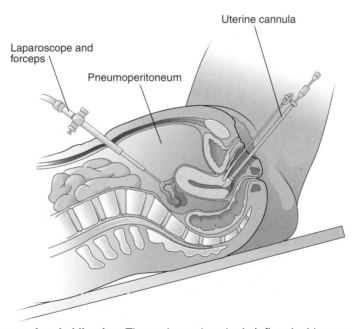

FIGURE 14-14 Laparoscopic tubal ligation. The peritoneal cavity is inflated with a gas, and the oviducts are cut laparoscopically through a small incision in the abdomen. From Cohen BJ. Medical Terminology: An Illustrated Guide, 5th Ed. Philadelphia: Lippincott Williams & Wilkins, 2007.

Abbreviation Table • The Reproductive System

ABBREVIATION	MEANING
BPH	benign prostatic hypertrophy
CS	cesarean section
D&C	dilation and curettage
DUB	dysfunctional uterine bleeding
EDC	estimated date of confinement (due date)
GC	gonorrhea
GYN	gynecology
HRT	hormone replacement therapy
HSG	hysterosalpingogram
HSV	herpes simplex virus
IUD	intrauterine device
IVF	in vitro fertilization
LMP	last menstrual period
OB	obstetrics
PID	pelvic inflammatory disease
PMS	premenstrual syndrome
STD	sexually transmitted disease
TAH	total abdominal hysterectomy
TURP	transurethral resection of the prostate
VD	venereal disease

Study Table • The Reproductive System

TERM AND PRONUNCIATION	ANALYSIS	MEANING
Structure and Function		
androgens (AN-droh-jehns)	from the Greek words *andros* (man) and *genein* (to produce)	hormones that promote the production of male gametes
cervix (SURV-ihks)	a Latin word meaning neck (as in the neck of the uterus)	common term for the uterine cervix
chromosome (KROM-oh-som)	from the Greek word *khroma* (color) and *soma* (body), so called because the structures contain a substance that stains readily with basic dyes	a gene-bearing bundle of DNA found in the nucleus of all cells

TERM AND PRONUNCIATION	ANALYSIS	MEANING
embryo (EHM-bree-oh)	from the Greek word *embryon* (young animal, literally, "that which grows")	name change from *zygote* after the first cell division until the eighth week of pregnancy
epididymis (ehp-ih-DIHD-ih-muhs)	from the Greek words *epi* (on) + *didymos* (testicle)	organ in which the male sperm become functional
fallopian (fah-LOH-pee-ahn) tubes; also called uterine (YU-teh-rihn) tubes	named after Gabriello Fallopio (1523–1562), an Italian anatomist who first described them	tubes between the ovaries and the uterus
fertilization (FUR-tih-ly-ZAY-shun)	from the Latin word *fertilis* (fruitful)	the joining of the male and female gametes (in the context of the human reproductive system)
fetus (FEE-tuhs)	a Latin word meaning the bearing, bringing forth, or hatching of young	name change from *embryo* after the eighth week of pregnancy to birth
gamete (GAH-meet)	a Greek word meaning a wife; also *gametes* (a husband), from *gamein* (to take a wife, to marry)	term given to both the female ovum and the male spermatozoon
gestation (jehs-TAY-shun)	from the Latin word *gestare* (to bear, carry, gestate)	development that occurs between the formation of the zygote and birth of the child
gonad (GOH-nad)	from the Greek word *gone* (seed, act of generation, race, family)	gamete-generating organ (ovary or testis)
gravida (GRA-vee-dah)	from the Latin word *gravis* (heavy, profound, important)	a pregnant woman
lactation (lack-TAH-shun)	from the Latin word *lactare* (to suckle, entice, lead on, induce); derived from the Latin word *lac* (milk)	milk production
mammary gland (MAM-mar-ry)	from the Latin word *mamma* (breast) + gland	breasts
menarche (meh-NAR-kee)	from the Greek words *men* (month) and *arkhe* (beginning)	beginning of menses
menopause (MEN-oh-pawz)	from the Latin words *men* (month) and *pausis* (a cessation, a pause)	normal stopping of the monthly period or menses
menses (MEN-seez)	plural form of the Latin word *mensis* (month)	end of one uterine cycle and the beginning of another

TERM AND PRONUNCIATION	ANALYSIS	MEANING
menstrual cycle (MEN-strew-ahl SY-kl); also called the uterine cycle (YU-tehr-in SY-kl)	from the Latin word *mensis* (month) + cycle	part of the reproductive system process in women, comprising three phases: secretory, proliferative, and menses
mitosis (my-TOH-sihs)	from the Greek word *mitos* (wrap, thread) + *-osis* (process)	process of cell division by which one cell becomes two, both of which contain the maternal and paternal chromosomes
ovary (OH-vah-ree)	from the Latin word *ovum* (egg)	small almond-shaped organ located on either side of the uterus
ovulation (OH-vyu-LAY-shun)	from the Latin word *ovum* (egg) + *atio* (process)	release of a mature ovum from the ovary
ovum (OH-vuhm); ova (OH-vah)	a Latin word meaning egg	the female gamete; ovum is singular; ova is plural
para (PAR-ah)	from the Latin verb *pario* (to bring forth, produce, create)	a woman who has given birth to a viable fetus
penis (PEE-nihs)	from the Latin *penis* (tail)	male sex organ that transports the male sperm into the female vagina
placenta (pla-SEN-tah)	a Latin word meaning cake	a spongy organ that is attached to the fetus by the umbilical cord and that provides nourishment to the fetus
pregnancy (PREG-nan-see)	from the prefix *pre-* (before) and the Latin word *gnascor* (to be born)	period of time when the fetus grows inside of the uterus
progestins (pro-JESS-tihns)	from *pro-* (before) and the Latin word *gestare* (to carry); + -in (suffix denoting chemical)	female hormones generated in the ovaries
prostate gland (PRAH-stayt)	from the Greek word *prostates* (one standing in front)	male gland that produces and stores prostatic fluid, a fluid medium that is part of semen
reproductive tract	from the Latin prefix *re-* (again) and the Latin word *producere* (to produce) + tract, common English word	in the male reproductive system, the ductwork leading from the epididymis to the outside of the body
scrotum (SKROH-tum)	Latin *scrotum* cognate with Old English *scrud* (garment, source of shroud)	the sac that encloses and protects the testicles

TERM AND PRONUNCIATION	ANALYSIS	MEANING
semen (SEE-mehn)	a Latin word meaning seed	combination of male gametes, their associated glandular secretions, and prostatic fluid
seminal vesicle (SEH-min-ahl)	from the Latin *semen* (seed) + vesicle from the Latin word *vesica* (bladder, balloon)	glands at the base of the urinary bladder that secrete a thick substance that nourishes sperm
sperm (spurm); spermatozoon (SPUR-mah-tah-ZOH-on); spermatozoa (SPUR-mah-tah-ZOH-ah)	from the Greek word *sperma* (seed) and *zoion* (animal)	the male gamete; sperm is singular or plural; spermatozoon is singular; spermatozoa is plural
spermatogenesis (SPUR-mah-toh-JEHN-ih-sihs)	*spermat/o* (sperm); *-genesis* (production)	production of sperm
testes (TEHS-teez); singular: testis (TEHS-tihs)	from the Latin word *testiculus* dim. of *testis* (witness) (the organ being evidence of virility)	the organs that produce and store the male gametes
testosterone (tehs-TOSS-teh-rohn)	from the Latin word *testis* (witness); *-sterone* (steroid hormone)	the male reproductive hormone (androgen) prominent in male gamete production
urethra (yu-REETH-rah)	from the Greek word *ourethra* (passage for urine)	male ductwork that acts as a part of both the male urinary and male reproductive systems
uterine cervix (YU-teh-rihn)	*uter/o* (uterus); *-ine* (adjective suffix) + cervix, Latin word for neck	the "neck" located at the lower end of the uterus
uterine cycle; also called the menstrual cycle	*uter/o* (uterus); *-ine* (adjective suffix) + cycle, common English word	part of the reproduction system process in women, comprising three phases: secretory, proliferative, and menses
uterine tubes (YU-teh-rihn); also called fallopian (fah-LOH-pee-ahn) tubes	*uter/o* (uterus); *-ine* (adjective suffix) + tubes, common English word	tubes between the ovaries and the uterus
uterus (YU-teh-ruhs)	a Latin word meaning womb, belly	reproductive organ in which the fertilized oocyte is implanted and in which the child develops
vas deferens (vas DEHF-eh rehnz)	from the Latin words *vas* (vessel) and *deferens* (carrying down)	duct leading out of the epididymis (also called the *ductus deferens*)

TERM AND PRONUNCIATION	ANALYSIS	MEANING
zygote (ZY-goht)	from the Greek word *zygotes* (yoked)	single cell formed at fertilization
Common Disorders		
amenorrhea (ah-MEN-oh-REE-ah)	*a-* (without); *men/o* (menses); *-rrhea* (flowing, discharge)	absence of menstruation
anorchism (an-OR-kism)	*an-* (without); *orch/o* (testes); *-ism* (condition)	congenital absence of one or both testes
anteflexion (an-tee-FLEX-shun)	*ante-* (something positioned in front of); from the Latin word *flectere* (to bend)	an exaggerated forward bend of the uterus
anteversion (an-tee-VER-shun)	*ante-* (something positioned in front of); from the Latin word *versio* (turning)	abnormal tipping forward of the entire uterus
azoospermia (ay-ZOH-oh-SPER-mee-ah)	from the Greek word *azoos* (lifeless) + *sperm/o* (sperm)	absence of sperm in the semen
balanitis (bal-ah-NIGH-tis)	*balan/o* (glans penis); *-itis* (inflammation)	inflammation of the glans penis
BPH, or benign prostatic hypertrophy	benign (common English word) + *prostat/o* (prostate) + -ic (adjective suffix); *hyper-* (above normal); *-trophy* (nourishment or development)	an enlarged, noncancerous prostate; *prostatomegaly*
cervicitis (sur-vih-SY-tihs); also trachelitis (trak-ih-LY-tihs)	*cervic/o* (cervix); *-itis* (inflammation)	inflammation of the uterine cervix
cryptorchism (kript-OR-kism); also cryptorchidism (kript-OR-kid-izm)	from the Greek word *kryptos* (hidden); *orch/o* (testes); *-ism* (condition)	undescended testicles or when one or both testes fail to descend into the scrotum
cystocele (SIS-toh-seel)	*cyst/o* (bladder); *-cele* (hernia)	protrusion of the bladder into the anterior wall of the vagina
dysmenorrhea (dis-MEN-oh-REE-ah)	*dys-* (bad, difficult); *men/o* (menses); *-rrhea* (flowing, discharge)	painful menstruation
endometriosis (EN-doh-MEE-tree-OH-sis)	from the Greek words *endon* (within) and *metra* (womb) + *-osis* (condition)	presence of endometrial tissue outside the uterus
epididymitis (ep-ih-did-ih-MY-tis)	from the Greek words *epi* (on) and *didymos* (testicle); *-itis* (inflammation)	inflammation of the epididymis

TERM AND PRONUNCIATION	ANALYSIS	MEANING
epispadias (ep-i-SPAY-dee-as)	from the Greek *epi* (on) and *spas* (something torn, rent)	congenital opening of the urethra on the top side of the penis
gonorrhea (gon-oh-REE-ah)	from the Greek *gonos* (offspring); *-rrhea* (discharge, flowing)	highly contagious sexually transmitted disease caused by bacteria
hydrocele (HIGH-droh-seel)	*hydro-* (water); *-cele* (hernia)	hernia filled with fluid in the testes
hypospadias (high-poh-SPAY-dee-as)	*hypo-* (below normal); from the Greek word *spas* (something torn, rent)	congenital defect where the opening of the urethra is on the underside of the penis
hysteralgia (HIHS-teh-RAL-jee-ah); also hysterodynia (HIHS-teh-roh-DIHN-ee-ah)	*hyster/o* (womb, uterus); *-algia/-dynia* (pain)	pain in the uterus
hysterectomy (HIS-ter-EK-toh-mee)	*hyster/o* (womb, uterus); *-ectomy* (excision)	removal of the uterus
hysteropathy (hiss-ter-ROP-ah-thee)	*hyster/o* (womb, uterus); *-pathy* (disease)	any disease of the uterus
mastitis (mast-EYE-tis)	*mast/o* (breast); *-itis* (inflammation)	inflammation of the breast
menorrhagia (MEN-oh-RAY-jee-ah)	*men/o* (menses); *-rrhagia* (rapid flow of blood)	increased amount and duration of flow
oligomenorrhea (oh-LIG-oh-MEN-oh-REE-ah)	*olig/o* (having little); *men/o* (menses); *-rrhea* (discharge, flowing)	markedly reduced menstrual flow along with abnormally infrequent menstruation
oligospermia (oh-LIG-oh-SPER-mee-ah)	*olig/o* (having little); *-sperm/o* (sperm); *-ia* (condition)	low sperm count
oophoritis (oo-foh-RY-tihs)	*oophor/o* (ovary); *-itis* (inflammation)	inflammation of an ovary
orchialgia (or-kee-AL-jee-ah)	*orchi/o* (testes); *-algia* (pain)	pain in the testes
orchiopathy (or-kee-OP-ah-thee)	*orchi/o* (testes); *-pathy* (disease)	any disease of the testes
orchitis (or-KY-tihs)	*orchi/o* (testes); *-itis* (inflammation)	inflammation of a testis
ovarialgia (oh-vahr-ee-AL-jee-ah)	*ovari/o* (ovary); *-algia* (pain)	pain in an ovary
ovaritis (ohv-ah-RY-tihs)	*ovari/o* (ovary); *-itis* (inflammation)	inflammation of an ovary (see also *oophoritis*)

TERM AND PRONUNCIATION	ANALYSIS	MEANING
PID, or pelvic inflammatory disease	common English words	acute or chronic suppurative inflammation of female pelvic structures (endometrium, uterine tubes, pelvic peritoneum) due to infection by *Neisseria gonorrhoeae*, *Chlamydia trachomatis*, or other organisms
phimosis (fi-MOH-sis)	from the Greek word *phimoo* (to muzzle); *-osis* (condition)	narrowing of the opening of the foreskin so it cannot be retracted or pulled back to expose the glans penis
prolapsed uterus	common English word; uterus is a Latin word meaning womb	descent of the uterus or cervix into the vagina
prostatitis (PROS-tah-TYE-tis)	*prostat/o* (prostate); *-itis* (inflammation)	inflammation of the prostate
rectocele (REK-toh-seel)	*rect/o* (rectum); *-cele* (hernia)	protrusion of the rectum into the posterior wall of the vagina
retroflexion (re-troh-FLEX-shun)	*retro-* (backward) + flexion, from the Latin word *flectere* (to bend)	abnormal tipping with the body of the uterus bent back on itself
retroversion (re-troh-VER-shun)	*retro-* (backward); from the Latin word *versio* (to turn)	an abnormal tipping of the entire uterus backward
salpingitis (sal-pin-JY-tiss)	*salping/o* (tube, fallopian tube); *-itis* (inflammation)	inflammation of the uterine tube
STD, or sexually transmitted disease	common English words	diseases that are transmitted through sexual intercourse or sexual contact (HIV, GC, syphilis, chlamydia)
syphilis (SIF-ih-lis)	from a poem *Syphilis sive Morbus Gallicus*, by Fracastorius, *Syphilus* being a shepherd and principal character	a highly contagious sexually transmitted disease that is caused by a bacterium
vaginitis (VAJ-ih-NIGH-tis)	*vagin/o* (vagina); *-itis* (inflammation)	inflammation of the vaginal tissues that may be infectious or due to several other causes
varicocele (VAR-ih-ko-seel)	*varic/o* (varix, varicose, varicosity); *-cele* (hernia)	a varicose vein of the testes

TERM AND PRONUNCIATION	ANALYSIS	MEANING
Practice and Practitioners		
gynecologist (guy-neh-KOL-oh-jist)	*gynec/o* (woman, female); *-logist* (one who studies a certain field)	a specialist of the female reproductive system
gynecology (guy-neh-KOL-oh-jee)	*gynec/o* (woman, female); *-logy* (study of)	the study of the female reproductive system
neonatology (NEE-oh-nay-TOL-oh-jee)	*neo-* (new); *nat/o* (birth); *-logy* (study of)	the medical specialty dealing with newborns
neonatologist (NEE-oh-nay-TOL-oh-jist)	*neo-* (new); *nat/o* (birth); *-logist* (one who studies a certain field)	the medical specialist dealing with newborns
obstetrician (OB-steh-trish-uhn)	from the Latin word *obstetricis* (midwife), derived from the Latin word *obstare* (to stand opposite to)	a physician who specializes in the medical care of women during pregnancy and childbirth
obstetrics (ob-STET-rihks)	from the Latin word *obstetricis* (midwife), derived from the Latin word *obstare* (to stand opposite to)	medical specialty concerned with the medical care of women during pregnancy and childbirth
pediatrician (pee-dee-a-TRISH-an)	from the Greek *paid-*, stem of *pais* (child) + *-iatr/o* (pertaining to medicine)	medical specialist of children
pediatrics (pee-dee-AT-riks)	from the Greek *paid-*, stem of *pais* (child) + *-iatr/o* (pertaining to medicine)	medical specialty dealing with children
Diagnostic and Surgical Procedures		
amniocentesis (am-nee-oh-sen-TEE-sihs)	*amni/o* (amnion); *-centesis* (surgical puncture for aspiration)	extraction and diagnostic examination of amniotic fluid from the amniotic sac
cervicectomy (surv-ih-SEK-toh-mee); also, rarely, trachelectomy (trak-eh-LEK-toh-mee)	*cervic/o* (cervix); *-ectomy* (excision); from the Greek word *trachelos* (neck)	excision of the uterine cervix
cervicoplasty (SURV-ih-ko-plass-tee) cervicotomy (surv-ih-KOT-oh-mee); also trachelotomy (trak-eh-LOT-oh-mee)	*cervic/o* (cervix); *-plasty* (surgical repair); *-tomy* (incision into); trachelotomy is from the Greek word *trachelos* (neck) + *-tomy* (incision into)	surgical repair of the uterine cervix OR the neck incision of the uterine cervix; *tracheotomy* is the term used to denote an incision into the neck (trachea); but *trachelotomy* refers to the uterine cervix and is synonymous with *cervicotomy*

TERM AND PRONUNCIATION	ANALYSIS	MEANING
cesarean section (c-section) (seh-SAYR-ee-ahn); other spellings are caesarean and caesarian	etymology uncertain	surgical operation through the abdominal wall and uterus for delivery of the baby
circumcision (SER-kum-SI-shun)	*circum/o* (around); from the Latin word *caedo* (cut)	a surgical procedure to remove the foreskin of the penis
colposcopy (kole-POSS-koh-pee)	*colp/o* (vagina); *-scopy* (use of an instrument for viewing)	using an endoscopic instrument to examine the vagina and cervix
D&C, or dilation and curettage	from the Latin word *dilatare* (to make wider, enlarge) + from the French word *curette* (scoop)	dilation of the cervix and curettage, which involves scraping of the lining of the uterus
hysterectomy (hiss-toh-REK-toh-mee)	*hyster/o* (uterus); *-ectomy* (excision)	surgical removal of the uterus
hysteropexy (HISS-teh-roh-pek-see)	*hyster/o* (uterus); *-pexy* (fixation)	surgical fixation of the uterus
hysteroplasty (HISS-teh-roh-plass-tee)	*hyster/o* (uterus); *-plasty* (surgical repair)	surgical repair of the uterus
hysterotomy (hiss-teh-ROT-oh-mee)	*hyster/o* (uterus); *-tomy* (incision into)	incision of the uterus
laparoscopy (lap-ah-RAH-sko-pee)	*lapar/o* (of or pertaining to the abdominal wall, flank); *-scopy* (use of an instrument for viewing)	direct visualization of the interior of the abdomen with the use of a laparoscope
mammography (mam-OG-rah-fee)	*mamm/o* (breast); *-graphy* (process of recording)	examination of the breast by means of an imaging technique, such as radiography
mastectomy (MAS-tek-toh-mee)	*mast/o* (breast); *-ectomy* (excision)	removal of a breast
oophorectomy (oo-foh-REK-toh-mee)	*oophor/o* (ovary); *-ectomy* (excision)	excision of an ovary; ovariectomy
oophoroplasty (OO-foh-roh-plass-tee)	*oophor/o* (ovary); *-plasty* (surgical repair)	surgical repair of an ovary
oophorotomy (oo-foh-ROT-oh-mee)	*oophor/o* (ovary); *-tomy* (incision into)	incision into an ovary
orchiectomy (or-kee-EK-toh-mee)	*orchi/o* (testes); *-ectomy* (excision)	removal of one or both testes (less commonly, *orchechtomy* or *orchidectomy*

TERM AND PRONUNCIATION	ANALYSIS	MEANING
orchioplasty (ORK-ee-oh-plass-tee)	*orchi/o* (testes); *-plasty* (surgical repair)	surgical repair of a testis
orchiotomy (or-kee-OT-ah-mee)	*orchi/o* (testes); *-tomy* (incision into)	incision into a testis
ovariectomy (oh-vahr-ee-EK-toh-mee)	*ovari/o* (ovary); *-ectomy* (excision)	excision of one or both ovaries
ovariotomy (oh-vahr-ee-OT-oh-mee)	*ovari/o* (ovary); *-tomy* (incision into)	incision of an ovary
Pap smear (Papanicolaou)	named after George Papanicolaou, who developed the technique	exfoliative biopsy or a scraping of the cervix to diagnose conditions of the cervix and surrounding tissues
salpingo-oophorectomy	*salping/o* (tube, fallopian tube) + *oophor/o* (ovary); *-ectomy* (excision)	removal of an ovary and fallopian tube
tubal ligation (TOO-ball lie-GAY-shun)	tube + *-al* (adjective suffix) + ligation, from the Latin word *ligare* (to bind)	surgical procedure performed for female sterilization where each fallopian tube is tied off or "ligated" to prevent the ovum from reaching the uterus
TURP, or transurethral resection of the prostate	from the Latin *trans* (across) + from the Greek word *ourethra* (urethra); + *re-* (again) from the Latin *secare* (to cut)	the removal of part or all of the prostate through the urethra
uteropexy (YU-teh-roh-pek-see)	*uter/o* (uterus); *-pexy* (fixation)	surgical fixation of the uterus (see also *hysteropexy*)
uteroplasty (YU-teh-roh-plass-tee)	*uter/o* (uterus); *-plasty* (surgical repair)	surgical repair of the uterus (see also *hysteroplasty*)
uterotomy (yu-teh-ROT-oh-mee)	*uter/o* (uterus); *-tomy* (incision into)	incision of the uterus (see also *hysterotomy*)
varicocelectomy (VAR-ee-coh-SEEL-ek-toh-mee)	*varic/o* (varix, varicose, varicosity); *-cele* (hernia); *-ectomy* (excision)	the removal of a portion of an enlarged vein to remove a varicocele
vasovasostomy (vay-soh-vay-ZOS-toh-mee)	*vas/o* (vessel, vas deferens); *-stomy* (creation of an opening)	procedure to restore fertility to a vasectomized male; reconnect the vas deferens

EXERCISES

EXERCISE 14-1   Figure Labeling: The Male Reproductive System

Label the figure of the male reproductive system.

bulbourethral gland	prepuce (foreskin)	urethra
ejaculatory duct	prostate	urinary bladder
epididymis	scrotum	ductus (vas) deferens
glans penis	seminal vesicle	
penis	testis	

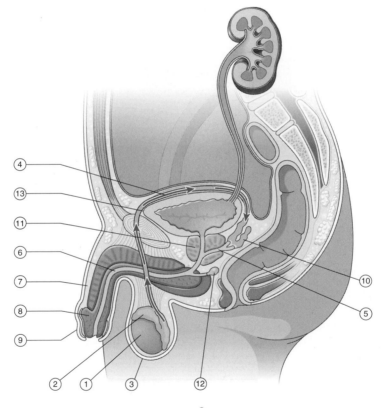

1. _____

2. _____

3. _____

4. _____

5. _____

6. _____

7. _____

8. _____

9. _____

10. _____

11. _____

12. _____

13. _____

EXERCISE 14-2   Figure Labeling: The Female Reproductive System

Label the figure of the female reproductive system.

anus	labium major	urethra
cervix	labium minor	urinary bladder
clitoris	rectum	uterus
fallopian tube	ovary	vagina

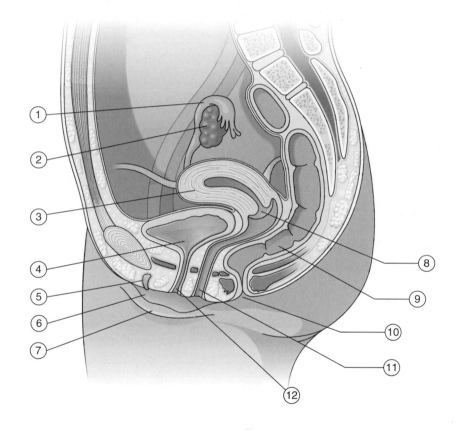

1. _____   7. _____
2. _____   8. _____
3. _____   9. _____
4. _____   10. _____
5. _____   11. _____
6. _____   12. _____

EXERCISE 14-3   Deciphering Medical Documents

Read the following excerpt from a hospital report, and answer the questions that follow.

A 27-year-old gravida II, para I woman without significant medical history. Blood work was normal before delivery of a stillborn 1-pound, 11-ounce infant during week 21. Although ultrasound studies during week 14 and amniocentesis during week 15 were unremarkable, intrauterine fetal demise had occurred during week 18.

1. What does gravida II, para I signify? _____

   _____

2. What is amniocentesis? _____

   _____

3. In the final sentence, both "fetal demise" and "stillborn" are self-evident terms. Using your knowledge of word elements, define intrauterine.

   _____

EXERCISE 14-4   Building Medical Terms

The combining form _hyster/o_ refers to the uterus. Use it to write a term that means:

1. surgical fixation of the uterus   _____

2. removal of the uterus   _____

3. rupture of the uterus   _____

4. suture of the uterus   _____

The combining form _metr/o_ also means uterus. Use it to write a term that means:

5. any uterine disease   _____

6. inflammation of the uterus   _____

7. uterine hemorrhage   _____

The combining form _vagin/o_ means vagina. Use it to write a term that means:

8. relating to the vagina   _____

9. vaginal hernia   _____

10. inflammation of the vagina   _____

11. relating to the vagina and labia   _____

The combining form *colp/o* also means vagina. Use it to write a term that means:

12. visual examination of the vagina using an instrument   _____

13. suture of the vagina   _____

The combining form *prostat/o* means prostate gland. Use it to write a term that means:

14. removal of the prostate   _____

15. pertaining to the prostate   _____

16. inflammation of the prostate   _____

The combining form *vesicul/o* means seminal vesicle. Use it to write a term that means:

17. disease of the seminal vesicle   _____

18. inflammation of the seminal vesicle   _____

The combining forms *orchid/o*, *orchi/o*, and *orch/o* refer to the testes. Write a term that means:

19. inflammation of the testes   _____

20. disease of the testes   _____

21. testicular pain   _____

....

EXERCISE 14-5   Surgical Procedure Term Identification

Name the anatomical parts operated on in the following procedures.

1. salpingectomy   _____

2. hysterectomy   _____

3. tubal ligation   _____

4. colporrhaphy   _____

5. mammoplasty   _____

6. oophorectomy _____

7. orchiectomy _____

8. vasectomy _____

9. balanoplasty _____

10. mastectomy _____

EXERCISE 14-6   Matching Terms with Definitions

Match the terms in Column 1 with the correct definitions in Column 2.

TERM

1. _____ vas deferens

2. _____ prostate gland

3. _____ spermatogenesis

4. _____ epididymis

5. _____ semen

6. _____ orchalgia

7. _____ testes

8. _____ hysterectomy and bilateral oophorectomy

9. _____ ovarialgia

10. _____ hysteropexy

11. _____ period of gestation

12. _____ oophoritis

13. _____ ovulation

14. _____ ovum

15. _____ cervicectomy

DEFINITION

A. combination of sperm and associated liquids that nourish the sperm

B. pain in the ovary

C. organs that produce and store male gametes

D. duct leading out of the epididymis

E. production of sperm

F. inflammation of an ovary

G. pain in the testes

H. release of the female gamete from the ovary

I. organ in which the male sperm become functional; lies on top of the testes

J. excision of the uterine cervix

K. surgical fixation of the uterus

L. the female gamete

M. surgical removal of the uterus and right and left ovaries

N. time lapse between zygote formation and birth

O. gland that surrounds the urethra; secretes alkaline fluid that assists in sperm motility

EXERCISE 14-7   Abbreviations

Identify the following abbreviations:

1. BPH   _____

2. D&C   _____

3. OB   _____

4. TURP   _____

EXERCISE 14-8   Crossword Puzzle: Reproductive System

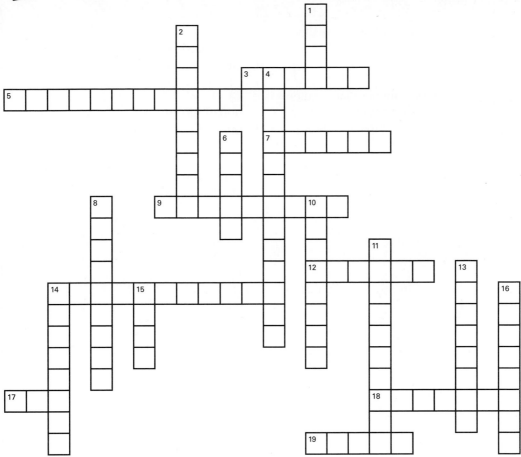

ACROSS

3. neck of the uterus
5. endoscopic examination of the abdomen
7. root word for ovary
9. cutting and sealing the vas deferens, male sterilization
12. dark pigmented area around nipple
14. inflammation of the prostate
17. root word for vas deferens and vessel
18. another term for fallopian tube
19. root word for woman

DOWN

1. root word for vulva
2. GC
4. growth of endometrial tissue outside of the uterus
6. tissue that partially covers the entrance to vagina
8. herniation of urinary bladder into vaginal wall
10. beginning of menstruation
11. instrument used to examine the vagina and cervix
13. area between the external vulva to the anus
14. narrowing of the opening of the prepuce so foreskin cannot be retracted
15. abbreviation for transurethral resection of the prostate
16. inflammation of the testis

CHAPTER 14 QUIZ

Multiple Choice

1. The surgical removal of testes is called:
   a. orchidectomy
   b. vasectomy
   c. circumcision
   d. cauterization

2. A prolapsed uterus means that the uterus is:
   a. bent backwards on itself
   b. descended down into the vagina
   c. tipped forward
   d. tipped backward

3. Menarche is:
   a. the beginning of menstruation
   b. the end of menopause
   c. part of the first trimester
   d. another name for gestation

4. Cryptorchidism is:
   a. underdeveloped testicles
   b. small ovaries
   c. ruptured ovaries
   d. undescended testicles

5. Removal of fluid from the area around the fetus to analyze is called:
   a. cervicentesis
   b. amniocentesis
   c. intrauterine analysis
   d. none of the above

6. The surgical procedure that removes the prostate gland is called a:
   a. vasectomy
   b. prostatectomy
   c. vasoligation
   d. circumcision

7. A Papanicolaou test is done to detect:
   a. fibroids
   b. metritis
   c. cancer of the cervix
   d. ovarian cancer

8. A difficult or painful monthly blood flow is termed:
   a. dysmenorrhea
   b. menorrhea
   c. dysmetrorrhagia
   d. menometrorrhagia

9. A colposcope is used to visualize the:
   a. testis
   b. epididymis
   c. cervix
   d. vagina

True or False

Place an X in the "True" or "False" column next to each statement. Write the correct answer in the "Correction, if False" column for any statements you identify as false.

Statement	True	False	Correction, if False
10. Fertilization is the development that occurs between the formation of the zygote and birth of the child.	____	____	_____

11. The tubes between the ovaries and the uterus are called the fallopian tubes.

_____ _____ _____

12. The joining of the male and female gametes is called ovulation.

_____ _____ _____

13. IVF is an abbreviation for intravenous filtration.

_____ _____ _____

14. The term for the release of the female gamete is proliferation.

_____ _____ _____

15. The male ductwork that acts as a part of both the male urinary and male reproductive systems is called the urethra.

_____ _____ _____

16. Hysteralgia is pain in the uterus.

_____ _____ _____

17. Obstetrician is the medical specialty concerned with the medical care of women during pregnancy and childbirth.

_____ _____ _____

18. Endometriosis is difficult or painful menses.

_____ _____ _____

19. Mammography is examination of cells from a mucosal surface, especially the uterine cervix.

_____ _____ _____

CHAPTER 15

The Special Senses of Sight and Hearing

LEARNING OBJECTIVES

Upon completion of this chapter, you should be able to:

- List the major organs and functions of the eyes and ears.
- Label diagrams of components of the eyes and ears.
- Identify and use the word elements relating to the eyes and ears.
- Describe symptoms, abnormal conditions, treatments, and surgical procedures relating to the eyes and ears.
- Name the major drug classifications used to treat disorders of the eyes and ears.
- Identify and interpret selected abbreviations relating to the eyes and ears.
- Analyze and define the new terms introduced in this chapter.

Word Elements • The Eye

WORD ELEMENT	REFERS TO
blephar/o	eyelid
conjunctiv/o	conjunctiva (plural: conjunctivae)
corne/o	cornea
dacry/o	tears; lacrima
dacryocyst/o	tears or lacrimal sac
dipl/o	two, double
irid/o, ir-, irit/o	iris
kerat/o	hard, cornea
lacrim/o	tear, lacrimal apparatus
ocul/o	eye
ophthalm/o	eye
-opia	suffix for eye vision
-opsia	suffix for vision
opt/o	light, eye, vision
phak/o, phac/o	lens
presby/o	old age
pupil/o	pupil
retin/o	retina
scler/o	sclera (also means hard)
uve/o	middle layer of the eye containing muscles and blood vessels

An Overview of Sight and Hearing

We get the English words *sense* and *sentience* from the Latin verb *sentire*, which refers to the human ability to perceive reality and thus to attain wisdom. Issuing from those two words, the phrase *special senses* refers to the five avenues along which the process begins, namely, the five senses: touch, taste, smell, sight, and hearing.

We have chosen to treat sight and hearing in a chapter of their own because, unlike smell, taste, and touch, which rely on chemical responses, sight and hearing include terminology associated with organs that process both electromagnetic energy (sight) and mechanical energy (hearing).

The eye is a unique, very complex sense organ that transmits a light image to the brain by way of the nervous system. It works pretty much the same way a video camera does (i.e., it can move to look at particular objects and focus on objects that are far away or close up). The eyes take continuous pictures and transmit them instantaneously to the brain, which converts them to

Word Elements • The Ear

WORD ELEMENT	REFERS TO
acous/o, acus/o, acoust/o	hearing
audi/o	sound
audit/o	hearing
aur/o	ear
auricul/o	ear
myring/o	tympanic membrane (eardrum)
ot/o	ear
staped/o	stapes
tympan/o	eardrum

images not only of the objects, but of their motions as well. The light energy that strikes the eyes is part of the electromagnetic spectrum, which also includes brain waves. However, brain waves have a different frequency, and so eyes must also change the detected light frequencies so that the brain can enable us to "see" objects and their motions.

The ear is the sense organ that detects sound waves and converts them into electromagnetic waves the brain uses to interpret audible information (e.g., music and spoken language). The difference between sight and hearing is interesting because, unlike light waves, sound waves are not part of the electromagnetic spectrum and, therefore, must be not only detected but also converted into a different kind of energy through a process called transduction. Therefore, whereas the eyes work pretty much the same way a camera does, the ears are more like a microphone, which detects sound waves and then converts them into electromagnetic waves for processing in the brain. Another huge difference, however, is that whereas a microphone signal must then be directed into an amplifier or some other electronic device that can convert electromagnetic energy waves back into sound waves, the brain merely creates, magically, the sense of hearing.

The study of the eye is called **ophthalmology** (ophthalm/o means "eye"; -logy means "the study of"), and the physician is called an **ophthalmologist** (ophthalm/o means "eye"; -logist means "one who studies or practices"). An ophthalmologist provides eye care ranging from examining and prescribing corrective lenses by determining refractive errors in the eye to performing surgery. This professional must have an undergraduate college degree, a degree from a medical school, a 1-year internship, and then at least 3 additional years of specialized clinical training in the field of ophthalmology, for a total of about 12 years,

An **optometrist** (opt/o means "light" or "eye"; -metry means "the act of measuring") is a health care professional who examines eyes and prescribes corrective lenses. In the United States, optometrists, also called doctors of optometry, must have an undergraduate college degree plus 4 years of training at an accredited school of optometry (opt/o means "light" or "eye"; -metry means "measurement of"). The technicians who fill eyeglass prescriptions and dispense eyewear are called **opticians**. This occupation requires a high school diploma and successful completion of an accredited optician program, which is usually about 1 year.

The physician who treats hearing disorders and performs surgery on the ears is called an **otologist** (ot/o means "ear"). Frequently, this specialist also diagnoses and treats disorders of the nose and throat and, in that case, is called an **otorhinolaryngologist** (ot/o means "ear"; rhin/o means "nose"; laryng/o means "throat"). The health care worker who measures hearing and treats

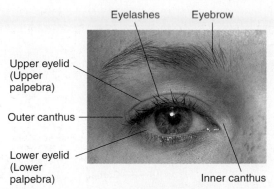

Eyelashes   Eyebrow

Upper eyelid (Upper palpebra)

Outer canthus

Lower eyelid (Lower palpebra)

Inner canthus

FIGURE 15-1 The protective structures of the eye. From Cohen BJ. Medical Terminology: An Illustrated Guide, 5th Ed. Philadelphia: Lippincott Williams & Wilkins, 2007.

hearing impairments is called an **audiologist** (audi/o means "to hear"). The field is called **audiology**.

Structure and Function

THE EYE

The main external structures of the eye include the **orbit**, the eyelids, the **conjunctiva**, and the **lacrimal** apparatus or tearducts. The orbit, also known as the eye socket, is a cavity formed by several bones that contain the eyeball. Each eye has a pair of eyelids (an upper **palpebra** and a lower palpebra) that protect the eyeball from dust, foreign particles, light, and impact. The edges of the eyelids have eyelashes and sebaceous glands that secrete an oily substance onto the inner side of the eyelids for lubrication. The **canthi** (singular **canthus**) are the corners of the eye where the upper and lower palpebrae join together. See Figure 15-1 for the protective structures of the eye.

The **conjunctiva** is the mucous membrane lining on the underside of the eyelid. This membrane acts as a protective covering for the exposed surface of the eyeball. The **lacrimal glands** produce and store tears that cleanse the eye. They are located above the outer corner of each eye and secrete tears, which may also be called **lacrimal fluid**. These glands help maintain moisture on the eyeball. The **lacrimal sac** is also known as a tear sac or **dacryocyst** (dacry/o means "tear"; -cyst means "sac"). Figure 15-2 illustrates the lacrimal gland and associated structures.

The eyeball is made up of three layers: the **sclera**, the **uveal tract** (contains the **choroid**, **iris**, and **ciliary body**), and the **retina** (Fig. 15-3). The sclera, also known as the white of the eye, helps maintain the shape of the eyeball and gives protection to it. The **cornea**, an extension of the sclera, is the transparent portion that provides most of the optical power of the eye through its ability to bend light rays to focus them on the surface of the retina.

The **iris** is the pigmented muscular ring that surrounds and controls the size of the pupil through which light enters the eye. The **ciliary body** is located within the choroid and consists of a group of muscles that suspend the lens and adjust it to direct the light entering the eye. The lens is responsible for focusing images on the retina. It is held in place by the suspensory ligaments of the ciliary body. These muscles control the shape of the lens to allow for far and near vision, a process called **accommodation** (Fig. 15-4). The choroid is the opaque layer of the eyeball that contains the many blood vessels that provide the blood supply to the eye.

The innermost layer, the **retina**, is the sensitive layer of the eye that contains the specialized light-sensitive cells called **rods** (black and white receptors that respond to dim light) and **cones** (color receptors that have a high visual acuity). These photosensitive cells receive the light waves that come in through the cornea and convert them into nerve impulses. The **fovea centralis** (fovea is a depression or pit; centralis means the central part) is a pit in

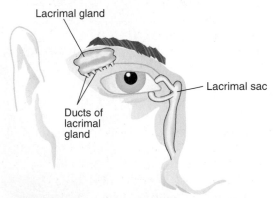

Lacrimal gland

Lacrimal sac

Ducts of lacrimal gland

FIGURE 15-2 Lacrimal glands. The right lacrimal gland and associated structures are shown. From Cohen BJ. Medical Terminology: An Illustrated Guide, 5th Ed. Philadelphia: Lippincott Williams & Wilkins, 2007.

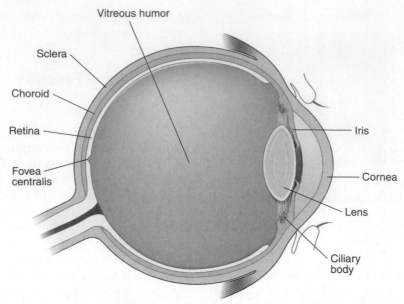

FIGURE 15-3   Structures of the eyeball. The innermost layer of the retina contains specialized cells called rods and cones. The rods have black and white receptors that respond to dim light. The cones have color receptors. Modified from Cohen BJ. Medical Terminology: An Illustrated Guide, 5th Ed. Philadelphia: Lippincott Williams & Wilkins, 2007.

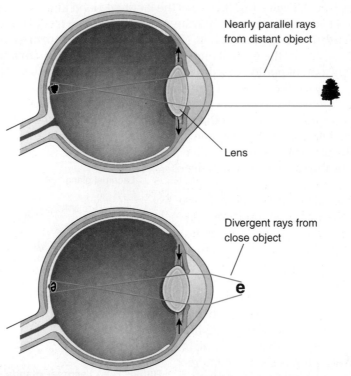

FIGURE 15-4   Accommodation. The muscles control the shape of the lens to allow for far and near vision. The top figure has an elongated lens allowing distant vision. The lower figure has a shortened lens, allowing the eye to focus on near objects. From Cohen BJ. Medical Terminology: An Illustrated Guide, 5th Ed. Philadelphia: Lippincott Williams & Wilkins, 2007.

the middle of the retina that is saturated with cone cells that permit the best possible color vision (see Fig. 15-3).

The interior spaces of the eyeball contain fluid. The space between the cornea and the lens is filled with a watery fluid called the **aqueous humor** (aqueous means water; humor comes from the Latin work *umor*, which means "clear fluid"), and the large open space between the lens and retina contains a semi-gelatinous liquid, the **vitreous humor** (vitreous means glassy or resembles glass; comes from the Latin word *vitreus*, which means "glassy").

THE EAR

The ear is responsible for both hearing and equilibrium. The outer ear is specially designed to bring sound waves into the inner parts of the ear where they are converted to electrical signals the brain can process. The ear is divided into three sections: the external, the middle, and the internal ear. The external ear, located along the sides of the head, is called the **pinna** or **auricle** (aur or auri means "ear"). Its purpose is to funnel sound waves into the auditory canal of the ear. Numerous glands line the auditory canal and secrete **cerumen**, better known as *earwax*. Cerumen protects the ear by preventing dust, insects, and some bacteria from entering the middle ear.

The sound waves entering the ear vibrate the **tympanic membrane** (tympan/o means "eardrum"), which separates the external and middle ear (Fig. 15-5). Just beyond the tympanic membrane is the middle ear. A tiny cavity in the skull houses three small bones or **ossicles**, called the **malleus**, **incus**, and **stapes** (Fig. 15-6). These are sometimes referred to as the hammer, anvil, and stirrup because of their shapes. Sound waves affect these tiny bones and cause them to transmit the sound vibrations to the inner ear. Also found inside of the middle ear are the **eustachian** or **auditory tubes**. They reach from the middle ear to the nasopharynx and help to equalize pressure in the ear to the outside atmosphere.

The inner ear is called a **labyrinth** or maze because of its complicated construction. It contains the sensory receptors for hearing and balance. One of the major structures in the labyrinth is the **cochlea**. Receptors in the cochlea change sound waves into electrical signals that the brain can interpret.

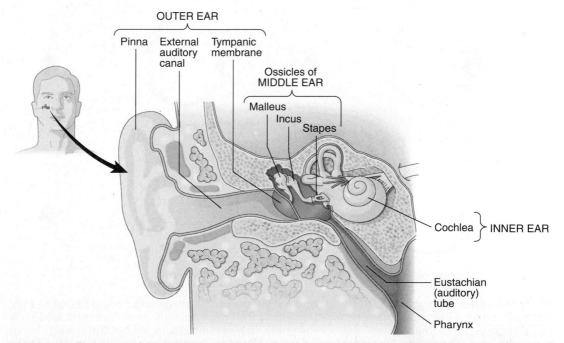

FIGURE 15-5 The ear and its internal structures. From Cohen BJ. Medical Terminology: An Illustrated Guide, 5th Ed. Philadelphia: Lippincott Williams & Wilkins, 2007.

Disorders and Treatments

DISORDERS OF THE EYE

Errors in refraction, infections, and disorders of the eyelids are common problems with the eye. Refractive errors can be corrected with glasses, contact lenses, or with newer surgical techniques that include the reshaping of the cornea. Some of the other eye conditions are treated with medications and, in some cases, surgery.

Refractory Errors

Visual acuity tends to diminish with age, and eyes often need corrective lenses to adjust their ability to focus. The lens becomes stiffer and may become opaque and yellow, and the ciliary muscles begin to weaken. All of these changes impair one's vision. Frequently, adults

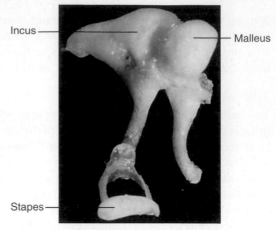

FIGURE 15-6   The ossicles.

may suffer from **presbyopia** (presby/o means "old"; -pia means "vision"), commonly called farsightedness. This condition occurs when the eyeball is too short and images fall behind the retina (**hyperopia**; hyper- means "excessive" or "above normal"; -opia means "vision"). When images fall in front of the retina, the condition is called nearsightedness or **myopia** (my/o means "muscle"; -opia means "vision")(Fig. 15-7). Another error of refraction is called **astigmatism** (a- means "without" or "not"; -stigmat comes from the Greek word *stigma*, which means "a point"). Astigmatism means the light coming into the eye does not focus on a single point; this condition is caused by an irregularity of the curve of the cornea that distorts the light entering the eye. Corrective lenses can usually compensate for refractive errors.

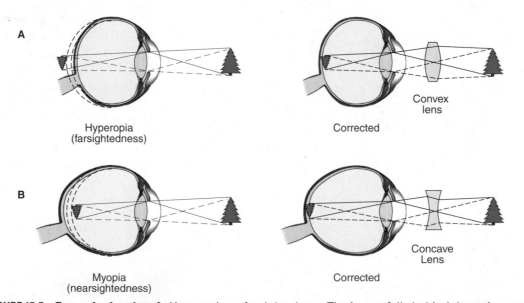

FIGURE 15-7   Error of refraction. A. Hyperopia or farsightedness. The image falls behind the retina making it difficult to see up close. The corrective lens places the image properly on the retina. **B.** Myopia or nearsightedness. The image falls in front of the retina making it difficult to see far. The corrective lens places the image properly on the retina. From Cohen BJ. Medical Terminology: An Illustrated Guide, 5th Ed. Philadelphia: Lippincott Williams & Wilkins, 2007.

Disorders of the Eyelids

Blepharoptosis (blephar/o means "eyelid") is the drooping of the upper eyelid. **Ectropion** is the turning outward (eversion) of the edge of the eyelid (ec- means "out"; trop means "turn"; -ion means "condition"). Entropion is the opposite, where the eyelid turns inward. A **hordeolum** is also known as a sty and is caused by an infection of the glands near the eyelid.

Infection

Conjunctivitis (conjunctiva is the mucous membrane of the anterior portion of the eye; -itis means "inflammation"; commonly known as pinkeye) is an inflammation of the transparent membrane (conjunctiva) that lines the eyelid and part of the eyeball. The inflammation causes small blood vessels in the conjunctiva to become more prominent, which gives a pink or red cast to the sclera or whites of the eyes. **Keratitis** (kerat/o means "cornea"; -itis means "inflammation") is an inflammation of the cornea that occurs when the cornea has been scratched or otherwise damaged. An inflamed tear sac is called **dacryocystitis**.

Other Disorders of the Eye

Xerophthamia, also known as dry eyes (xer/o means "dry"), occurs when the surface of the eye becomes dry. This is commonly seen in people who wear daily contact lens or who have a diminished tear flow.

Glaucoma is a disease characterized by an increase in intraocular pressure that causes damage to the optic nerve. If left untreated, it can result in permanent blindness. Symptoms frequently go unnoticed by the patient until the optic nerve has been damaged.

A cloudiness or opacity of the lens is called a **cataract** (Fig. 15-8). Cataracts may be caused by disease, injury, chemicals, or exposure to various physical elements. Surgery to replace the clouded lens with an artificial intraocular lens has become common.

DISORDERS OF THE EAR

Hearing loss is the major disorder of the ear. It may range from a partial loss of hearing that involves only certain frequencies to complete **deafness**. A **conductive** hearing loss is defined as one in which the outer or middle ear cannot conduct sound vibrations to the inner ear. A **sensorineural** (sensori refers to the sensory; neural refers to the nerve) hearing loss involves nerve deafness. **Presbycusis** (presby means "old"; -cusis comes from the Greek word *acousis*, which means "hearing") is a progressive hearing loss that may occur as one ages. **Anacusis** (a- means "without"; -cusis comes from the Greek word *acousis*, which means "hearing") is total deafness.

Ear disorders can occur in any of the three parts of the ear—the outer, middle, or inner ear. **Impacted cerumen**, or accumulation of earwax or cerumen in the external auditory canal, may cause a hearing loss. An earache, termed **otalgia** or **otodynia** (ot/o means "ear"; -algia and -dynia both mean "pain"), may be caused by trauma or infections. **Otitis** (ot/o means "ear"; -itis means "inflammation") is any inflammation of the ear, while **otitis media** (media means middle) is an inflammation that pertains to the middle ear. The latter inflammatory process can be painful and is frequently seen in children.

Other inflammations that may occur are **myringitis** (myring/o means "tympanic membrane"; -itis means "inflammation"); **mastoiditis** (mastoid is part of the temporal bone of the skull), which is an inflammation of the mastoid process; and **labyrinthitis** (labyrinth/o means "labyrinth"), which is an inflammation of the labyrinth and may cause dizziness.

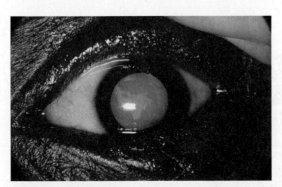

FIGURE 15-8   Clouded cataract lens. From Cohen BJ. Medical Terminology: An Illustrated Guide, 5th Ed. Philadelphia: Lippincott Williams & Wilkins, 2007.

Two other disorders of the ear include **otosclerosis** (ot/o means "ear"; -sclerosis means "hardening") and **Ménière syndrome**. With otosclerosis, sound is unable to travel from the outer to the inner ear where it is converted from mechanical to nervous stimulation. Hardened spongy bone tissue forms in the ear preventing the necessary vibrations from occurring. This frequently involves the stapes. Ménière syndrome is a chronic disease of the inner ear characterized by vertigo, tinnitus, and periodic hearing loss. **Vertigo** is a dizziness and possibly a loss of balance that is frequently seen in patients with Ménière syndrome. **Tinnitus**, or a ringing, buzzing, or roaring sound in the ears, is also a common complaint.

Many disorders of the ear are treated by surgical intervention. Some of these procedures include the following:

- **Otoplasty** (ot/o means "ear"; -plasty means "surgical repair"): surgical repair of the pinna of the ear
- **Mastoidectomy** (mastoid is part of the temporal bone of the skull; -ectomy means "removal of"): surgical removal of the mastoid process
- **Myringectomy** or **tympanectomy** (myring/o and tympan/o both are roots meaning "eardrum"): surgical removal of all or part of the tympanic membrane
- **Myringotomy** (myring/o is a root meaning "eardrum"): surgical incision of the eardrum to create an opening for placement of tubes (ventilating ear tubes to provide ongoing drainage for fluids)
- **Tympanoplasty** (tympan/o means "eardrum"; -plasty means "surgical repair"): surgical correction of a damaged tympanic membrane
- **Stapedectomy** (staped/o means "stapes"; -ectomy means "removal of"): surgical removal of the stapes
- **Labyrinthotomy** (labyrinth/o means "labyrinth"; -tomy means "incision into"): a surgical incision into the labyrinth

Pharmacology

Pharmacologic treatment of the eye is usually done with the topical administration of eye drops or ointments. The most common drug classifications prescribed include antibiotics for infections; **corticosteroids** (cortico means "cortex"; ster/o means "solid"; -oid means "resembling" or "like") for eye inflammations that result from allergies, trauma, or surgery; **cycloplegics** (cyclo means "circle" or "ciliary"; -plegic means "to paralyze") that paralyze the ciliary muscles to dilate the pupil; **mydriatics** that dilate the pupil to facilitate eye examinations; **miotics** that constrict the pupils; and **beta-adrenergic drugs** that lower the intraocular pressure to treat glaucoma.

The most common types of drugs given for ear disorders include antibiotics for infections and antiemetics (anti- means "against"; emetic means "to vomit") for help in controlling the nausea and vomiting accompanying vertigo.

Abbreviation Table • Sight and Hearing

ABBREVIATION	MEANING
AD	right ear [spell out "right ear"]
AS	left ear [spell out "left ear"]
ASL	American Sign Language
AU	both ears [spell out "both ears"]
dB	decibel

ABBREVIATION	MEANING
ECCE	extracapsular cataract extraction
EOM	extraocular movement
ERG	electroretinography
ICCE	intracapsular cataract extraction
IOP	intraocular pressure
OD	right eye [spell out "right eye"]
OM	otitis media
OS	left eye [spell out "left eye"]
OU	both eyes [spell out "both eyes"]
PVD	posterior vitreous detachment (referring to the vitreous body)

Study Table • Sight and Hearing

TERM AND PRONUNCIATION	ANALYSIS	MEANING
Structure and Function: Eye		
accommodation (ah-KOM-moh-DAY-shun)	common English word	the process that allows the shape of the lens to change for near and far vision
aqueous humor (A-kwee-us HUE-mor)	from the Latin word *aqua* (water) + humor, from the Latin word *umor* (body fluid)	thick watery substance filling the space between the lens and the cornea
canthus (KAN-thus)	from the Greek word *kanthus* (corner of the eye)	angle where the upper and lower eyelids meet
choroid (KOH-royd)	derived from the Greek words *chorion* (skin, leather; a spot or plot of ground) and *eidos* (form, likeness, appearance, resemblance)	opaque middle layer of the eyeball
ciliary body (SIL-ee-her-ee)	from the Latin word *ciliaris* (pertaining to eyelashes) + body	set of muscles and suspensory ligaments that adjust the lens
cones	from the Greek word *konos* (cone)	color receptors on the retina that have high visual acuity
conjunctiva (kon-JUNK-tih-vuh); plural: conjunctivae (kon-JUNK-tih-vay)	from the Latin words *con* (with) and *jungere* (to join)	the mucous membrane covering the anterior of the eyeball and inner eyelid

(continued)

TERM AND PRONUNCIATION	ANALYSIS	MEANING
cornea (KOR-nee-uh)	from the Latin word *cornus* (horn)	transparent shield of tissue forming the outer wall of the eyeball
dacryocyst (DACK-ree-oh-sist)	from the Greek words *dakryon* (tear) and *kytis* (bag)	tear sac; lacrimal sac
extraocular (EX-trah-AWK-yu-lahr)	*extra-* (outside); *ocul/o* (eye); *-ar* (adjective suffix)	situated outside the eye
fovea centralis (FOH-avee-ah sen-TRAH-lis)	*fovea*, a Latin word meaning small pit + *centralis*, a Latin word meaning central	a pit in the middle of the retina that is the area of sharpest vision
iris (EYE-rihs); plural: irides (IHR-ih-deez)	a Greek word meaning lily, iris of the eye, originally "messenger of the gods," personified as the rainbow	the anterior part of the vascular tunic; it is the colored part of the eye
lacrimal apparatus (LAK-rih-mahl app-ah-RAT-uhs)	from the Latin words *lacrima* (tear) + *ad* (toward) and *parare* (to make ready)	collectively: the lacrimal gland, lake, canaliculi (small canals), and sac, along with the nasolacrimal duct
lens (lenz)	common English word	the refractive structure of the eye, lying between the iris and the vitreous body
ocular (OK-yoo-lahr)	*ocul/o* (eye); *-ar* (adjective suffix)	adjective referring to the eye
optic nerve (OP-tik nuhrv)	*opt/o* (light, eye, vision); *-ic* (adjective suffix) + nerve	the cranial nerve responsible for vision
orbit (OR-biht)	from the Latin word *orbita* (wheel track, course, orbit)	bony depression in the skull that houses the eyeball
palpebra (pal-PEE-brah)	a Latin word meaning eyelid	eyelid
photoreceptors (FOH-toh-ree-SEPP-tohrs)	from the Greek word *phos* (light) and the Latin word *recipere* (to receive)	retinal cones and rods
pupil (PYOO-pihl)	from the Latin word *pupilla* (little girl-doll) so called from the tiny image one sees of oneself reflected in the eye of another	the dark part in the center of the iris through which light enters the eye
retina (RETT-ih-nah)	from Medieval Latin *retina* probably from the Latin word *rete* (net)	light-sensitive membrane forming the innermost layer of the eyeball

TERM AND PRONUNCIATION	ANALYSIS	MEANING
rods	a common English word	black and white receptors on the retina that respond to dim light
sclera (SKLER-ah); plural: sclerae (SKLER-ay)	from the Greek word *skleros* (hard)	the outer surface of the eye; part of the fibrous tunic
uvea (YOO-vee-ah)	from the Latin word *uva* (grape)	vascular layer of the eye
vitreous body (VIH-tree-uhs BOD-ee)	from the Latin word *vitreus* (of glass, glassy) + body	a transparent jelly-like substance filling the interior of the eyeball
vitreous humor (VIH-tree-uhs HYU-mohr)	from the Latin word *umor* (body fluid)	the fluid component of the vitreous body
Common Disorders: Eye		
amblyopia (am-blee-OH-pee-ah)	from the Greek word *ambly* (dim); *-opia* (eye, vision)	condition that occurs when visual acuity is not the same in both eyes; also called "lazy eye"
astigmatism (ah-STIG-mah-tizm)	*a-* (without) + from the Greek word *stigmatos* gen. of *stigma* (a mark, spot, puncture)	fuzzy vision caused by the irregular shape of one or both eyeballs
blepharitis (bleff-ah-RY-tiss)	*blephar/o* (eyelid); *-itis* (inflammation)	inflammation of the eyelid
blepharoconjunctivitis (BLEFF-ah-roh-kon-junk-tih-VY-tiss)	*blephar/o* (eyelid); *conjunctiv/o* (mucous membrane covering the anterior surface of the eyeball and inner eyelid); *-itis* (inflammation)	inflammation of the palpebral conjunctiva, the inner lining of the eyelids
blepharoplegia (BLEFF-ah-roh-pleej-ee-uh)	*blephar/o* (eyelid); *-plegia* (paralysis)	paralysis of an eyelid
blepharoptosis (BLEFF-ahr-opp-TOH-sis)	*blephar/o* (eyelid); *-ptosis* (falling, downward placement, prolapse)	drooping eyelid
blepharospasm (BLEFF-ahr-oh-SPAZ-um)	*blephar/o* (eyelid); from the Greek *spasmos* (spasm, convulsion)	involuntary contraction of the eyelid
cataract (KAT-ah-rakt)	from the Latin word *cataracta* (waterfall)	complete or partial opacity of the ocular lens
conjunctivitis (kon-junk-tih-VY-tiss)	*conjunctiv/o* (mucous membrane covering the anterior surface of the eyeball); *-itis* (inflammation)	inflammation of the conjunctiva; pinkeye

(continued)

TERM AND PRONUNCIATION	ANALYSIS	MEANING
dacryocele (DAKK-ree-oh-seel)	*dacry/o* (tears); *-cele* (hernia)	herniated lacrimal sac (filled with fluid); often called a *dacryocystocele*, because *dacryocyst* is a synonym for *lacrimal sac*
dacryocystitis (DAKK-ree-oh-SIST-it is)	*dacryocyst/o* (tear sac); *-itis* (inflammation)	inflammation of the tear sac
dacryolith (DAKK-ree-oh-lith)	*dacry/o* (tears); *-lith* (stone)	a "stone" in the lacrimal apparatus
dacryorrhea (DAK-ree-uh-REE-yuh)	*dacry/o* (tears); *-rrhea* (discharge)	excessive discharge of tears
glaucoma (glaw-KOH-mah)	from the Greek word *glaucoma* (cataract, opacity of the lens) (note: cataracts and glaucoma not distinguished until around 1705)	disease of the eye characterized by increased intraocular pressure and atrophy of the optic nerve
hordeolum (hor-DEE-oh-lum)	from the Latin word *hordeum* (barley)	a sty on the eyelid; a sty is an infection of a gland in the eye
hyperopia (hy-pur-OH-pee-ya) or presbyopia (pres-be-OH-pee-ah)	*hyper-* (above normal); *-opia* (eye, vision)	farsightedness
iridomalacia (IHR-ih-doh-muh-LAY-shee-uh)	*irid/o* (iris); *-malacia* (softening)	softening of the iris
iritis (eye-RY-tiss)	*ir/o* (iris); *-itis* (inflammation)	inflammation of the iris
keratitis (ker-ah-TYE-tis)	*kerat/o* (hard, cornea); *-itis* (inflammation)	inflammation of the cornea
lacrimal (LAK-rih-muhl)	*lacrim/o* (tear, lacrimal apparatus); *-al* (adjective suffix)	referring to or related to tears or the tear ducts and glands
lacrimation (LAK-rih-MAY-shun)	*lacrim/o* (tear, lacrimal apparatus); *-ation* (noun suffix)	excessive tearing; synonym for *dacryorrhea*
myopia (my-OHP-ee-ah)	from the Greek word *myops* (nearsighted)	nearsightedness
oculodynia (AWK-yu-loh-DIN-ee-ah)	*ocul/o* (eye); *-dynia* (pain)	pain in the eyeball
oculopathy (AWK-yu-loh-path-ee)	*ocul/o* (eye); *-pathy* (disease)	generic term for eye disease; synonym for *ophthalmopathy*

TERM AND PRONUNCIATION	ANALYSIS	MEANING
ophthalmolith (off-THAL-moh-lith)	*ophthalm/o* (eye); *-lith* (stone)	a stone in the lacrimal apparatus; synonym for *dacryolith*
ophthalmomalacia (off-THAL -moh-muh-LAY-shee-uh)	*ophthalm/o* (eye); *-malacia* (softening)	softening of the eyeball
ophthalmopathy (off-THAL-moh-path-ee)	*ophthalm/o* (eye); *-pathy* (disease)	generic term for eye disease; synonym for oculopathy
presbyopia (prez-bee-OH-pee-ah)	from the Greek word *presbys* (old man); *-opia* (eye, vision)	farsightedness resulting from loss of elasticity of the lens due to aging
retinitis (rett-ih-NY-tiss)	*retin/o* (retina); *-itis* (inflammation)	inflammation of the retina
retinopathy (rett-ihn-AWP-uh-thee)	*retin/o* (retina); *-pathy* (disease)	disease of the retina
scleroiritis (skler-oh-EYE-RY-tiss)	*sclera/o* (sclera); *ir/o* (iris); *-itis* (inflammation)	inflammation of the sclera and iris
strabismus (stra-BIZ-muhs)	from the Greek word *strabismos*, from *strabos* (squinting, squint-eyed)	lack of parallelism in the visual axes; crossed eyes
xerophthalmia (zee-roh-OFF-thal-mee-ah)	from the Greek word *xeros* (dry); *ophthalm/o* (eye); *-ia* (condition)	dry eyes

Practice and Practitioners: Eye

ophthalmologist (off-thul-MAWL-uh-jist)	*ophthalm/o* (eye); *-logist* (one who studies a specific field)	physician whose specialty is the diagnosis and treatment of eye disorders
ophthalmology (off-thul-MAWL-uh-jee)	*ophthalm/o* (eye); *-logy* (study of)	medical specialty dealing with the eye
optician (opp-TISH-ihn)	*opt/o* (light, eye, vision)	a maker of lenses
optometrist (opp-TOM-uh-trist)	*opt/o* (light, eye, vision); *-metrist* (one who measures)	one trained in examining the eyes and prescribing corrective lenses
optometry (opp-TOM-uh-tree)	*opt/o* (light, eye, vision); *-metry* (measurement)	science of examining eyes for impaired vision and other disorders

Diagnosis and Treatment: Eye

ophthalmoscope (OFF-THAL-moh-skope)	*ophthalm/o* (eye); *-scope* (instrument for viewing)	device for examining the interior of the eyeball by looking through the pupil
ophthalmoscopy (OFF-thal-MAW-skuh-pee)	*ophthalm/o* (eye); *-scopy* (use of instrument for viewing)	examination of the eye with an ophthalmoscope

(continued)

TERM AND PRONUNCIATION	ANALYSIS	MEANING
refraction (re-FRAK-shun)	from the Latin wod *refractus*, pp of *refringere* (to break up)	deflection of a ray of light into the eye for accommodation or correction of vision as it passes from one medium to another of different density

Surgical Procedures: Eye

blepharectomy (bleff-ah-REK-tuh-mee)	*blephar/o* (eyelid); *-ectomy* (excision)	surgical removal of part or all of an eyelid
blepharoplasty (BLEFF-ah-roh-plass-tee)	*blephar/o* (eyelid); *-plasty* (surgical repair)	surgery to correct a defective eyelid
blepharotomy (BLEFF-uh-rot-uh-mee)	*blephar/o* (eyelid); *-tomy* (incision into)	surgical incision of an eyelid
conjunctivoplasty (kon-JUNK-tih-voh-plass-tee)	*conjunctiv/o* (conjunctiva); *-plasty* (surgical repair)	surgery on the conjunctiva
dacryocystectomy (dakk-ree-oh-sist-EKK-toh-mee)	*dacryocyst/o* (tear sac); *-ectomy* (excision)	surgical removal of the lacrimal sac
dacryocystotomy (dakk-ree-oh-sist-AW-toh-mee)	*dacryocyst/o* (tear sac); *-tomy* (incision into)	incision into the lacrimal sac
lacrimotomy (lakk-rih-MAW-toh-mee) (uncommon)	*lacrim/o* (tear, lacrimal apparatus); *-tomy* (incision into)	incision into the lacrimal sac; rarely used synonym for dacryocystotomy
phacolysis (fah-KAWL-uh-sis)	*phac/o* (lens); *-lysis* (destruction)	operative removal of the lens in pieces
retinectomy (ret-ihn-EK-tuh-mee)	*retin/o* (retina); *-ectomy* (excision)	surgical removal of part of the retina
retinopexy (RETT-ihn-oh-pexx-ee)	*retin/o* (retina); *-pexy* (surgical fixation	surgical fixation of a detached retina
retinotomy (rett-ihn-AW-tuh-mee)	*retin/o* (retina); *-tomy* (incision into)	incision through the retina

Structure and Function: Ear

auricle (AW-rik-uhl)	*auri-* (ear)	one of the two parts of the external ear (the other part is the auditory canal)
cerumen (seh-ROO-men)	from the Latin word *cera* (wax)	wax-like secretion occurring in the external auditory canal
cochlea (KOK-lee-uh)	a Latin word meaning snail shell	part of the bony labyrinth
eustachian tube (yu-STAY-shun)	named after Bartolomeo Eustachia (died 1574), who discovered the passages from the ears to the throat	the auditory tube that connects the middle ear to the pharynx

TERM AND PRONUNCIATION	ANALYSIS	MEANING
external auditory canal (ODD-ih-tor-ee)	from the Latin word *auditorius* (pertaining to hearing)	one of the two parts of the external ear (the other part is the auricle)
incus (INK-uhs)	a Latin word meaning anvil	one of the auditory ossicles (the anvil)
labyrinth (LAB-uh-rinth)	from the Greek word *labyrinthos* (maze, large building with intricate passages)	canals of the inner ear
malleus (MAL-ee-uhs)	a Latin word meaning hammer	one of the auditory ossicles (the hammer)
ossicles (OSS-ih-kulz)	from the Latin word *ossiculum* (a small bone)	three small bones in the middle ear: the malleus (hammer), the incus (anvil), and the stapes (stirrup)
pinna (PIN-ah)	a Latin word meaning feather, wing, fin, lobe	another term for *auricle*
stapes (STAY-peez)	a Modern Latin word meaning stirrup	one of the auditory ossicles (the stirrup)
tympanic cavity (tim-PAN-ik)	*tympan/o* (ear drum); *-ic* (adjective suffix) + cavity	the middle ear
tympanic membrane (tim-PAN-ik MEM-brayn)	*tympan/o* (ear drum); *-ic* (adjective suffix)	the eardrum
Common Disorders: Ear		
anacusis (ann-ah-KU-sis)	*a-* (without); cusis, from the Greek word *akousis* (hearing)	totál deafness
conductive hearing loss (kon-DUK-tihv)	common English words	hearing loss caused by interference with sound transmission in the external auditory canal, middle ear, or ossicles
labyrinthitis (lab-ih-rin-THIGH-tis)	*labyrinth/o* (internal ear); *-itis* (inflammation)	inflammation of the labyrinth
mastoiditis (mas-toy-DYE-tis)	mastoid (mastoid process); *-itis* (inflammation)	inflammation of any part of the mastoid process
Ménière syndrome (men-YEHRS)	named for Prosper Ménière, the French physician who first described the illness in 1861	chronic disease of the inner ear characterized by vertigo, tinnitus, and periodic hearing loss
myringitis (mir-in-JIGH-tis)	*myring/o* (tympanic membrane); *-itis* (inflammation)	inflammation of the tympanic membrane

(continued)

TERM AND PRONUNCIATION	ANALYSIS	MEANING
otalgia (oh-TAHL-jee-ah)	*ot/o* (ear); *-algia* (pain)	pain in the ear
otitis (oh-TY-tihs)	*ot/o* (ear); *-itis* (inflammation)	inflammation of the ear (otitis externa = the outer ear; otitis media = the middle ear; otitis interna = the inner ear)
otodynia (oh-toh-DIN-ee-uh)	*ot/o* (ear); *-dynia* (pain)	earache
otopathy (oh-TOP-ahth-ee)	*ot/o* (ear); *-pathy* (disease)	any disease of the ear
otoplasty (oh-toh-PLAS-tee)	*ot/o* (ear); *-plasty* (surgical repair)	surgical repair of the pinna of the ear
otorrhea (oh-toh-REE-uh)	*ot/o* (ear); *-rrhea* (discharge)	fluid discharge from the ear
otosclerosis (OH-toh-skler-OH-sihs)	*ot/o* (ear); *scler/o* (hardening); *-osis* (abnormal condition)	formation of spongy bone in the inner ear producing hearing loss
presbycusis (PREZ-be-KOO-sihs)	*presby-* (old); cusis, from the Greek word *akousis* (hearing)	hearing loss that occurs with aging
sensorineural hearing loss (SENTZ-oh-rih-NOO-rahl)	*sensor-* (sensory); *neur/o* (nervous system); *-al* (adjective suffix)	hearing loss caused by a neural condition
tinnitus (TIN-nih-tuhs)	from the Latin word *tinnire* (to ring)	sensation of noises (such as ringing) in the ears
vertigo (VUR-tih-go)	a Latin word meaning dizziness	sensation of spinning or whirling; can be caused by infection or other disorder in the inner ear

Practice and Practitioners: Ear

audiologist (awd-ee-AWL-oh-jist)	*audi/o* (sound, hearing); *-logist* (one who studies a certain field)	specialist who measures hearing efficiency and treats hearing impairment
audiology (awd-ee-AWL-oh-jee)	*audi/o* (sound, hearing); *-logy* (the study of a certain field)	specialty dealing with hearing and hearing disorders
otologist (oh-TOL-oh-jist)	*ot/o* (ear); *-logist* (one who studies a certain field)	specialist in otology, the branch of medical science concerned with the study, diagnosis, and treatment of diseases of the ear and its related structures

TERM AND PRONUNCIATION	ANALYSIS	MEANING
otology (oh-TOL-oh-jee)	*ot/o* (ear); *-logy* (the study of a certain field)	branch of medical science concerned with the study, diagnosis, and treatment of diseases of the ear and its related structures
otorhinolaryngologist (oh-TOH-REYE-no-lair-in-GOL-oh-jist)	*ot/o* (ear); *rhin/o* (nose); *laryng/o* (throat); *-logist* (one who studies a certain field)	physician who specializes in the diagnosis and treatment of ear, nose, and throat disorders
Diagnosis and Treatment: Ear		
audiogram (AW-dee-oh-gram)	*audi/o* (sound, hearing); *-gram* (record or picture)	automatically recorded results of a hearing test with an audiometer
audiometer (aw-dee-AWM-ih-tehr)	*audi/o* (sound, hearing); *-meter* (measurement)	electrical device for measuring hearing
audiometry (aw-dee-AWM-ih-tree)	*audi/o* (sound, hearing); *-metry* (process of measuring)	measuring hearing with an audiometer
cochlear implant (KOK-lee-ahr IM-plant)	from the Latin word *cochlea* (snail shell); *-ar* (adjective suffix) + implant	surgically implanted hearing aid in the cochlea
otoscope (OH-toh-skope)	*ot/o* (ear); *-scope* (instrument for viewing)	device for looking into the ear
otoscopy (oh-TOSS-kuh-pee)	*ot/o* (ear); *-scopy* (use of an instrument for viewing)	looking into the ear with an otoscope
Rinne test (rihn-eh)	named after Heinrich A. Rinne, German otologist (1819–1868)	hearing test using a tuning fork; checks for differences in bone conduction and air conduction
tuning fork (TOO-ning)	common English words	an instrument that vibrates when struck
Weber test (VAY-behr)	named after Wilhelm Edward Weber, German physicist (1804–1891)	hearing test using a tuning fork; distinguishes between conductive and sensorineural hearing loss
Surgical Procedures: Ear		
labyrinthotomy (lab-ih-rin-THAH-toh-mee)	*labyrinth/o* (internal ear); *-tomy* (incision into)	a surgical incision into the labyrinth
mastoidectomy (mas-toy-DECK-toh-mee)	mastoid (mastoid process) + *-ectomy* (excision)	surgical removal of the mastoid process

(continued)

TERM AND PRONUNCIATION	ANALYSIS	MEANING
myringectomy (mir-ini-JECK-toh-mee) or tympanectomy	*myring/o* (tympanic membrane); *-ectomy* (excision)	surgical removal of all or part of the tympanic membrane
myringoplasty (mih-RIN-go-PLASS-tee)	*myring/o* (tympanic membrane); *-plasty* (surgical repair)	surgical repair of the tympanic membrane (eardrum)
myringotomy (mih-rin-GOT-uh-mee)	*myring/o* (tympanic membrane); *-tomy* (incision into)	incision or surgical puncture of the eardrum
otoplasty (OH-toh-plass-tee)	*ot/o* (ear); *-plasty* (surgical repair)	surgical repair of the pinna of the ear
stapedectomy (stay-peh-DECK-toh-mee)	*staped/o* (stapes); *-ectomy* (excision)	surgical removal of the stapes
tympanectomy (TIM-puh-NEK-tuh-mee)	*tympan/o* (eardrum); *-tomy* (incision into)	surgical removal of the eardrum
tympanocentesis (TIM-puh-noh-senn-TEE-sihs)	*tympan/o* (eardrum); *-centesis* (surgical puncture for aspiration)	puncture of the tympanic membrane with a needle to aspirate middle ear fluid
tympanoplasty (TIM-puh-no-plass-tee)	*tympan/o* (eardrum); *-plasty* (surgical repair)	surgery performed on the eardrum
tympanotomy (TIM-puh-NOT-oh-mee);	*tympan/o* (eardrum); *-tomy* (incision)	synonyms for *myringotomy*

EXERCISES

EXERCISE 15-1   Figure Labeling: The Eye

Use the following terms to label the diagram:

choroid	fovea centralis	retina
ciliary body	iris	sclera
cornea	lens	vitreous humor

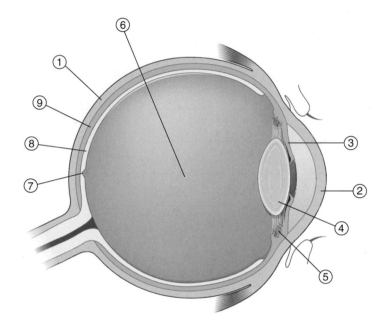

1. _____   6. _____

2. _____   7. _____

3. _____   8. _____

4. _____   9. _____

5. _____

EXERCISE 15-2   Operative Report

Read the following report and define the italicized terminology in the spaces below.

PREOPERATIVE DIAGNOSIS: Chronic (1) *otitis media*

OPERATIVE PROCEDURE: Bilateral (2) *myringotomy* and placement of tubes

INDICATIONS: Recurrent ear infections with persistent fluid buildup despite prolonged medical treatment

PROCEDURE: The patient was brought to the operating suite and placed under general mask anesthesia. The ear canals were cleaned of dry (3) *cerumen* and crust. Myringotomies were placed bilaterally. Cultures were taken of the fluid present in the middle ear spaces. Ear tubes were placed in the myringotomy sites bilaterally. (4) *Antibiotic* drops and cotton balls were placed in the ear canal.

The patient tolerated the procedure well and was taken to the recovery room.

1. _____

2. _____

3. _____

4. _____

EXERCISE 15-3   Matching Terms with Definitions: Eye

Match the terms in Column 1 with the correct definitions in Column 2.

TERM

1. _____ ophthalmology

2. _____ vitreous humor

3. _____ pupil

4. _____ iris

5. _____ sclera

6. _____ cornea

7. _____ conjunctiva

8. _____ ophthalmoscope

9. _____ retina

10. _____ lacrimal

DEFINITION

A. transparent shield of tissue covering the iris

B. adjective associated with tears

C. sensitive inner nerve layer of the eye that contains the rods and cones

D. the "colored" part of the eye

E. the dark part in the very center of the eye

F. mucous membrane that covers the anterior surface of the eyeball and lines the underside of each eyelid

G. gelatinous liquid between the lens and retina

H. part of the outermost layer of the eye, which is white in color

I. a device for examining the interior of the eyeball by looking through the pupil

J. name of the medical specialty dealing with the eye

EXERCISE 15-4   Matching Terms with Definitions: Ear

Match the terms in Column 1 with the correct definitions in Column 2.

TERM

1. _____ audiologist

2. _____ cerumen

3. _____ otoscope

4. _____ tympanoplasty

5. _____ labyrinth

6. _____ auditory ossicles

7. _____ otitis media

8. _____ tympanic membrane

9. _____ Eustachian tube

10. _____ cochlea

DEFINITION

A. the eardrum

B. maze-like portion of the inner ear

C. specialist treating abnormal hearing

D. device for looking in the ear

E. inflammation of the middle ear

F. part of the bony labyrinth (inner ear)

G. wax-like secretion in the external auditory canal

H. auditory tube that connects the middle ear to the nasopharynx

I. surgical repair on the tympanic membrane

J. three small bones in the middle ear: the malleus, incus, and stapes

EXERCISE 15-5   Fill in the Blank

Select a term from the list and complete the statements. Note that not all terms will be used.

antiemetic	cataract	hordeolum	OD	presbycusis
astigmatism	cycloplegic	keratitis	otalgia	presbyopia
audiometry	diplopia	labyrinthitis	otosclerosis	tinnitus
blepharoptosis	glaucoma	Ménière disease	pinna	vertigo
xerophthalmia				

1. A cloudiness or opacity of the lens is called _____.

2. Difficulty hearing due to the aging process is termed _____.

3. The medical term for double vision is _____.

4. Another name for dizziness due to an inner ear disturbance is _____.

5. _____ is a ringing or buzzing of the ears.

6. The external ear component is called the auricle or _____.

7. Another name for a sty is _____.

8. _____ means pain in the ear or an earache.

9. An irregularity of the curve of the cornea that distorts the light entering the eye is called _____.

10. An inflammation of the cornea is called _____.

11. The medical term for "dry eyes" is _____.

12. The drug classification that is prescribed for nausea and vomiting is _____.

13. An ankylosis (fixation) of the bones of the middle ear resulting in a conductive hearing loss is called _____.

14. _____ is the proper term for a drooping eyelid.

15. The measurement of hearing is called _____.

EXERCISE 15-6   Crossword Puzzle: Eye and Ear

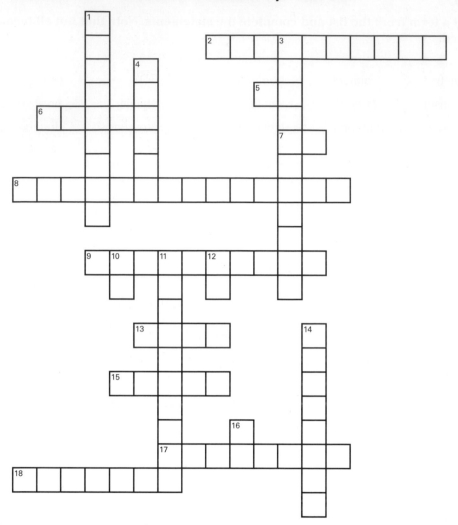

ACROSS

2. deviation of the visual lines of the eye so that the eyes are not directed at the same object
5. abbreviation for right eye
6. root of cornea
7. abbreviation for left eye
8. instrument used to examine the eye
9. tear sac
13. colored muscular ring that surrounds the pupil
15. lay term for ossicle is anvil
17. root for eye
18. earwax

DOWN

1. inner ear maze like struture
3. health care professional that measures hearing, treats hearing disorder
4. innermost layer of the eye, actual visual receptor
10. abbreviation for left ear
11. bending of light rays
12. abbreviation for both eyes
14. small bones in the ear
16. root for ear

CHAPTER 15 QUIZ

Multiple Choice

1. The medical specialist who treats ear disorders is called a(n):
   a. ophthalmologist
   b. otologist
   c. audiologist
   d. optometrist

2. A term for eardrum is:
   a. tympanic membrane
   b. malleus
   c. oval window
   d. none of the above

3. The function(s) of the ear include:
   a. equilibrium
   b. hearing
   c. sound vibrations
   d. both A and B

4. The ability of the eye to adjust to variations in distance is:
   a. eversion
   b. strabismus
   c. accommodation
   d. presbycusis

5. An inflammation of the tear sac is:
   a. dacryocystitis
   b. scleritis
   c. blepharitis
   d. keratitis

6. The layer of the eye that contains the rods and cones is the:
   a. sclera
   b. choroid
   c. uvea
   d. retina

7. Hearing loss that is due to nerve damage is a:
   a. conductive loss
   b. sensorineural loss
   c. tympanitis
   d. tinnitus

8. The cornea is the transparent part of the eye and is an extension of the:
   a. choroid
   b. iris
   c. sclera
   d. both A and C

9. The ciliary body is:
   a. a group of muscles that suspends the lens
   b. the curved portion of the eye that refracts light
   c. the area between the lens and retina
   d. the protective layer of the eye

10. Farsightedness is called:
    a. myopia
    b. hyperopia
    c. presbyopia
    d. both B and C

Fill in the blank with the correct term.

11. The root word for *stapes* is _____.

12. _____ is an inflammation of the tympanic membrane.

13. _____ is a disease characterized by an increase in intraocular pressure.

14. The tube that goes from the middle ear to the nasopharynx is the _____.

15. The abbreviation for right eye is _____.

16. An inflammation of the mastoid process is _____.

17. A _____ hearing loss is one in which the outer or middle ear cannot conduct the sound vibrations to the inner ear.

18. A surgical incision into the labyrinth is called a _____.

19. The abbreviation for left ear is _____.

20. The _____ contains the sensory receptors for hearing.

APPENDIX A
Answers to Chapter Exercises

CHAPTER 1
EXERCISE 1-1   Word Elements

1. append/o (CF)	append (R)	-ectomy (S)
2. post- (P)	nat (R)	-al (S)
3.	mast (R)	-itis (S)
4. colon/o (CF)		-scope (S)
5. enter/o (CF)	col(R)	-itis (S)
6. pre- (P)	nat (R)	-al (S)
7. oste/o, (CF)	arthr (R)	-itis (S)
8. arthr/o (CF)		-tomy (S)
9.	thyroid (R)	-ectomy(S)
10. amni/o (CF)		-centesis (S)

EXERCISE 1-2   Combining Roots and Suffixes

1. -logy	psychology;	-pathy	psychopathy			
2. -logy	pathology					
3. -dynia	cardiodynia;	-pathy	cardiopathy			
4. -logy	hematology;	-pathy	hematopathy			
5. -itis	dermatitis;	-pathy	dermatopathy			
6. -dynia	arthrodynia;	-algia	arthralgia;	-itis	arthritis
7. -algia	neuralgia;	-dynia	neurodynia;	-pathy	neuropathy
8. -itis	osteitis;	-pathy	osteopathy			

EXERCISE 1-3   Matching Word Elements with Meanings

1. F	6. B
2. G	7. E
3. A	8. C
4. D	9. J
5. H	10. I

CHAPTER 1 QUIZ

1. root, prefix, suffix
2. inflammation of the skin
3. heart
4. tumor of a nerve
5. nuclei
6. gerontology
7. root and combining vowel
8. arthroscope
9. gastrectomy
10. hepatomegaly

CHAPTER 2

EXERCISE 2-1   Combining Roots and Suffixes That Signify Medical Conditions

1. card/i/o
   a. cardiocele; herniation of the heart
   b. cardiodynia; heart pain
   c. cardiectasia; dilation of the heart
   d. carditis; inflammation of the heart
   e. cardiomalacia; softening of the heart
   f. cardiomegaly; enlargement
      of the heart
   g. cardioptosis; drooping of the heart
   h. cardioplegia; paralysis of the heart
   i. cardiorrhexis; rupture of the heart
   j. cardiospasm; spasm of the heart
2. dermat/o
   a. dermatitis; inflammation of the skin
   b. dermatoma; tumor of the skin
   c. dermatomegaly; enlargement
      of the skin
   d. dermatosis; abnormal condition
      of the skin
3. hem/o, hemat/o
   a. hemolysis; destruction of the blood cells
   b. hematogenesis; produced
      by the blood
   c. hematoma; localized mass of blood
   d. hematosis; abnormal condition of
      the blood

4. neur/o
   a. neuralgia; nerve pain
   b. neurectasis; dilation of a nerve
   c. neuritis; inflammation of a nerve
   d. neuroma; tumor of a nerve
5. oste/o
   a. osteodynia; bone pain
   b. osteoma; bone tumor
   c. osteomalacia; softening of the bone
   d. osteopenia; decreased bone density
   e. osteoporosis; reduction in the quantity
      of bone
   f. osteitis; inflammation of the bone
6. psych/o
   a. psychosis; severe mental
      and behavioral disorder

EXERCISE 2-2   Combining Roots and Suffixes That Signify Diagnostic Terms, Test Information, or Surgical Procedures

1. card/i/o
   a. cardiogenic; originating in the heart
   b. cardiogram; graphic record
      of the heart
   c. cardiograph; machine that produces
      a cardiogram
   d. cardiography; process of electrically
      measuring heart function
   e. cardiopathy; heart disease
   f. cardiorrhaphy; suture of the wall
      of the heart
2. dermatoplasty; surgical repair of the skin
3. hemat/o
   a. hematogenesis; originating with
      or in the blood
   b. hematometry; examination of blood

4. neur/o
   a. neurectomy; removal of a nerve
      or part of a nerve
   b. neurogenic; adjectival from of
      neurogenesis
   c. neurogenesis; originating
      in the nervous system
5. oste/o
   a. osteorrhaphy; suturing broken bone
      together
   b. osteoplasty; surgical repair of the bone
   c. osteogenesis; formation of bone
   d. ostectomy; excision of bone
   e. osteotomy; cutting of bone

6. path/o
   a. pathogen; a disease-causing agent
   b. pathogenic; adjectival form of
      pathogen
   c. pathogenesis; development
      of a disease

7. psych/o
   a. psychogenic; adjectival form of
      psychogenesis
   b. psychogenesis; mental development
   c. psychometry; mental testing
   d. psychopath; mentally ill person

EXERCISE 2-3   Combining Roots and Suffixes Associated with a Medical Specialist or Specialty

1. card/i/o
   a. cardiology; medical specialty that
      diagnoses and treats heart diseases
   b. cardiologist; heart specialist
2. derm/o, dermat/o
   a. dermatology; medical specialty that
      diagnoses and treats skin disorders
   b. dermatologist; skin specialist
3. ger/o/, geront/o
   a. geriatrics; medical specialty that
      diagnoses and treats the aged
   b. gerontology; the study of the process
      and results of aging
   c. gerontologist; specialist in gerontology
4. hem/o, hemat/o
   a. hematology; medical specialty that
      diagnoses and treats blood disorders
   b. hematologist; a specialist who treats
      blood disorders
5. neur/o
   a. neurology; medical specialty that diag-
      noses and treats the nervous system
   b. neurologist; specialist who treats
      the nervous system

6. oste/o
   a. osteology; medical specialty that
      diagnoses and treats disorders of the
      skeletal system; orthopedics
   b. osteologist; a bone specialist or
      orthopedic surgeon
7. path/o
   a. pathology; study of disease
   b. pathologist; a medical specialist
      who studies pathology
8. ped/o, pedi/o, pedia/o
   a. pediatrics; medical specialty dealing
      with children
   b. pediatrician; specialist in childhood
      development and disease
9. psych/o
   a. psychology; study of the mind
   b. psychiatry; the medical specialty that
      diagnoses and treats mind disorders
   c. psychiatrist; a medical specialist
      in psychiatry

EXERCISE 2-4   Combining Roots and Suffixes That Denote Adjectives

1. card/i/o
   a. cardiac, cardial; refers to the heart
2. hemat/o, hem/o
   a. hematic; refers to the blood
3. derm/o, dermat/o
   a. dermal; adjective denoting skin
   b. dermatic; adjective denoting skin
4. ger/o, geront/o
   a. geriatric; adjectival form of *geriatrics*
   b. gerontal; adjective meaning
      "old-age related"

5. neur/o
   a. neural; adjective meaning
      "related to the nervous system"
   b. neurotic; adjectival form of *neurosis*
6. spin/o
   a. spinal; adjective referring to spinal
      column
   b. spinous; adjective meaning
      "having spines"
7. oste/o
   a. osteal; adjective meaning "bone"
   b. osteoid; adjective meaning
      "resembling bone"

EXERCISE 2-5   Matching Suffixes with Meanings

1. G	6. D	11. A
2. I	7. C	12. O
3. B	8. H	13. N
4. M	9. F	14. K
5. J	10. E	15. L

EXERCISE 2-6   Adding Prefixes of Time or Speed

1. anteroom; outer room that leads into another room
2. neoclassic; new classic work
3. postglacial; following the glacial period
4. predominant; important
5. tachymeter; instrument used to compute speed based on travel time or measure distance based on speed

EXERCISE 2-7   Adding Prefixes of Direction

1. abnormal; adjective meaning "away from normal"
2. adjoining; adjective meaning "next to"
3. concentric; having the same center
4. contralateral; the other side
5. diagram; illustration that gives an overall view
6. sympathetic; sharing emotions with another person
7. synthesis; assembling parts into a whole

EXERCISE 2-8   Adding Prefixes of Position

1. eccentric; outside the center; unusual
2. ectomorph; slightly built person
3. enslave; to make a slave of
4. endocardial; adjective meaning "inside the heart"
5. epidemic; great number of occurrences of a particular disease
6. exchange; give something in return for another
7. exosphere; the far reaches of the atmosphere
8. extraterrestrial; beyond the earth
9. hypersensitive; highly sensitive
10. hypothesis; a possible explanation underlying the facts
11. infrastructure; the internal framework of a system or organization
12. intercollegiate; participation involving at least two colleges
13. intramural; inside the walls; often applied to sports teams within a school
14. mesosphere; the middle part of the earth's atmosphere
15. metaphysics; beyond physics
16. panorama; a wide expansive view of everything
17. paralegal; a trained assistant to a lawyer
18. retrorocket; a rocket that provides thrust in the direction of motion to slow a vehicle

EXERCISE 2-9   Adding Prefixes of Size or Number

1. biannual; occurring twice a year
2. hemisphere; half of a sphere
3. macrocosm; the universe
4. microscope; a device for viewing objects invisible to the human eye
5. monorail; a railway system on which the vehicle travels on one rail
6. oligarchy; rule by a small group of people
7. quadrilateral; having four sides
8. semiannual; twice a year
9. triangle; three-sided geometric shape
10. unicycle; a vehicle having one wheel

EXERCISE 2-10   Crossword Puzzle

1. across: prefix, big–MACRO
   down: prefix, one–MONO
2. prefix, above or beyond normal–HYPER
3. suffix, study of–LOGY
4. across: prefix, away from–AB
   down: prefix, against–ANTI
5. prefix, total or everywhere–PAN
6. across: prefix, between or across–INTER
   down: suffix, inflammation–ITIS
7. suffix, pictorial recording–GRAPH
8. prefix, before–PRE
9. suffix, narrowing–STENOSIS
10. prefix, abnormally fast–TACHY
11. suffix, act of viewing–SCOPY
12. suffix, device for measuring–METER
13. across: suffix, cell–CYTE
    down: suffix, protrusion–CELE
14. suffix, pain–DYNIA
15. suffix, removal of–ECTOMY
16. prefix, four–QUADRI

CHAPTER 2 QUIZ

SUFFIXES

1. -algia, -dynia
2. angiectasis
3. adjective
4. suture of a blood vessel
5. -graphy
6. tumor of the blood vessel
7. surgical repair;
8. dermatologist
9. old
10. gerontology is a noun
    geriatrics is an adjective

PREFIXES

1. ad-
2. ante-
3. abnormally slow
   heartbeat
4. beyond
5. hyper-
6. radar used to prevent
   a collision
7. three
8. the instrument will make
   visible the objects that
   are too small to see
9. endocarditis; inflammation
   of the inside of the heart
10. tachypnea is rapid
    breathing; dyspnea is
    difficulty or painful
    breathing

CHAPTER 3
EXERCISE 3-1   Matching

A. PLANES OF THE BODY

1. C   2. B   3. A

B. DIRECTIONAL TERMS

1. F   3. H   5. I   7. A   9. C
2. G   4. J   6. E   8. D   10. B

EXERCISE 3-2   Fill in the Blank

1. distal
2. distal
3. anterior, ventral
4. ventral, anterior
5. superior
6. lateral
7. posterior, dorsal
8. inferior

EXERCISE 3-3   Word Building

1. hypo-, -ic hypogastric
2. -al dorsal
3. -itis chondritis
4. trans-, -ic transthoracic
5. -itis neuritis
6. epi-, -al epicardial

EXERCISE 3-4   Crossword Puzzle

1. umbilicus
2. chromosome
3. organ
4. anterior
5. transverse
6. hypogastric
7. respiratory
8. five
9. epithelial
10. connective
11. digestive
12. posterior
13. cytoplasm

CHAPTER 3 QUIZ

1. lateral
2. towards the back
3. proximal
4. anterior or forward
5. muscle pain
6. guts, internal organs
7. False, face down
8. True
9. False, lateral to the big toe
10. True
11. True
12. False, coccyx is the tailbone
13. True

CHAPTER 4
EXERCISE 4-1   Case Study

1. antibiotic; medication used to kill bacteria or treat an infection
2. Benadryl; medication used to relieve itching
3. impetigo; contagious superficial skin infection that presents with vesicles
4. dermatologist; medical specialist who diagnoses and treats disorders of the skin
5. dermatitis; inflammation of the skin
6. erythematous; redness of the skin
7. pustules; small elevated area of skin that contains pus
8. edema; swelling in the tissues
9. antipruritic; medication used to reduce or stop itching
10. pruritus; itching

EXERCISE 4-2   Labeling the Skin

1. epidermis
2. dermis (corium)
3. subcutaneous layer
4. adipose tissue
5. hair follicle
6. vein
7. nerve
8. artery
9. sudoriferous gland
10. sebaceous gland
11. nerve endings
12. hair

EXERCISE 4-3   Word Building

1. dermatitis
2. melanoma
3. epidermis
4. onychopathy
5. dermatology
6. ichthyosis
7. subcutaneous
8. percutaneous
9. intradermal
10. epidermis

EXERCISE 4-4   Matching

1. D
2. E
3. I
4. F
5. B
6. C
7. G
8. J
9. H
10. A

EXERCISE 4-5   Pronunciation

There are no right/wrong answers. The student can select ANY terms from the CD they want and pronounce them.

EXERCISE 4-6   Integumentary System Crossword Puzzle

1. cuticle
2. pustule
3. dermis
4. shingles
5. melanoma
6. adipose
7. scabies
8. necr
9. tinea
10. lesion
11. paronychia
12. melanin
13. alopecia
14. erythematous
15. cry
16. onych
17. vitiligo

CHAPTER 4 QUIZ

1. B	8. C	15. alopecia
2. B	9. B	16. albinism
3. B	10. B	17. vitiligo
4. D	11. keloid	18. urticaria
5. D	12. fissure	19. biopsy
6. B	13. cyanosis	20. polyp
7. A	14. scleroderma	

CHAPTER 5

EXERCISE 5-1   Figure Labeling: Skeleton

1. cranium	10. calcaneous	19. scapula
2. facial bones	11. metatarsals	20. humerus
3. mandible	12. phalanges	21. ribs
4. sternum	13. tarsals	22. radius
5. costal cartilage	14. tibia	23. ulna
6. vertebral column	15. fibula	24. carpals
7. ilium or pelvis	16. patella	25. metacarpals
8. pelvis or ilium	17. femur	26. phalanges
9. sacrum	18. clavicle	

EXERCISE 5-2   Figure Labeling: Long Bone

1. proximal epiphysis	5. epiphyseal line	9. yellow marrow
2. diaphysis	6. spongy bone	10. periosteum
3. distal epiphysis	7. compact bone	
4. cartilage	8. medullary	

EXERCISE 5-3   Word Building

1. osteomyelitis	6. kinesiology	11. arthroplasty
2. arthroscopy	7. chondroplasty	12. myelogram
3. chondromalacia	8. intercostal	13. chondritis
4. arthrogram	9. osteitis	14. osteoporosis
5. arthrodesis	10. osteosarcoma	15. costalgia

EXERCISE 5-4   Matching: Terms of Joint Movement

1. E	5. A
2. D	6. F
3. B	7. G
4. C	

EXERCISE 5-5   Matching: Types of Fractures

1. C	4. G	7. A
2. H	5. D	8. B
3. F	6. E	

EXERCISE 5-6   Fill in the Blank

1. osteoporosis
2. rickets
3. polydactylism
4. osteosarcoma
5. scoliosis
6. rheumatoid arthritis
7. arthroplasty

EXERCISE 5-7   Case Study

1. orthopedic
2. comminuted
3. range of motion
4. impacted
5. reduction
6. traction
7. narcotic
8. anti-inflammatory

EXERCISE 5-8   Crossword Puzzle: The Skeletal System

1. osteoplasty
2. maxilla
3. arthroscope
4. ROM
5. mandible
6. arthrodynia
7. CT
8. arthritis
9. carpals
10. phalanges
11. chondr
12. crani
13. across: calcaneus;
    down: coccyx
14. costalgia

CHAPTER 5 QUIZ

1. C
2. B
3. C
4. D
5. A
6. A
7. D (all the terms are conditions except for diaphysis)
8. B (all are bones in the upper extremity except for the fibula)
9. D (all are bones in the lower extremity except for the ulna)
10. A (all are bones except for deltoid)
11. A (all are abnormal curvatures of the spine except for sclerosis)
12. B (all are parts of the spine except for parietal)
13. D (all are bones except for diaphragm)
14. B (all are fractures except for insertion)
15. thoracotomy
16. arthritis
17. arthrocentesis
18. orthopedics
19. set, repair, or realign broken bones
20. orthopedic surgeon

CHAPTER 6
EXERCISE 6-1   Case Study

1. neck flexion, extension and rotation
2. inflammation of the tendon
3. ROM is range of motion; total degrees of joint movement
4. drug used to decrease inflammation, promote healing, enable joint movement without pain; Motrin (non-steriodal anti-inflammatories)
5. treat pain, disease, or injury by physical means; promote health and prevent physical diability

EXERCISE 6-2   Word Building

1. hemiparesis
2. kinesialgia
3. tenotomy
4. myoitis
5. myopathy, musculopathy
6. fibromyalgia
7. myocele
8. neurologist
9. paraplegia
10. fasciitis

EXERCISE 6-3   Fill in the Blank

1. skeletal, smooth, cardiac
2. orthopedic surgeons, neurologist
3. paraplegic is a person who has paralysis of both legs and the lower part of the body (para- is a prefix meaning "alongside" and -plegia means "paralysis"); a hemiplegic has total paralysis of one side of the body (hemi- means "half")
4. a- is a prefix meaning "without"; my/o is the combining form meaning "muscle"; troph is a root meaning "nutrition or growth"; -ic is an adjective suffix
5. muscles that contract and produce movement
6. epicondylitis
7. electromyography
8. a group of inherited muscle disorders that cause muscle weakness
9. RICE: rest, ice, compress, elevation
10. They are ordered to help reduce muscle spasms and or tension.

EXERCISE 6-4   True or False

1. True
2. False; it is a type of muscular dystrophy
3. True
4. False; it is epicondylitis
5. True
6. False, weakness or partial paralysis
7. True
8. True
9. False, attach muscles to bones
10. True

EXERCISE 6-5   Crossword Puzzle: Muscular System

1. deltoid
2. paresis
3. atrophy
4. quadri
5. fibromyalgia
6. DMD
7. antagonist
8. hemi
9. tendon
10. plegia
11. fascia
12. atony
13. epicondylitis
14. IM
15. hamstring
16. my
17. ROM
18. smooth (down)
18. SLR (across)
19. myocardium

CHAPTER 6 QUIZ

1. C
2. C
3. B
4. D
5. A
6. A
7. C
8. plantar flexion
9. asthenia
10. myocele
11. plantar fasciitis
12. EMG
13. tenoplasty, tenotoplasty, tendinoplasty, tendoplasty
14. myology
15. myodynia, myalgia
16. a muscle that counteracts the action of another muscle
17. weakness or slight paralysis of a muscle
18. deep tendon reflex
19. rest, ice, compression, elevation
20. moving away from a central point

CHAPTER 7
EXERCISE 7-1   Figure Labeling: Neuron

1. dendrites
2. cell body
3. nucleus
4. axon covered with myelin sheath
5. axon branch
6. myelin sheath
7. muscle

EXERCISE 7-2   Case Study

1. transient ischemic attack; sometimes called a mini-stroke
2. cerebrovascular accident
3. dys- means "difficult"; -phasia- means "speak"
4. partial or incomplete paralysis
5. hemiparesis means "partially paralyzed on half the body"; hemiplegia means "complete paralysis on half the body"
6. hemi- means "half"; -plegia means "paralysis"

EXERCISE 7-3   Word Parts

1. neur/o
2. myel/o
3. tom/o
4. cephal/o
5. -phasia
6. schiz/o
7. psych/o, -phrenia, ment/o

EXERCISE 7-4   Word Parts

1. psych–root
   o–CV
   sis–suffix
   a severe condition of the mind
2. electr–root
   o–CV
   encephal–root
   o–CV
   graphy–suffix
   the process of recording the electrical record of the brain
3. astr–root
   o–CV
   cyt–root
   oma–suffix
   a tumor of the brain cell (astrocyte)
4. cerebr–root
   o–CV
   vascul–root
   ar–suffix
   pertaining to the blood vessels in the brain
5. hemi–root
   plegia–suffix
   paralysis on one side of the body
6. hydr-root
   o–CV
   cephal–root
   us–suffix
   pertaining to fluid on the brain
7. encephal–root
   itis–suffix
   inflammation of the brain
8. epi–prefix
   dur–root
   al–suffix
   pertaining to the outer surface of the brain
9. psych–root
   iatr–root
   ist–suffix
   a specialist who treats disorders of the mind
10. meningi–root
    oma–suffix
    tumor of the meninges

EXERCISE 7-5   Matching

1. K
2. F
3. C
4. N
5. H
6. J
7. E
8. B
9. M
10. G
11. D
12. A
13. L
14. I

EXERCISE 7-6 Spell Check

1. Aphasia
2. Schizophrenia
3. Neurotransmitters
4. Subdural hematoma

EXERCISE 7-7 Crossword Puzzle

1. phobia
2. cerebrum
3. delusions
4. psychologist
5. brainstem
6. hallucination
7. OCD
8. depression
9. bipolar
10. LOC
11. pons
12. MRI
13. schizophrenia
14. subarachnoid
15. sedative
16. (across) midbrain
16. (down) myelin
17. neuroglia

CHAPTER 7 QUIZ

1. transient ischemic attack
2. pupils equal, round, and reactive to light and accommodation
3. lumbar puncture
4. electroencephalography
5. multiple sclerosis
6. organic brain syndrome
7. D
8. C
9. A
10. B
11. A
12. B
13. C
14. C
15. C
16. hyperesthesia
17. poliomyelitis
18. dementia
19. multiple sclerosis
20. myelomeningocele
21. cerebral thrombosis
22. ataxia
23. epilepsy
24. syncope
25. neuralgia

CHAPTER 8
EXERCISE 8-1 Figure Labeling: The Endocrine System

1. pineal
2. pituitary (hypophysis)
3. thyroid
4. parathyroids
5. thymus
6. adrenals
7. pancreatic islets
8. ovaries
9. testes

EXERCISE 8-2 Case Study

1. Graves disease; toxic goiter
2. difficulty speaking
3. goiter; thyromegaly
4. thyroid-stimulating hormone
5. exophthalmos; ex- means "out from" or "away from"; ophthalm/o means "eye"

EXERCISE 8-3 Spell Check

1. endocrinologist
2. hypoglycemic
3. insulin
4. diabetes mellitus

EXERCISES 8-4 Disorders and Symptoms of the Endocrine System

1. thyromegaly
2. DM or diabetes mellitus
3. polyuria
4. hyperglycemia
5. endogenous
6. acromegaly
7. glycosuria
8. Cushing syndrome

EXERCISE 8-5   Word Building: The Endocrine System

1. adrenomegaly
2. adrenalectomy
3. adrenopathy
4. hypothyroidism
5. thyroiditis
6. thyroidotomy
7. thyromegaly
8. pancreatoma
9. pancreatitis
10. pancreatogenic

EXERCISE 8-6   Crossword Puzzle: The Endocrine System

1. thyroid
2. testosterone
3. ovary
4. (across) GH
4. (down) glycosuria
5. (across) hypoglycemic
5. (down) hypoglycemia
6. FBS
7. pituitary
8. insulin
9. Graves
10. Cushing
11. hormone
12. goiter
13. gigantism
14. adenoma
15. testes
16. parathyroids
17. adrenal
18. LH

CHAPTER 8 QUIZ

1. A
2. B
3. B
4. C
5. B
6. A
7. D
8. A
9. D
10. D
11. K
12. G
13. I
14. A
15. E
16. F
17. M
18. J
19. B
20. C
21. L
22. H

CHAPTER 9
EXERCISE 9-1   Figure Labeling: The Blood Flow Through the Heart

1. superior and inferior venae cavae
2. right atrium
3. tricuspid valve
4. right ventricle
5. pulmonary valve
6. pulmonary arteries
7. pulmonary veins
8. left atrium
9. mitral valve
10. left ventricle
11. aortic valve
12. aorta

EXERCISE 9-2   Case Study

1. pain in the chest due to ischemia
2. shortness of breath
3. high blood pressure
4. electrocardiogram; record of the heart's electrical activity
5. aspirin–anticoagulant affect; anti-arrhythmics–decrease abnormal atrial heart beats; diuretics–decrease fluid volume by increasing urine volume output; vasodilators–increase diameter of blood vessels to help decrease blood pressure and increase blood flow
6. heart attack, lack of blood supply (infarction) to the heart muscle (my/o means "muscle"; cardi/o means "heart")
7. irregular atrial contractions; frequently a rapid irregular rhythm

EXERCISE 9-3   Word Building: The Cardiovascular System

1. cardiogenic
2. atriotomy
3. erythrocyte
4. hemophilia
5. vasospasm
6. thrombectomy
7. vasodilation
8. cardiomegaly
9. arteriostenosis
10. atheroma
11. leukocyte
12. valvectomy
13. cardiac
14. hemolysis, erythrolysis
15. interventricular
16. anemia
17. myocardium
18. atherectomy
19. arrhythmia

EXERCISE 9-4   Spelling

1. thrombocytopenia
2. oxygen
3. myocardial
4. ischemia
5. arterectomy
6. atrioventricular
7. leukemia
8. atherosclerosis
9. semilunar
10. diastolic

EXERCISE 9-5   Matching

1. D
2. C
3. H
4. J
5. I
6. E
7. A
8. F
9. B
10. G

EXERCISE 9-6   Crossword Puzzle

1. coagulation
2. thrombocyte
3. venules
4. arterioles
5. vasoconstriction
6. thrombus
7. edema
8. plasma
9. CHF
10. aortic
11. ischemia
12. capillaries
13. ather
14. erythrocyte
15. hematology
16. leukemia
17. dyscrasia
18. HB
19. phagocytosis
20. emia

CHAPTER 9 QUIZ

1. C
2. C
3. B
4. A
5. B
6. B
7. D
8. A
9. A
10. C
11. A
12. B
13. B
14. D
15. B
16. D
17. D
18. D
19. D
20. D

CHAPTER 10
EXERCISE 10-1   Case Study

1. disease of the lymph nodes
2. analgesics reduce pain; Tylenol
3. splenomegaly

EXERCISE 10-2   Matching

1. E	5. A	9. D
2. G	6. B	10. F
3. J	7. C	
4. H	8. I	

EXERCISE 10-3   Word Building

1. adenitis
2. lymphoma
3. thymomegaly
4. lymphangiitis or lymphangitis
5. lymphadenopathy
6. immunologist
7. lymphography
8. phagocytosis

EXERCISE 10-4   Crossword Puzzle: The Lymphatic System and Immunity

1. phag	6. erythema	11. AIDS
2. leuk	7. autoimmune	12. emia
3. hemolysis	8. thymus	13. aden
4. chemotherapy	9. immunity	
5. splen	10. Hodgkin	

CHAPTER 10 QUIZ

1. True
2. False; The tonsils are one of four protective organs in the immune system.
3. False; A reaction to poison ivy is an example of dermatitis.
4. True
5. False; Hemolysis is the destruction of red blood cells.
6. True
7. True
8. True
9. False; Peyer's patches are located on the walls of the small intestine.
10. True

CHAPTER 11

EXERCISE 11-1   Figure Labeling: The Respiratory System

1. nares	8. larynx	15. terminal bronchiole
2. nasal cavity	9. esophagus	16. alveolar duct
3. pharynx	10. trachea	17. alveoli
4. nasopharynx	11. left lung	18. capillaries
5. oropharynx	12. right lung	19. diaphragm
6. laryngopharynx	13. right bronchus	
7. epiglottis	14. mediastinum	

EXERCISE 11-2   Case Study

1. A   2. E

EXERCISE 11-3 Matching

1. E	7. B	13. O
2. D	8. J	14. H
3. C	9. K	15. M
4. F	10. L	16. Q
5. A	11. R	17. I
6. G	12. N	18. P

EXERCISE 11-4 Definitions

1. inspiration	4. sinusitis	7. pleurotomy
2. hemoptysis	5. dysphonia	8. pleuralgia
3. thoracopathy	6. pneumothorax	9. pleurocele

EXERCISE 11-5 Word Building

1. bronchitis	5. laryngitis	9. tachypnea
2. bronchodilator	6. bronchitis	10. bradypnea
3. bronchoconstrictor	7. sinusitis	11. dyspnea
4. bronchiectasis	8. epiglottitis	12. orthopnea

EXERCISE 11-6 Case Study

1. a. crackling sounds caused by mucus in airways; abnormal breath sounds heard with a stethoscope
   b. discomfort in breathing that is brought on or aggravated by lying flat
   c. shortness of breath

2. procedure to remove liquid used in bronchiectasis and lung abscess; the patient's body is positioned so that the trachea is inclined downward and below the affected chest area

EXERCISE 11-7 Crossword Puzzle: Respiratory System

1. bronchiole	8. sputum	15. pharynx
2. emphysema	9. pulmonology	16. bronchitis
3. pnea	10. trachea	17. rhinitis
4. laryngitis	11. mediastinum	18. alveolus
5. ABG	12. atelectasis	19. bronchoscope
6. asthma	13. bronchus	20. thoracentesis
7. pneumonia	14. larynx	

CHAPTER 11 QUIZ

1. C	8. B	15. A
2. B	9. D	16. B
3. C	10. A	17. C
4. B	11. C	18. C
5. C	12. D	19. B
6. D	13. C	20. C
7. B	14. B	

CHAPTER 12
EXERCISE 12-1   Figure Labeling: The Digestive System

1. mouth
2. pharynx
3. esophagus
4. stomach
5. duodenum
6. small intestine
7. cecum
8. ascending colon
9. transverse colon
10. descending colon
11. sigmoid colon
12. rectum
13. anus
14. parotid gland
15. sublingual gland
16. submandibular gland
17. liver
18. gallbladder
19. pancreas

EXERCISE 12-2   Chart Note

1. gastroenterologist
2. constipation
3. cholelithiasis
4. cholecystectomy
5. GERD (gastroesophageal reflux disease)
6. ascites
7. barium enema X-ray
8. polyps
9. colonoscopy
10. sigmoid colon
11. colectomy

EXERCISE 12-3   Word Building

1. oral
2. stomatitis
3. buccal
4. cheilosis
5. gingivectomy
6. glossotomy
7. lingual
8. gastrodynia; gastralgia
9. pharyngeal
10. enteritis
11. duodenal
12. jejunal
13. ileitis
14. colectomy
15. rectocele
16. anal
17. proctologist
18. hepatomegaly
19. bilirubin
20. cholecystectomy

EXERCISE 12-4   Abbreviations

1. barium enema
2. bowel movement
3. gastrointestinal
4. irritable bowel
   syndrome
5. gastroesophageal
   reflux disorder

EXERCISE 12-5   Crossword Puzzle: Digestive System

1. dysphagia
2. peritonitis
3. saliva
4. stomatitis
5. polyp
6. alimentary
7. bulimia
8. cirrhosis
9. flatus
10. ulcer
11. melena
12. across: gastr; down: gloss
13. sial
14. eructation
15. anorexia
16. hyperemesis
17. buccal
18. cecum
19. jejunum
20. anus

CHAPTER 12 QUIZ

MATCHING

1. B
2. F
3. I
4. G
5. H
6. D
7. E
8. A
9. C
10. J

MULTIPLE CHOICE

11. B	15. C	18. D
12. C	16. C	19. B
13. C	17. B	20. A
14. A		

CHAPTER 13

EXERCISE 13-1   Figure Labeling: The Urinary System

1. left kidney
2. left ureter
3. urethra
4. right kidney
5. right ureter
6. urinary bladder

EXERCISE 13-2   Case Study

1. urologist
2. dysuria
3. hematuria
4. urinalysis
5. KUB
6. calculi
7. bladder
8. UTI
9. calculi
10. antibiotic
11. cystoscopy

EXERCISE 13-3   Definitions

1. incision into the kidney
2. condition of stones in the kidney
3. filtration to remove wastes from the kidney
4. continuous ambulatory peritoneal dialysis
5. pus in the urine
6. plastic repair of the ureter
7. urinary tract infection
8. suture repair of the ureter
9. around the urethra
10. enlarged kidney

EXERCISE 13-4   Matching Terms with Definitions

1. G	7. H	13. N
2. D	8. F	14. Q
3. K	9. E	15. L
4. A	10. R	16. I
5. B	11. P	17. C
6. J	12. M	18. O

EXERCISE 13-5   Word Building

1. nephritis
2. pyelonephritis
3. nephrolithiasis
4. nephrotomy
5. urolith
6. uremia
7. urinalysis
8. polyuria
9. hematuria
10. anuria

EXERCISE 13-6   True or False

1. True
2. True
3. False; two tubes are the ureters
4. False, the renal fascia is a thin layer of connective tissue that forms each kidney's outer covering
5. True
6. True
7. False; one who studies
8. False; nephrotomy
9. False; ureterotomy
10. False; cystitis

EXERCISE 13-7 Crossword Puzzle: Urinary System

1. dysuria
2. dialysis
3. IVP
4. nephron
5. pyuria
6. hematuria
7. BUN
8. diuretic
9. bladder
10. enuresis
11. cystectomy
12. UA
13. nephroptosis
14. ureters
15. uremia
16. void
17. anuria
18. cystitis
19. ren
20. nocturia

CHAPTER 13 QUIZ

1. renal transplant
2. nephropexy
3. pyelolithotomy
4. ureterectomy
5. cystoscopy
6. drug used to kill bacterial growth
7. drug used to decrease spasms of the bladder
8. blood urea nitrogen
9. bedwetting
10. overgrowth of the kidney

MULTIPLE CHOICE

11. D
12. B
13. B
14. B
15. D
16. A
17. C
18. D
19. B
20. C

CHAPTER 14
EXERCISE 14-1 Figure Labeling: The Male Reproductive System

1. testis
2. epididymis
3. scrotum
4. vas deferens
5. ejaculatory duct
6. urethra
7. penis
8. glans penis
9. foreskin
10. seminal vesicle
11. prostate
12. bulbourethral gland
13. urinary bladder

EXERCISE 14-2 Figure Labeling: The Female Reproductive System

1. fallopian tube or oviduct
2. ovary
3. uterus
4. urinary bladder
5. clitoris
6. labia minora
7. labia majora
8. cervix
9. rectum
10. anus
11. vagina
12. urethra

EXERCISE 14-3 Deciphering Medical Documents

1. second pregnancy, 1 child or live birth
2. transabdominal puncture of the amniotic sac to remove amniotic fluid for testing
3. within the uterus

EXERCISE 14-4   Building Medical Terms

1. hysteropexy
2. hysterectomy
3. hysterorrhexis
4. hysterorrhaphy
5. metropathy
6. metritis
7. metrorrhagia
8. vaginal
9. vaginocele
10. vaginitis
11. vaginolabial or labiovaginal
12. colposcopy
13. colporrhaphy
14. prostatectomy
15. prostatic
16. prostatitis
17. vesiculopathy
18. vesiculitis
19. orchitis
20. orchidopathy
21. orchalgia, orchodynia

EXERCISE 14-5   Surgical Procedure Term Identification

1. fallopian tube
2. uterus
3. fallopian tube
4. vagina
5. breast
6. ovary
7. testis
8. vas deferens
9. glans penis
10. breast

EXERCISE 14-6   Matching Terms with Definitions

1. D
2. O
3. E
4. I
5. A
6. G
7. C
8. M
9. B
10. K
11. N
12. F
13. H
14. L
15. J

EXERCISE 14-7   Abbreviations

1. benign prostatic hypertrophy
2. dilation and curettage
3. obstetrics
4. transurethral resection of the prostate

EXERCISE 14-8   Crossword Puzzle: Reproductive System

1. vulv
2. gonorrhea
3. cervix
4. endometriosis
5. laparoscopy
6. hymen
7. oophor
8. cystocele
9. vasectomy
10. menarche
11. colposcope
12. areola
13. perineum
14. phimosis (down)
14. prostatitis (across)
15. TURP
16. orchitis
17. vas
18. oviduct
19. gynec

CHAPTER 14 QUIZ

1. A
2. B
3. A
4. D
5. B
6. B
7. C
8. A
9. D
10. False; gestation
11. True
12. False; fertilization
13. False; in vitro fertilization
14. False; ovulation
15. True
16. True
17. False; obstetrics
18. False; dysmenorrhea
19. False; Pap smear

CHAPTER 15

EXERCISE 15-1   Figure Labeling: The Eye

1. sclera
2. cornea
3. iris
4. lens
5. ciliary bodies
6. vitreous humor
7. fovea centralis
8. retina
9. choroid

EXERCISE 15-2   Operative Report

1. middle ear infection or inflammation
2. incision into the tympanic membrane
3. earwax
4. medication given to combat the growth of bacteria

EXERCISE 15-3   Matching Terms with Definitions: Eye

1. J
2. G
3. E
4. D
5. H
6. A
7. F
8. I
9. C
10. B

EXERCISE 15-4   Matching Terms with Definitions: Ear

1. C
2. G
3. D
4. I
5. B
6. J
7. E
8. A
9. H
10. F

EXERCISE 15-5   Fill in the Blank

1. cataract
2. presbycusis
3. diplopia
4. vertigo
5. tinnitus
6. pinna
7. hordeolum
8. otalgia
9. astigmatism
10. keratitis
11. xerophthalmia
12. antiemetic
13. otosclerosis
14. blepharoptosis
15. audiometry

EXERCISE 15-6   Crossword Puzzle: Eye and Ear

1. labyrinth
2. strabismus
3. audiologist
4. retina
5. OD
6. kerat
7. OS
8. ophthalmoscope
9. dacryocyst
10. AS
11. refraction
12. OU
13. iris
14. ossicles
15. incus
16. OT
17. ophthalm
18. cerumen

CHAPTER 15 QUIZ

1. B	8. C	15. OD
2. A	9. A	16. mastoiditis
3. D	10. D	17. conductive
4. C	11. staped	18. labyrinthotomy
5. A	12. tympanitis, myringitis	19. AS
6. D	13. glaucoma	20. cochlea
7. B	14. eustachian tube	

APPENDIX B
Glossary of Prefixes, Suffixes, and Combining Forms

a-	without
ab-	away from
abdomin/o	abdomen
-ac	pertaining to
acr/o	extremity or topmost
acous/o; acust/o	hearing
ad-	to, toward, or near
aden/o	gland
adip/o	fat
adren/o; adrenal/o	adrenal
-al	pertaining to
albin/o	albino
-algia; -alges	pain
alimen/o	digestive tract
alveol/o	alveolus (air sac)
amni/o	amnion
amphi-	on both sides
an-	without
ana-	up, apart
andr/o	male
-aneous	converts noun to adjective: pertaining to
angi/o	vessel
ankyl/o	crooked
ante-	before
anter/o	anterior
anti-	against or opposed to
aort/o	aorta
appendic/o	appendix
-ar	pertaining to
arachn/o	spider
arteri/o	artery
arthr/o	joint
-ary	pertaining to
-asthen	weakness
astr/o	star-shaped
ather/o	fatty, or lipid, paste
atri/o	atrium
audi/o; audit/o	hearing
aur/o; auricul/o	ear
auto-	self
bacteri/o	bacteria
balan/o	glans penis
bi-	two or both
bi/o	life
blephar/o	eyelid
brachi/o	arm
brady-	slow
bronch/o; bronchi/o	bronchus (airway)
bucc/o	cheek
bulb/o	bulb-like
calcane/o	heel
calc/i	calcium
cardi/o	heart
carp/o	wrist
-cele	pouching or hernia
-centesis	puncture for aspiration
cephal/o	head
cerebell/o	cerebellum
cerebr/o	largest part of the brain, cerebrum
cerv/o; cervic/o	neck
cheil/o	lip
chem/o	chemical
chir/o	hand
cholangi/o	bile duct
chol/o; chole/o	bile
cholecyst/o	gallbladder
choledoch/o	common bile duct
chondr/o	cartilage
-cidal; -cide	to kill
circum/o	around
cirrh/o	yellow
coagul/o	clotting
col/o; colon/o	colon (large intestine)
colp/o	vagina
con-	with, together
condyl-	rounded end surface of a bone
conjunctiv/o	conjunctiva
contra-	against or opposed to
corne/o	cornea
coron/o	circle or crown
cortic/o	outer layer or covering
cost/o	rib

crani/o	skull	**esophag/o**	esophagus
-crasia	blending; mixture	**esthesi/o**	sensation
crin/o	to secrete	**eu-; ex-; ex/o**	out or away
cry/o	to freeze	**extra-**	outside
crypt-	hidden	**fasci/o**	fibrous membrane
-cusis	hearing	**femur/o**	femur, thigh bone
cutane/o	skin	**fibr/o**	fiber
cyan/o	blue	**gangli/o; ganglion/o**	ganglia (singular:
cyst/o	bladder or sac		ganglion)
-cyte; cyt/o	cell	**gastr/o**	stomach
dacry/o	tear	**gen-; -genesis**	origin or produc-
dacryocyst/o	lacrimal sac		tion
dactyl/o	finger, toe	**-genic**	pertaining to origin
de-	from, down, or not	**ger/o; geront/o**	aged
dent/i; dent/o	teeth	**gingiv/o; gli/o**	glue
derm/o; dermat/o	skin	**-globin**	protein
-desis	binding	**glomerul/o**	glomerulus
di-	two	**gloss/o**	tongue
dia-	across or through	**gluc/o; glyc/o**	sugar (glucose)
-dilator	increase diameter;	**gonad/o**	gonad
	open up	**-gram**	record
dipl/o; dipl-	two, double	**-graph**	instrument for
dips/o	thirst		recording
dors/o	dorsal	**-graphy**	process of recording
duoden/o	duodenum	**gyn/o; gynec/o**	female
dur/o	dura	**hem/o; hemat/o**	blood
-dynia	painful	**hemi-**	half
dys-	painful, difficult, or	**hep/o; hepat/o**	liver
	faulty	**herni/o**	hernia
ec-, ecto	out or away	**hormon/o**	hormone
-ectasia	dilation of a tubular	**humer/o**	humerus, upper
	structure		arm bone
-ectasis	dilation of a tubular	**hydr/o**	water
	structure	**hyper-**	above or excessive
-ectomy	excision or removal	**hypn/o**	sleep
-edema	collection of watery	**hypo-**	below or deficient
	fluid in tissues	**hypophys/o**	pituitary gland
electr/o	electricity	**hyster/o**	uterus
-emesis	vomiting	**-ia**	condition of
-emetic	pertaining to	**iac; -ian**	specialist
	vomiting	**-iasis**	formation or
-emia	blood condition		presence of
encephal/o	entire brain	**-iatric**	medical specialty
en-, endo-	within	**-iatrist**	specialist
endocrin/o	endocrine	**iatr/o**	treatment
enter/o	small intestine	**-iatry**	medical specialty
-eous	upon, following,	**-ic, -ical**	pertaining to
	subsequent to	**ichthy/o**	fish scales, very dry
epi-	upon	**-ics**	medical specialty
erythr/o	red	**ile/o**	ileum
erythemat/o	redness	**immun/o**	safe

-ine	suffix used in the formation of names of chemical substances
infra-	inside or below
inguin/o	inguinal
inter-	between
intra-	within
-iole	smaller
-ion	condition
ir/o; irid/o; irit/o	iris (colored circle)
isch/o	to hold back
-ism	condition of
-ist	one who specializes in
-itis	inflammation
-ium	structure or tissue
jaund/o	yellow
jejun/o	jejunum
kerat/o	cornea
kine-; kinesi/o; -kinesia	movement
kyph/o	humpbacked
labi/o	lips
labyrinth/o	labyrinth
lacrim/o	tear
lact/o	milk
lapar/o	abdomen
laryng/o	larynx (voice box)
-lepsy	seizure
leuk/o	white
ligament/o	ligament
-lipid;	fatty
lith/o; -lith	stone
-lithiasis	condition of having stones
-logist	one who specializes in the study or treatment of
-logy	study of
lord/o	bent
lumb/o	loin (lower back)
lymph/o; lymphat/o	clear fluid
lymphaden/o	lymph nodes
lymphangi/o	lymph vessels
-lysis	breakdown or dissolution
macro-	large (prefix)
-malacia	softening
mamm/o	breast
-mania	condition of abnormal impulse toward or frenzy

mast/o	breast
-megaly	enlargement
melan/o	black
men/o	month (menstruation)
mening/o	membrane (meninges)
ment/o	referring to the mind
meso-	middle, mean
meta-	beyond, after, or change
-meter	instrument for measuring
metr/o	uterus
-metry	process of measuring
micro-	small
-mnesia	memory
mono-	one
muc/o	mucus
muscul/o	muscle
myc/o	fungus
my/o	muscle
myel/o	bone marrow or spinal cord
myring/o	eardrum or tympanic membrane
narc/o	stupor or sleep
nas/o	nose
nat/o	birth
necr/o	dead
neo-	new
nephr/o	kidney
neur/o	nerve
noct/o	night
ocul/o	eye
-oid	resembling
-ole	small
olig-, oligo-	scanty
-oma	tumor
onc/o	tumor
-one	chemical compound
onych/o	nail
oo	ovary, egg
oophor/o	ovary
ophthalm/o	eye
-opia	eye, vision
-opsia	vision
-opsy	process of viewing
opt/o	eye
or/o	mouth

orch/o; orchi/o, orchid/o	testis or testicle	-physis	to grow
orth/o-	straight, normal, or correct	pil/o	hair
		-plasia	formation
-ory	pertaining to	-plasty	surgical repair or reconstruction
-osis	abnormal condition or increase	-plegia	paralysis
osse/o	bone, bony	pleur/o	pleura
oste/o	bone	-pnea	breathing
ot/o	ear	pneum/o	air or lung
-otic	pertaining to	-poiesis	formation
-ous	pertaining to	poly-	many
ov/i; ov/o	egg	-porosis	porous
ovari/o	ovary	post-	after
ox/o; -oxia	oxygen	poster/o	posterior
pan-	all	pre-	before
pancreat/o	pancreas	presby/o	old age
para-	alongside of or abnormal	proct/o	rectum and anus
parathyr/o; parathyroid/o	parathyroid	prostat/o	prostate gland
		proxim/o	proximal
pariet/o	a wall of the body	prurit/o	to itch
-paresis	weakness, loss of movement	psych/o	mind
		-ptosis	falling or downward displacement
path/o; -pathy	disease	-ptysis	spitting
pector/o	chest	pulmon/o	lung
pedicul/o	lice	pupil/o	pupil
-penia	abnormal reduction	py/o	pus
ped/o	foot, child	pyel/o	pelvis
pelv/o	pelvis	pylor/o	pylorus
-penia	deficiency	pyret/o	fever
-pepsia	digestion	quadri-	four
peri-	around	rect/o	rectum
-pexy	suspension or fixation	ren/o	kidney
		retin/o	retina
phag/o; -phagia	eat or swallow	retro-	behind, backward
phak/o; phac/o	lens	rheum/o; rheumat/o	to flow
phalang/o	bones of fingers and toes	rhin/o	nose
		-rrhage, -rrhagia	to burst forth (usually blood)
pharm/o; pharmacy/o	drug	-rrhaphy	suture
		-rrhea	discharge
pharyng/o	pharynx or throat	-rrhexis	rupture
phas/o; -phasia	speech	salping/o	uterine or fallopian tube
-phil	attraction for		
phleb/o	vein	sarc/o	flesh
-phobia	condition of abnormal fear or sensitivity	scab/o	to scratch
		schiz/o	split
		scler/o	hard or sclera
phon/o; -phonia	voice	-sclerosis	hardness
phot/o	light	scoli/o	twisted
phren/o	diaphragm, mind	-scope	instrument for examination
-phylaxis	protection		

-scopy	process of examination
seb/o	sebaceous
semi-	half
-septic	decay or breaking
sial/o	salivary glands
sigmoid/o	sigmoid colon
sinus/o	sinus
-spasm	involuntary contraction
sperm/o	sperm
spermat/o-	sperm
sphygm/o	pulse
spin/o	thorn
spir/o	breathing
splen/o	spleen
spondyl/o	vertebra
staped/o	stapes
-stasis	stop or stand
sten/o	narrow
-stenosis	narrowed, block
stern/o	chest
steth/o	chest
sthen/o	strength
stomat/o	mouth
-stomy	creation of an opening
sub-	below or under
sudor/o	sweat gland
super/o; super-; supra-	above or excessive
sym-	together
syn-	together or with
tachy-	fast
temper/o	temper
tend/o; tendin/o	tendon
tens-	pressure
test/o; testost/o	testis or testicle
tetra-	four
thorac/o; thorac/i; thoracic/o	chest
thromb/o	clot
thym/o	thymus gland

thyr/o, thyroid/o	thyroid gland (shield)
tom/o	to cut
-tome	cutting instrument
-tomy	incision
ton/o	tone or tension
tonsill/o	tonsil
trache/o	trachea (windpipe)
trans-; trans/o	across or through
tri-	three
-tripsy	crushing
troph/o; tropin; -trophy	nourishment or development
tympan/o	eardrum or tympanic membrane
-ular	converts a root or noun to an adjective
-um	singular noun ending
uni-	one
ur/o, urin/o	urine
ureter/o	ureter
urethr/o	urethra
-us	condition
uter/o	uterus
uve/o	uvea
vagin/o	vagina
valv/o; valvul/o	valve
varic/o	swollen, twisted vein
vas/o; vascul/o	vessel
ven/o	vein
ventricul/o	ventricle (belly or pouch)
-version	to turn
vertebr/o	vertebra
vesic/o	bladder or sac
vulv/o	vulva
xanth/o	yellow
xer/o	dry
-y	adjective suffix
zyg/o	yoke, to join

APPENDIX C
Glossary of Medical Abbreviations

A	anterior; assessment
A&P	auscultation and percussion
A&W	alive and well
a.c.	before meals
a.m.	morning
a.m.	before noon
ACL	anterior cruciate ligament
ACTH	adrenocorticotrophin hormone
AD	right ear [spell out right ear]
ad lib.	as desired
ADH	antidiuretic hormone
ADHD	attention-deficit/ hyperactivity disorder
A-fib	atrial fibrillation
Ag	antigen; [L.] *argentum*, silver
AID	artificial insemination donor
AIDS *(ādz)*	acquired immunodeficiency syndrome
AIH	artificial insemination by husband; artificial insemination, homologous
AJCCS	American Joint Committee on Cancer Staging (criteria)
AKA	above-knee amputation
Al	aluminum
alb	albumin
ALL	acute lymphocytic leukemia
ALS	amyotrophic lateral sclerosis
ALT	alanine aminotransferase (enzyme)
AMA	antimitochondrial antibody
AML	acute myelogenous leukemia
amt	amount
Amu	atomic mass unit
ANA	antinuclear antibody
ANS	autonomic nervous system
AP	anteroposterior
APAP	acetaminophen
Apgar *(ap'gär)*	appearance, pulse, grimace, activity, respiration
aq	water
ARF	acute renal failure; acute rheumatic fever
As	arsenic
AS	[L.] *auris sinistra*, left ear [spell out left ear]
ASA	acetylsalicylic acid (aspirin); antisperm antibodies
ASD	atrial septal defect
ASHD	arteriosclerotic heart disease
ASL	American Sign Language
AST	aspartate aminotransferase (enzyme)
at. wt.	atomic weight
ATP	adenosine 5′-triphosphate
Au	[L.] *aurum*, gold
AU	[L.] *auris utraque*, each ear, both ears (spell out both ears)
AV; A-V	arteriovenous; atrioventricular
AVN	atrioventricular node
AW	atomic weight
ax.	axis
b	blood (subscript)
B	barometric pressure (subscript); boron
Ⓑ	bilateral
b.i.d.	[L.] *bis in die*, twice a day
Ba	barium
BADL	basic activities of daily living
BAEP	brainstem auditory evoked potential
BAER	brainstem auditory evoked response
BBB	blood-brain barrier
BCC	basal cell carcinoma
BD	bipolar disorder

BE	barium enema	**CAD**	coronary artery disease
B-E	below-the-elbow amputation	**cal**	calorie (small)
		Cal	calorie (large)
Bi	Bismuth	**CAM**	complementary and alternative medicine
BIPAP	bilevel positive airway pressure	**cap**	capsule
BKA	below-knee amputation	**CAPD**	continuous ambulatory peritoneal dialysis
BM	bowel movement		
BMI	body mass index	**CAT *(kat)***	computerized axial tomography
BMP	basic metabolic panel		
BP	blood pressure; boiling point; British Pharmacopoeia	**CBC**	complete blood (cell) count
		CC	chief complaint
BPH	benign prostatic hypertrophy; benign prostatic hyperplasia	**cc**	cubic centimeter [use the metric equivalent mL]
		CCK	cholecystokinin
Br	bromine	**CCU**	cardiac care unit; coronary care unit; critical care unit
BRAT	diet of banana, rice cereal, applesauce, toast		
BRCA	breast cancer antigen	**Cd**	cadmium
BRP	bathroom privileges	**CEA**	carcinoembryonic antigen
BS	blood sugar		
BSA	body surface area	**CF**	complement fixation; cystic fibrosis; coupling factor
BT	bleeding time		
BTU	British thermal unit		
BUN	blood urea nitrogen	**CHF**	congestive heart failure
BUN:Cr	blood urea nitrogen to creatinine ratio	**CHO**	carbohydrate
		CI	color index
Bx	biopsy	**CIB**	[L.] *cibus*, food
C	calorie (large); carbon; Celsius; centigrade; cervical; clearance rate, renal (as subscript); compliance; concentration; cylindrical lens; cytidine	**CIS**	carcinoma in situ
		CJD	Creutzfeldt-Jakob disease
		Cl	chlorine
		CL	cardiolipin
		CLIA	Clinical Laboratory Improvement Amendments
c	calorie (small); capillary blood (subscript); centi-	**CLL**	chronic lymphocytic leukemia
c̄	with	**cm**	centimeter
C&S	culture and sensitivity	**Cm**	curium
C. diff	*Clostridium difficile*	**CMC**	carpometacarpal
c/o	complains of	**CML**	chronic myelogenous leukemia
CA	cancer; carcinoma; cardiac arrest; chronologic age; croup-associated (virus); cytosine arabinoside; cancer antigen; carbohydrate antigen	**CMP**	comprehensive metabolic panel
		CMV	controlled mechanical ventilation; cytomegalovirus
ca.	[L.] *circa*, about, approximately	**CNS**	central nervous system
		Co	cobalt
CABG	coronary artery bypass graft	**CO**	cardiac output
		CO₂	carbon dioxide

CoA	coenzyme A	**D&E**	dilation and evacuation
COG	center of gravity	**db, dB**	decibel
COPD	chronic obstructive pulmonary disease	**DC, D/C**	discharge; discontinue [spell out discharge or discontinue]
CP	cerebral palsy; chest pain; costophrenic	**D-dimer**	fibrin degradation product
CPPB	continuous (or constant) positive-pressure breathing	**DDS**	doctor of dental surgery
		def	decayed, extracted, or filled (deciduous teeth)
CPPV	continuous positive-pressure ventilation	**DEF**	decayed, extracted, or filled (permanent teeth)
CPR	cardiopulmonary resuscitation	**df**	decayed and filled (deciduous teeth)
cps	cycles per second	**DF**	decayed and filled (permanent teeth)
Cr	chromium; creatinine		
CR	conditioned reflex; crown-rump length	**DIC**	disseminated intravascular coagulation
CRD	chronic respiratory disease	**DJD**	degenerative joint disease
CRP	cross-reacting protein	**DKA**	diabetic ketoacidosis
CRST	calcinosis cutis, Raynaud phenomenon, sclerodactyly, and telangiectasia syndrome	**DM**	diabetes mellitus
		DMD	Duchenne muscular dystrophy
CS	cesarean section	**dmf**	decayed, missing, or filled (deciduous teeth)
CSD	cat scratch disease	**DMF**	decayed, missing, or filled (permanent teeth)
CSF	cerebrospinal fluid		
CT	computed tomography	**DNA**	deoxyribonucleic acid
CTA	computed tomographic angiography	**DNR**	do not resuscitate
		DOA	dead on arrival
CTD	cumulative trauma disorder	**DPI**	dry powder inhaler
		DPT	dipropyltryptamine; diphtheria, pertussis, and tetanus (vaccines)
CTS	carpal tunnel syndrome		
cu mm, mm³	cubic millimeter		
CV	cardiovascular		
CVA	cerebrovascular accident	**dr**	dram
CVP	central venous pressure	**DRE**	digital rectal examination
CVS	chorionic villus sampling	**DRG**	diagnosis-related group
CXR	chest X-ray	**DSA**	digital subtraction angiography
Cys	cysteine		
Cyt	cytosine	**dsDNA**	double-stranded DNA
d	deci-; day	**DT**	delirium tremens; duration of tetany
D	dead space gas (subscript); deciduous; deuterium; diffusing capacity; dihydrouridine (in nucleic acids); diopter; [L.] *dexter*, right (opposite of left); vitamin D potency of cod liver oil	**DTP**	diphtheria and tetanus toxoids and pertussis vaccine; distal tingling on percussion (Tinel sign)
		DTR	deep tendon reflex
		DUB	dysfunctional uterine bleeding
D&C	dilation and curettage	**DVT**	deep vein thrombosis

EB, EBV	Epstein-Barr virus
ECCE	extracapsular cataract extraction
ECF	extracellular fluid
ECG	electrocardiogram
echo	echocardiogram
ECT	electroconvulsive therapy
ECU	emergency care unit
EDC	estimated date of confinement
EDD	estimated date of delivery
EEG	electroencephalogram
EENT	eye, ear, nose, and throat
EGD	esophagogastroduodenoscopy
EGR	electroretinopathy
EKG	[German] *Elektrokardiogramme*, electrocardiogram
ELISA (*ē-lī′să*)	enzyme-linked immunosorbent assay
EM	electron microscopy
EMG	electromyogram
EMS	emergency medical services
ENT	ear, nose, and throat
EOM	extraocular movement; extraocular muscles
EP	electrophysiology
EPAP	expiratory positive airway pressure
EPS	electrophysiologic study
ER	endoplasmic reticulum; emergency room; estrogen receptor
ERBF	effective renal blood flow
ERV	expiratory reserve volume
ESP	extrasensory perception
ESR	electron spin resonance; erythrocyte sedimentation rate
ESRD	end-stage renal disease
ESWL	extracorporeal shock wave lithotripsy
ETOH	ethyl alcohol
EUS	endoscopic ultrasonography
F	Fahrenheit; Faraday constant; fertility factor; field of vision; fluorine; force; fractional concentration; free energy
FB	foreign body
FBS	fasting blood sugar
Fe	[L.] *ferrum*, iron
FEF	forced expiratory flow
FET	forced expiratory time
FEV	forced expiratory volume
FGT	female genital tract
FH	family history
FHR	fetal heart rate
FHT	fetal heart tones
fl oz	fluid ounce
FOBT	fecal occult blood test
Fr	francium; French (gauge, scale)
FRC	functional residual capacity (of lungs)
Fru	fructose
FS	frozen section
FSH	follicle-stimulating hormone
FU	fluorouracil
FUO	fever of unknown origin
FVC	forced vital capacity
Fw	F wave (fibrillary wave, flutter wave)
Fx	fracture
g	gram
Ga	gallium
GAD	generalized anxiety disorder
GB	gallbladder
GBS	gallbladder series
GC	gonococcus, gonorrhea
GERD (*gĕrd*)	gastroesophageal reflux disease
GFR	glomerular filtration rate
GH	glenohumeral; growth hormone
GI	gastrointestinal; Gingival Index
GIST (*jist*)	gastrointestinal stromal tumor
gm	gram
gr	grain
gt	drop
gt.	[L.] *gutta*, a drop
GTT	glucose tolerance test
gtt.	[L.] *guttae*, drops
GU	genitourinary
GVHD	graft-versus-host disease
Gy	gray (unit of absorbed dose of ionizing radiation)

GYN	gynecology	**HSV-2**	herpes simplex virus type 2
h	hecto-; hour	**Ht**	height
H	henry; hydrogen; hyperopia; hyperopic	**HTN**	hypertension
		Hx	medical history
H&H	hemoglobin and hematocrit	**Hz**	hertz
H&P	history and physical	**I**	inspired gas (subscript); iodine
H. pylori	*Helicobacter pylori*	**I&D**	incision and drainage
h. s., HS	[L.] *hora somni*, at bedtime	**I&O**	(fluid) intake and output
H⁺	hydrogen ion	**I, II, III, IV, V, VI, VII, VIII, IX, X**	uppercase Roman numerals 1–10
HAART *(hart)*	highly active antiretroviral therapy	**IBD**	inflammatory bowel disease
HAV	hepatitis A virus	**IBS**	irritable bowel syndrome
Hb, Hbg	hemoglobin	**ICCE**	intracapsular cataract extraction
HbA1c	hemoglobin A1c	**ICD**	*International Classification of Diseases*; implantable cardioverter defibrillator
HBV	hepatitis B virus		
HCG, hCG	human chorionic gonadotropin		
HCl	hydrochloric acid		
HCT, Hct	hematocrit	**ICF**	intracellular fluid
HCV	hepatitis C virus	**ICP**	intracranial pressure
HD	Huntington's disease	**ICU**	intensive care unit
HDL	high-density lipoprotein	**ID**	intradermal
He	helium	**IDDM**	insulin-dependent diabetes mellitus
HEENT	head, eyes, ears, nose, and throat		
Hg	[L.] *hydrargyrum*, mercury	**IF**	initiation factor; intrinsic factor
HGB, Hgb	hemoglobin	**IFN**	interferon
HGH	human (pituitary) growth hormone	**Ig**	immunoglobulin
		IgG	immunoglobulin G
HHV	human herpesvirus	**IgM**	immunoglobulin M
HIPAA *(hip'ă)*	Health Insurance Portability and Accountability Act of 1996	**IH**	infectious hepatitis
		IL	interleukin
		IM	internal medicine; intramuscular(ly); infectious mononucleosis
HIV	human immunodeficiency virus		
HLA	human leukocyte antigen	**IMP**	impression
HMO	health maintenance organization	**INR**	International Normalized Ratio (prothrombin time)
hpf, HPF	high-power field	**IOP**	intraocular pressure
HPI	history of present illness	**IP**	interphalangeal; intraperitoneal(ly); inpatient
HPV	human papilloma virus		
HR	heart rate		
HRT	hormone replacement therapy	**IPAP**	inspiratory positive airway pressure
HSG	hysterosalpingogram	**IPPV**	intermittent positive-pressure ventilation
HSV	herpes simplex virus		
HSV-1	herpes simplex virus type 1	**IPV**	inactivated poliovirus vaccine

IQ	intelligence quotient
Ir	iridium
IRV	inspiratory reserve volume
ISMP	Institute for Safe Medication Practices
ITP	idiopathic thrombocytopenic purpura; inosine 5'-triphosphate
IU	International Unit
IUCD	intrauterine contraceptive device
IUD	intrauterine device
IV	intravenous
IVF	in vitro fertilization
IVP	intravenous pyelogram
IVU	intravenous urogram
J	joule
JCAHO	Joint Commission on Accreditation of Healthcare Organizations
k	kilo-
K	[Modern L.] *kalium*, potassium; Kelvin
kcal	kilocalorie
kg	kilogram
KJ	knee jerk
KS	Kaposi's sarcoma
KUB	kidneys, ureters, bladder
kV	kilovolt
L	inductance; left; [L.] *limes*, boundary, limit; liter; lumbar
Ⓛ	left
L&W	living and well
LA	lupus antibody, lupus anticoagulant
LASER *(lā'zĕr)*	light amplification by stimulated emission of radiation
LASIK *(lā'sik)*	laser *in situ* keratomileusis
lb	pound
LBT	lupus band test
LC	lethal concentration
LD	lethal dose
LDL	low-density lipoprotein
LE	left eye; lower extremity; lupus erythematosus
LEEP *(lēp)*	loop electrosurgical excision procedure
LES	lower esophageal sphincter
LFA	left frontoanterior (fetal position)
LFP	left frontoposterior (fetal position)
LFT	left frontotransverse (fetal position)
LH	luteinizing hormone
Li	lithium
LLQ	left lower quadrant
LMA	left mentoanterior (fetal position)
LMP	left mentoposterior (fetal position); last menstrual period
LMT	left mentotransverse (fetal position)
LOA	left occipitoanterior (fetal position)
LOC	level of consciousness
LOP	left occipitoposterior (fetal position)
LOT	left occipitotransverse (fetal position)
LP	lumbar puncture
lpf, LPF	low-power field
Lr	lawrencium
LSA	left sacroanterior (fetal position)
LSP	left sacroposterior (fetal position)
LST	left sacrotransverse (fetal position)
LTB	laryngotracheobronchitis
LTH	luteotropic hormone
LTM	long-term memory
LUQ	left upper quadrant
LVET	left ventricular ejection time
LVH	left ventricular hypertrophy
lytes	electrolytes
ⓜ	mass; meter; milli-; minim; molar; moles (per liter)
M	mega-, meg-; molar; moles (per liter); morgan; myopic; myopia
m	murmur
mA	milliampere
MA	mental age

MAC *(mak)*	monitored anesthesia care
MAP	morning-after pill
mA-S	milliampere-second
Mb	myoglobin
MBC	maximum breathing capacity
MCH	mean cell hemoglobin
MCHC	mean cell hemoglobin concentration
MCP	metacarpophalangeal
MCV	mean corpuscular (cell) volume
MCV	mean cell volume
MD	medical doctor; muscular dystrophy
MDI	metered-dose inhaler
MEDLARS	Medical Literature Analysis and Retrieval System
MEP	maximal expiratory pressure
meq, mEq	milliequivalent
MET	metabolic equivalent of task
MEV	million electron-volts (10 ev)
mg	milligram
Mg	magnesium
MG	myasthenia gravis
MHA	microhemagglutination
MHC	major histocompatibility complex
MHz	megahertz
MI	myocardial infarction
MICU *(mik′yū)*	medical intensive care unit
MID	minimal infecting dose
MIP	maximum inspiratory pressure
MIS (mis)	minimally invasive surgery
MJD	Machado-Joseph disease
ml or mL	milliliter
MLD	minimal lethal dose
mm	millimeter
mm³	cubic millimeter
mmol	millimole
MMPI	Minnesota Multiphasic Personality Inventory
MMR	measles-mumps-rubella (vaccine)
Mn	manganese
MO	medical officer; mineral oil
MODS *(mods)*	multiple organ dysfunction syndrome
mol	mole
mol wt	molecular weight
MOM	milk of magnesia
mono	infectious mononucleosis
MOPP	Mustargen (mechlorethamine hydrochloride), Oncovin (vincristine sulfate), procarbazine hydrochloride, and prednisone
mor. sol.	[L.] *more solito*, as usual, as customary
MPD	maximal permissible dose
MRA	magnetic resonance angiography
mrd, MRD	minimal reacting dose
MRI	magnetic resonance imaging
mRNA	messenger RNA
MRSA	methicillin-resistant *Staphylococcus aureus*
MS	multiple sclerosis; morphine sulfate; musculoskeletal
ms, msec	millisecond
MSG	monosodium glutamate
MSH	melanocyte-stimulating hormone
MTP	metatarsophalangeal (joint)
MUGA *(myū′ga)*	multiple-gated acquisition (imaging)
mV	millivolt
MVP	mitral valve prolapse
MVV	maximal voluntary ventilation
MW	molecular weight
My	myopia
mμ	millimicron
N	Newton; nitrogen; normal concentration
n	normal (small caps)
Na	[Modern L.] *natrium*, sodium
NA	*Nomina Anatomica*

NAD	nicotinamide adenine dinucleotide; no acute distress
NCV	nerve conduction velocity
Ne	neon
NE	norepinephrine; not examined
NEEP	negative end-expiratory pressure
NF	National Formulary
ng	nanogram
NG	nasogastric
NGT	nasogastric tube
Ni	nickel
NICU *(nik'yū)*	neonatal intensive care unit
NIDDM	noninsulin-dependent diabetes mellitus
NK	natural killer (cell)
NKA	no known allergies
NKDA	no known drug allergy
nm	nanometer
noc.	night
NPO	nothing by mouth
NREM	nonrapid eye movement (sleep)
nRNA	nuclear RNA
NSAID	nonsteroidal anti-inflammatory drug
NSR	normal sinus rhythm
O	[L.] *oculus*, eye; opening (in formulas for electrical reactions); oxygen; objective
o-	ortho-
Ø	none; negative
O&P	ova and parasites
O_2	oxygen
OA	osteoarthritis
OB	obstetrics
OB/GYN	obstetrics and gynecology
OBS	organic brain syndrome
OC	oral contraceptive
OCD	obsessive-compulsive disorder
OCP	oral contraceptive pill
OD	right eye [spell out right eye]
OH	occupational history
OM	otitis media
OMS	organic mental syndrome
OP	osmotic pressure; outpatient
OPV	oral poliovirus vaccine
OR	operating room
ORIF	open reduction, internal fixation
OS	[L.] *oculus sinister*, left eye [spell out left eye]
OT	occupational therapy
OTC	over the counter (nonprescription drug)
OU	both eyes [spell out both eyes]
OXT	oxytocin
oz	ounce
p	pico-; pupil
p-	para-
P	partial pressure; peta-; phosphorus, phosphoric residue; plasma concentration; pressure; para (obstetric history); plan; posterior; pulse; blood group (PI antigen)
p̄	after
p.c.	[L.] *post cibum*, after a meal
p.m.	after noon
p.o., PO	[L.] *per os*, by mouth
p.r.n., PRN	as needed
p24	HIV antibody
PA	posterior-anterior
$PaCO_2$	partial pressure of carbon dioxide
PACS *(paks)*	picture archival communications system
PACU *(pak'yū)*	postanesthetic care unit
PALS *(pals)*	pediatric advanced life support
PaO_2	partial pressure of arterial oxygen
Pap	Papanicolaou (smear)
PAR	postanesthetic recovery
Pb	[L.] *plumbum*, lead
Pco_2	partial pressure of carbon dioxide
PD	prism diopter; panic disorder
PDA	patent ductus arteriosus
PDLL	poorly differentiated lymphocytic lymphoma

PE	physical examination; pulmonary embolism; polyethylene	**ppm**	parts per million
		PPPPPP	pain, pallor, pulselessness, paresthesia, paralysis, prostration
PEFR	peak expiratory flow rate		
PEG *(peg)*	percutaneous endoscopic gastrostomy	**PPV**	positive pressure ventilation
per	by or through	**PR**	per rectum; progesterone receptor
PERRLA	pupils equal, round, and reactive to light and accommodation		
		pre-op, preop	preoperative
		PRL	prolactin
PET	positron emission tomography	**pro time**	prothrombin time
		PSA	prostate-specific antigen
PF	peak flow	**PSG**	polysomnography
PFT	pulmonary function test	**psi**	pounds per square inch
PG	prostaglandin	**PSV**	pressure-supported ventilation
pH	hydrogen ion concentration; p (power) of $[H^+]_{10}$; potential of hydrogen		
		pt	patient
		PT	physical therapy; prothrombin time
PH	past history		
PI	present illness	**PTA**	plasma thromboplastin antecedent; phosphotungstic acid; prior to admission
PICC	peripherally inserted central catheter		
PICU *(pik'yū)*	pediatric intensive care unit	**PTCA**	percutaneous transluminal coronary angioplasty
PID	pelvic inflammatory disease	**PTH**	parathyroid hormone
		PT-INR	prothrombin time internal normalized ratio
PIH	pregnancy-induced hypertension		
		PTP	posttransfusion purpura
PIP *(pip)*	proximal interphalangeal (joint)	**PTSD**	posttraumatic stress disorder
PKU	phenylketonuria	**PTT**	partial thromboplastin time
PLT	platelet	**Pu**	plutonium
PM	postmortem	**PUD**	peptic ulcer disease
PMH	past medical history	**PUO**	pyrexia of unknown origin
PMN	polymorphonuclear (leukocyte)	**PUVA** *(pū-vă)*	psoralen ultraviolet A
		PV	per vagina
PMS	premenstrual syndrome	**PVD**	posterior vitreous detachment
PND	paroxysmal nocturnal dyspnea; postnasal drip		
		Px	physical examination
PNPB	positive-negative pressure breathing	**Q**	volume of blood flow
		q	every
PNS	peripheral nervous system	**q.d.**	every day, daily [spell out every day or daily]
PO₂, Po₂	partial pressure of oxygen		
POMP	prednisone, Oncovin (vincristine sulfate), methotrexate, and Purinethol (6-mercaptopurine)	**q.i.d.**	four times a day
		q.o.d.	every other day [spell out every other day]
POR	problem-oriented medical record	**q.s.**	[L.] *quantum satis*, as much as is enough; [L.] *quantum sufficiat*, as much as may suffice; quantity sufficient
post-op, postop	postoperative		
PPBS	postprandial blood sugar		

Note: PO_2, Po_2 = partial pressure of oxygen

q2h	every 2 hours	**RLQ**	right lower quadrant
qh	every hour	**RMA**	right mentoanterior (fetal
QNS	quantity not sufficient		position)
Qo₂	oxygen consumption	**RML**	right middle lobe
qt	quart	**RMP**	right mentoposterior
r	racemic; roentgen		(fetal position)
R	gas constant	**RMT**	right mentotransverse
	(8.315 joules); organic		(fetal position)
	radical; Réamur (scale);	**Rn**	radon
	[L.] *recipe*, take;	**RNA**	ribonucleic acid
	resistance determinant	**RNase**	ribonuclease
	(plasmid); resistance	**RNP**	ribonucleoprotein
	(electrical); resistance	**R/O**	rule out
	(unit; in the cardiovascu-	**ROA**	right occipitoanterior
	lar system); resolution;		(fetal position)
	respiration; respiratory	**ROM**	range of motion
	(exchange ratio); respira-	**ROP**	right occipitoposterior
	tory rate; roentgen		(fetal position)
Ⓡ	right	**ROS**	review of symptoms
Ra	radium	**ROT**	right occipitotransverse
RA	rheumatoid arthritis		(fetal position)
RAI	radioactive iodine	**rpm**	revolutions per minute
RBC	red blood cell; red blood	**rRNA**	ribosomal RNA
	count	**Rs**	resolution
RBF	renal blood flow	**RSA**	right sacroanterior
RD	reaction of degeneration;		(fetal position)
	reaction of denervation	**RSP**	right sacroposterior
RDA	recommended daily		(fetal position)
	allowance	**RST**	right sacrotransverse
rDNA	ribosomal DNA		(fetal position)
RDS	respiratory distress	**RTC**	return to clinic
	syndrome	**RTO**	return to office
REM *(rem)*	rapid eye movement	**RUQ**	right upper quadrant
	(sleep); reticular	**RV**	residual volume
	erythematous mucinosis	**RVH**	right ventricular
RF	release factor;		hypertrophy
	rheumatoid factor	**Rx**	[L.] *recipe*, (the first word
RFA	right frontoanterior (fetal		on a prescription), take;
	position)		prescription; treatment
RFP	right frontoposterior	**S**	[L.] *sinister*, left; sacral;
	(fetal position)		saturation of hemoglobin
RFT	right frontotransverse		(percentage of; followed
	(fetal position)		by subscript O₂ or CO₂);
Rh	Rhesus (Rh blood		siemens; spherical; spheri-
	group); rhodium		cal lens; sulfur; Svedberg
RH	releasing hormone		unit; subjective
RhD	rhesus antigen D typing	**s̄**	without
RIA	radioimmunoassay	**SA; S-A**	sinoatrial
RICE	rest, ice, compression,	**SAB**	spontaneous abortion
	elevation	**SAD *(sad)***	seasonal affective
RLL	right lower lobe		disorder

SaO$_2$	oxygen saturation of arterial (oxyhemoglobin)	**sp. gr., SpGr**	specific gravity
SARS *(sarz)*	severe acute respiratory syndrome	**SPECT**	single-photon emission computed tomography
sat.	saturated	**SPF**	sun protection factor
sat. sol.	saturated solution	**SpGr**	specific gravity
sc	subcutaneous(ly)	**spm**	suppression and mutation
SC	sternoclavicular; subcutaneous(ly) [spell out subcut or subcutaneously]	**spp.**	species (plural)
		SQ	subcutaneous [spell out subcut or subcutaneously]
SCC	squamous cell carcinoma	**Sr**	strontium
Se	selenium	**SR**	systems review
SERM *(serm)*	selective estrogen receptor modulator	**ssDNA**	single-stranded DNA
		ssp.	subspecies
SGOT	serum glutamic-oxaloacetic trans-aminase (aspartate aminotransferase)	**ST**	scapulothoracic
		stat, STAT	[L.] *statim*, immediately, at once
SGPT	serum glutamic-pyruvic transaminase (alanine aminotransferase)	**STD**	sexually transmitted disease
		STM	short-term memory
SH	serum hepatitis; social history	**STSG**	split-thickness skin graft
		sub-Q	subcutaneous [spell out subcut or subcutaneously]
Si	silicon		
SIDS *(sids)*	sudden infant death syndrome	**SUI**	stress urinary incontinence
Sig:	label; instruction to patient	**suppos**	suppository
		SV	stroke volume
SIMV	spontaneous intermittent mandatory ventilation; synchronized intermittent mandatory ventilation	**SVT**	supraventricular tachycardia
		Sx	symptom
		t	metric ton
SIRS (sĕrs)	systemic inflammatory response syndrome	**T**	temperature, absolute (Kelvin); tension (intraocular); tera-; tesla; tetanus (toxoid); thoracic; tidal (volume) (subscript); tocopherol; transverse (tubule); tritium; tumor (antigen)
SK	streptokinase		
SL	sublingual		
SLE	systemic lupus erythematosus		
SLR	straight leg raising		
SMAC *(smak)*	sequential multiple ana-lyzer computer	**T&A**	tonsillectomy and adenoidectomy
Sn	[L.] *stannum*, tin	**T&C**	type and crossmatch
SOAP *(sōp)*	subjective data, objective data, assessment, and plan (problem-oriented medical record)	**t.i.d.**	three times a day
		T$_3$, T3	3,5,5′-triiodothyronine
		T$_4$, T4	tetraiodothyronine (thyroxine)
SOB	shortness of breath	**TA**	*Terminologia Anatomica*
sol., soln.	solution	**tab**	tablet
sp.	species		

TAB	therapeutic abortion
TAF	tumor angiogenesis factor
TAH	total abdominal hysterectomy
TB	tuberculosis
Tc	technetium
TCN	talocalcaneonavicular (joint)
Td	tetanus-diphtheria (toxoids, adult type)
TEDS	thromboembolic disease stockings
TEE	transesophageal echocardiogram
TENS *(tens)*	transcutaneous electrical nerve stimulation
THR	total hip replacement
TKA	total knee arthroplasty
TKR	total knee replacement
Ti	titanium
TIA	transient ischemic attack
TIBC	total iron-binding capacity
tinct.	tincture
TKO	to keep (venous infusion line) open
Tl	thallium
TLC	thin-layer chromatography; total lung capacity; tender loving care
TLV	threshold-limit value
TM	transport maximum; tympanic membrane
TMJ	temporomandibular joint
TMT	tarsometatarsal
TNF	tumor necrosis factor
TNM	tumor, node, metastasis (tumor staging)
t-PA, tPA, TPA	tissue plasminogen activator
TPN	total parenteral nutrition
TPR	temperature, pulse, and respirations
Tr	treatment
tr.	tincture
tRNA	transfer RNA
TRUS *(trŭs)*	transrectal ultrasound
TSH	thyroid-stimulating hormone

TSS	toxic shock syndrome
TTP	thrombotic thrombocytopenic purpura
TU	toxic unit
TURP	transurethral resection of the prostate
TV	tidal volume
Tx	treatment; traction
U	unit; uranium; uridine (in polymers); urinary (concentration)
UA	urinalysis
UCHD	usual childhood diseases
UGI	upper gastrointestinal
UGIS	upper gastrointestinal series
ung.	[L.] *unguentum*, ointment
u-PA	urokinase
URI	upper respiratory infection
US, U/S	ultrasound
UTI	urinary tract infection
UV	ultraviolet
v	venous (blood); volt
V	vanadium; vision; visual (acuity); volt; volume (frequently with subscripts denoting location, chemical species, and conditions)
V̇	ventilation; gas flow (frequently with subscripts indicating location and chemical species); ventilation
V̇/Q̇	ventilation/perfusion
VA	viral antigen
V-A	ventriculoatrial
VATS *(vats)*	video-assisted thoracic surgery
VC	vision, color; vital capacity
VCE	vagina, (ecto)cervix, endocervical canal
VCU, VCUG	voiding cystourethrogram
V$_D$	(physiologic) dead space
VD	venereal disease
VDRL	Venereal Disease Research Laboratory (test)

VHDL	very-high-density lipoprotein	γ	gamma; Ostwald solubility coefficient; the third in a series; heavy chain class corresponding to IgG
VLDL	very-low-density lipoprotein		
V_{max}	maximal velocity		
VP	vasopressin; Voges-Proskauer	**Δ**	delta; change; heat
		μ	mu; micro-; heavy chain class corresponding to IgM
VS	volumetric solution; vital signs		
V_T	tidal volume	**μl, μL**	microliter
W	watt; [German] *Wolfram*, tungsten	**μm**	micrometer
		μμ	micromicro-
w.a.	while awake	**Σ**	sigma; reflection coefficient; standard deviation; 1 millisecond (0.001 sec)
WBC	white blood cell; white blood count		
WDLL	well-differentiated lymphocytic (or lymphatic) lymphoma	**Ω**	omega; ohm
		#	number; pound
		<	less than [spell out less than]
WDWN	well-developed, well-nourished		
wk	week	**>**	greater than [spell out greater than]
WN	well nourished		
WNL	within normal limits	**×**	times; for
WNV	West Nile virus	**↑**	increased
Wt	weight	**↓**	decreased
x	times; for	**°**	degree; hour
X-ray, x-ray	radiography	**μg**	microgram
y/o or y.o.	year old	**¹²³I**	iodine-123 (radioisotope)
yr	year	**¹²⁵I**	iodine-125
β	beta, second in a series; blood (subscript)	**¹³¹I**	iodine-131
		^{99m}Tc	technetium-99m

APPENDIX D
ISMP's List of Error-Prone Abbreviations, Symbols, and Dose Designations

The abbreviations, symbols, and dose designations found in this table have been reported to ISMP through the USP-ISMP Medication Error Reporting Program as being frequently misinterpreted and involved in harmful medication errors. They should NEVER be used when communicating medical information. This includes internal communications, telephone/verbal prescriptions, computer-generated labels, labels for drug storage bins, medication administration records, as well as pharmacy and prescriber computer order entry screens.

The Joint Commission (TJC) has established a National Patient Safety Goal that specifies that certain abbreviations must appear on an accredited organization's do-not-use list; we have highlighted these items with a double asterisk (**). However, we hope that you will consider others beyond the minimum TJC requirements. By using and promoting safe practices and by educating one another about hazards, we can better protect our patients.

ABBREVIATIONS	INTENDED MEANING	MISINTERPRETATION	CORRECTION
μg	Microgram	Mistaken as "mg"	Use "mcg"
AD, AS, AU	Right ear, left ear, each ear	Mistaken as OD, OS, OU (right eye, left eye, each eye)	Use "right ear," "left ear," or "each ear"
OD, OS, OU	Right eye, left eye, each eye	Mistaken as AD, AS, AU (right ear, left ear, each ear)	Use "right eye," "left eye," or "each eye"
BT	Bedtime	Mistaken as "BID" (twice daily)	Use "bedtime"
cc	Cubic centimeters	Mistaken as "u" (units)	Use "mL"
D/C	Discharge or discontinue	Premature discontinuation of medications if D/C (intended to mean "discharge") has been misinterpreted as "discontinued" when followed by a list of discharge medications	Use "discharge" and "discontinue"
IJ	Injection	Mistaken as "IV" or "intrajugular"	Use "injection"
IN	Intranasal	Mistaken as "IM" or "IV"	Use "intranasal" or "NAS"
HS	Half-strength	Mistaken as bedtime	Use "half-strength" or "bedtime"
hs	At bedtime, hours of sleep	Mistaken as half-strength	
IU**	International unit	Mistaken as IV (intravenous) or 10 (ten)	Use "units"
o.d. or OD	Once daily	Mistaken as "right eye" (OD-oculus dexter), leading to oral liquid medications administered in the eye	Use "daily"
OJ	Orange juice	Mistaken as OD or OS (right or left eye); drugs meant to be diluted in orange juice may be given in the eye	Use "orange juice"

ABBREVIATIONS	INTENDED MEANING	MISINTERPRETATION	CORRECTION
Per os	By mouth, orally	The "os" can be mistaken as "left eye" (OS-oculus sinister)	Use "PO," "by mouth," or "orally"
q.d. or QD**	Every day	Mistaken as q.i.d., especially if the period after the "q" or the tail of the "q" is misunderstood as an "i"	Use "daily"
qhs	Nightly at bedtime	Mistaken as "qhr" or every hour	Use "nightly"
qn	Nightly or at bedtime	Mistaken as "qh" (every hour)	Use "nightly" or "at bedtime"
q.o.d. or QOD**	Every other day	Mistaken as "q.d." (daily) or "q.i.d. (four times daily) if the "o" is poorly written	Use "every other day"
q1d	Daily	Mistaken as q.i.d. (four times daily)	Use "daily"
q6PM, etc.	Every evening at 6 PM	Mistaken as every 6 hours	Use "6 PM nightly" or "6 PM daily"
SC, SQ, sub q	Subcutaneous	SC mistaken as SL (sublingual); SQ mistaken as "5 every;" the "q" in "sub q" has been mistaken as "every" (e.g., a heparin dose ordered "sub q 2 hours before surgery" misunderstood as every 2 hours before surgery)	Use "subcut" or "subcutaneously"
ss	Sliding scale (insulin) or ½ (apothecary)	Mistaken as "55"	Spell out "sliding scale;" use "one-half" or "½"
SSRI	Sliding scale regular insulin	Mistaken as selective-serotonin reuptake inhibitor	Spell out "sliding scale (insulin)"
SSI	Sliding scale insulin	Mistaken as Strong Solution of Iodine (Lugol's)	
i/d	One daily	Mistaken as "tid"	Use "1 daily"
TIW or tiw	3 times a week	Mistaken as "3 times a day" or "twice in a week"	Use "3 times weekly"
U or u**	Unit	Mistaken as the number 0 or 4, causing a 10-fold overdose or greater (e.g., 4U seen as "40" or 4u seen as "44"); mistaken as "cc" so dose given in volume instead of units (e.g., 4u seen as 4cc)	Use "unit"

DOSE DESIGNATIONS AND OTHER INFORMATION	INTENDED MEANING	MISINTERPRETATION	CORRECTION
Trailing zero after decimal point (e.g., 1.0 mg)**	1 mg	Mistaken as 10 mg if the decimal point is not seen	Do not use trailing zeros for doses expressed in whole numbers"

(continued)

DOSE DESIGNATIONS AND OTHER INFORMATION	INTENDED MEANING	MISINTERPRETATION	CORRECTION
"Naked" decimal point (e.g., .5 mg)**	0.5 mg	Mistaken as 5 mg if the decimal point is not seen	Use zero before a decimal point when the dose is less than a whole unit
Drug name and dose run together (especially problematic for drug names that end in "l" such as Inderal 40 mg; Tegretol300 mg)	Inderal 40 mg Tegretol 300 mg	Mistaken as Inderal 140 mg Mistaken as Tegretol 1300 mg	Place adequate space between the drug name, dose, and unit of measure
Numerical dose and unit of measure run together (e.g., 10mg, 100mL)	10 mg 100 mL	The "m" is sometimes mistaken as a zero or two zeros, risking a 10- to 100-fold overdose	Place adequate space between the dose and unit of measure
Abbreviations such as mg. or mL. with a period following the abbreviation	mg mL	The period is unnecessary and could be mistaken as the number 1 if written poorly	Use mg, mL, etc. without a terminal period
Large doses without properly placed commas (e.g., 100000 units; 1000000 units)	100,000 units 1,000,000 units	100000 has been mistaken as 10,000 or 1,000,000; 1000000 has been mistaken as 100,000	Use commas for dosing units at or above 1,000, or use words such as 100 "thousand" or 1 "million" to improve readability

DRUG NAME ABBREVIATIONS	INTENDED MEANING	MISINTERPRETATION	CORRECTION
ARA A	vidarabine	Mistaken as cytarabine (ARA C)	Use complete drug name
AZT	zidovudine (Retrovir)	Mistaken as azathioprine or aztreonam	Use complete drug name
CPZ	Compazine (prochlorperazine)	Mistaken as chlorproma-zine	Use complete drug name
DPT	Demerol-Phenergan-Thorazine	Mistaken as diphtheria-pertussis-tetanus (vaccine)	Use complete drug name
DTO	Diluted tincture of opium, or deodorized tincture of opium (Paregoric)	Mistaken as tincture of opium	Use complete drug name
HCl	hydrochloric acid or hydrochloride	Mistaken as potassium chloride (The "H" is misinterpreted as "K")	Use complete drug name unless expressed as a salt of a drug
HCT	hydrocortisone	Mistaken as hydrochlorothiazide	Use complete drug name
HCTZ	hydrochloro-thiazide	Mistaken as hydrocortisone (seen as HCT250 mg)	Use complete drug name

DRUG NAME ABBREVIATIONS	INTENDED MEANING	MISINTERPRETATION	CORRECTION
MgSO4**	magnesium sulfate	Mistaken as morphine sulfate	Use complete drug name
MS, MSO4**	morphine sulfate	Mistaken as magnesium sulfate	Use complete drug name
MTX	methotrexate	Mistaken as mitoxantrone	Use complete drug name
PCA	procainamide	Mistaken as patient controlled analgesia	Use complete drug name
PTU	propylthiouracil	Mistaken as mercaptopurine	Use complete drug name
T3	Tylenol with codeine No. 3	Mistaken as liothyronine	Use complete drug name
TAC	triamcinolone	Mistaken as tetracaine, Adrenalin, cocaine	Use complete drug name
TNK	TNKase	Mistaken as "TPA"	Use complete drug name
ZnSO4	zinc sulfate	Mistaken as morphine sulfate	Use complete drug name

STEMMED DRUG NAMES	INTENDED MEANING	MISINTERPRETATION	CORRECTION
"Nitro" drip	nitroglycerin infusion	Mistaken as sodium nitroprusside infusion	Use complete drug name
"Norflox"	norfloxacin	Mistaken as Norflex	Use complete drug name
"IV Vanc"	intravenous vancomycin	Mistaken as Invanz	Use complete drug name

SYMBOLS	INTENDED MEANING	MISINTERPRETATION	CORRECTION
℥	Dram	Symbol for dram mistaken as "3"	Use the metric system
ℳ	Minim	Symbol for minim mistaken as "mL"	
x3d	For three days	Mistaken as "3 doses"	Use "for three days"
> and <	Greater than and less than	Mistaken as opposite of intended; mistakenly use incorrect symbol; "< 10" mistaken as "40"	Use "greater than" or "less than"
/ (slash mark)	Separates two doses or indicates "per"	Mistaken as the number 1 (e.g., "25 units/10 units" misread as "25 units and 110" units)	Use "per" rather than a slash mark to separate doses
@	At	Mistaken as "2"	Use "at"
&	And	Mistaken as "2"	Use "and"
+	Plus or and	Mistaken as "4"	Use "and"
°	Hour	Mistaken as a zero (e.g., q2° seen as q 20)	Use "hr," "h," or "hour"

**These abbreviations are included on TJC's "minimum list" of dangerous abbreviations, acronyms and symbols that must be included on an organization's "Do Not Use" list, effective January 1, 2004. Visit www.jointcommission.org for more information about this TJC requirement.

Reprinted with permission from the Institute for Safe Medication Practices. List originally appeared at www.ismp.org. Report medication errors or near misses to the ISMP Medication Errors Reporting Program (MERP) at 1-800-FAIL-SAF(E) or online at www.ismp.org.

INDEX

....

Page numbers followed by an *"f"* indicates figures; page numbers followed by a *"t"* indicates tables.

A

Abbreviations, 387–399
   body organization, 47t
   cardiovascular system, 193t–194t
   digestive system, 264t
   endocrine system, 164t–165t
   error-prone, ISMP list of, 400–403
   immune and lymphatic system, 216t
   integumentary system, 61t
   muscular system, 116t
   nervous system, 136t–137t
   reproductive system, 315t ·
   respiratory system, 237t–238t
   sight and hearing, 342t–343t
   skeletal system, 90t
   urinary system, 288t
Abdominal cavity, 44–45, 44f–45f, 45t–46t
Abdominopelvic cavity, 44–45, 44f–45f, 45t–46t
ABGs. *See* Arterial blood gases
Ablation therapy, 192
Absorption, 257
Accessory organs, of digestive system, 257, 257f, 259–260, 260f, 263
Accommodation, 337, 338f
Acne, 59
Acquired immunity, 214
Acromegaly, 161t, 162, 162f
Addison's disease, 161t, 163
Adenohypophysis, 158
ADH. *See* Antidiuretic hormone
Adjectives, suffixes that denote, 15–16, 16t, 26–27
Adrenal glands, 156f, 157t, 158f, 159–160, 160f, 161t, 163, 163f
Alimentary canal. *See* Gastrointestinal tract
Allergist, 214
Alopecia, 59
ALS. *See* Amyotrophic lateral sclerosis
Alveoli, 227, 228f, 229–230
Amniocentesis, 308, 308f, 313
Amniotic fluid, 307f, 308
Amniotic sac, 307f, 308
Amyotrophic lateral sclerosis (ALS), 113
Anacusis, 341
Anatomic position, 41–42, 42f
Anatomy, 38
Androgens, 304
Anemia, 188, 192
Aneurysm, 133, 133f
Ankles, bones of, 82f, 83, 83f
Anorexia, 263
Anteflexion, of uterus, 310, 310f
Anteversion, of uterus, 310, 310f

Antidiuretic hormone (ADH), 157t, 158, 158f
Anuria, 285
Aortic semilunar valve, 183
Apex, of lungs, 230
Apnea, 232
Appendicitis, 262
Appendicular skeleton, 76, 76f, 81–83, 81f–83f
Appendix, 214, 215f, 259, 259f
Aqueous humor, 339
Arachnoid layer, 131–132, 131f
Areola, 306
Arm, bones of, 81, 81f
Arrhythmias, 192
Arterial blood gases (ABGs), 236
Arterial stent, 189, 190f
Arteries, 186
Arterioles, 186
Arteriosclerosis, 192
Arthritis, 88
Arthroscopy, 85, 85f
Artificial immunity, 214
Ascending colon, 259, 259f
Ascites, 263
Asthma, 234
Astigmatism, 340
Atelectasis, 234, 236
Atheroma, 190
Atherosclerosis, 188, 188f
Atrial fibrillation, 191
Atrioventricular (AV) node, 183, 185f
Atrium, 182
Audiologist, 337
Auditory tube. *See* Eustachian tube
Auricle. *See* Pinna
Autonomic nervous system, 128, 128f, 129f, 132
AV node. *See* Atrioventricular node
Axial skeleton, 76–80, 76f–80f
Axon, 128, 129f
Azotemia, 285

B

Back, divisions of, 46, 46f, 47t
Balanitis, 309
Barium swallow upper GI series, 261
Barrel chest, 235f
Bartholin's glands, 305–306, 305f–306f
Behavioral disorders, 134–135
Beta-adrenergic drugs, 342
Bicuspid valve. *See* Mitral valve
Bile duct. *See* Common bile duct

Bilirubin, 263
Biopsy
    cone, 313, 313*f*
    of skin, 59–60
Bladder. *See* Gallbladder; Urinary bladder
Blepharoptosis, 341
Blood, 184–187, 187*f*, 188*t*
Blood disorders, 192
Blood elements, 186–187, 187*f*
Blood groups, 187, 188*t*
Blood urea nitrogen (BUN), 285
Blood vessels, 184–187, 187*f*, 188*t*
Body cavities, 44–46, 44*f*–45*f*, 45*t*–46*t*
Body organization, 37–52
    abbreviations, 47*t*
    anatomic position and direction, 41–42, 42*f*, 43*t*
    cavities and divisions of, 44–47, 44*f*
    exercises and quiz, 49–52
        answers to, 365–366
    levels of, 38–41, 39*f*
    planes, 43–44, 43*f*
    study table, 47*t*–48*t*
    word elements related to, 38
Bradycardia, 191
Bradypnea, 232
Brain stem, 130*f*, 131
Brain trauma, 132, 133*f*
Breasts. *See* Mammary glands
Bronchi, 227, 228*f*, 229–230
Bronchiectasis, 234
Bronchioles, 227, 228*f*, 229–230
Bronchoconstriction, 234
Bronchodilators, 234, 237
Bronchoscopy, 236–237, 237*f*
Bruxism, 261
Bulbourethral glands, 303–304, 303*f*
Bulimia, 263
Bulla, 56, 57*f*
BUN. *See* Blood urea nitrogen
Bundle of His, 183, 185*f*
Burns, 59, 59*t*
Bursae, 83
Bursitis, 83

C
CABG. *See* Coronary artery bypass graft
CAD. *See* Coronary artery disease
Calculi, renal, 286, 287*f*
Cancer. *See also* Tumors
    of digestive system, 263
    of skin, 59
Canthi, 337
CAPD. *See* Continuous ambulatory peritoneal dialysis
Capillaries, 186
Cardiac catheterization, 191
Cardiac glycosides, 193
Cardiac muscles, 109, 110*f*, 111
Cardiac sphincter, 258
Cardiologists, 188
Cardiovascular surgeons, 188

Cardiovascular system, 179–210
    abbreviations, 193*t*–194*t*
    disorders and treatments of, 188–192, 188*f*–191*f*
        arrhythmias, 191–192
        blood disorders, 192
        congestive heart failure, 192
        coronary artery disease, 188–189, 188*f*–190*f*
        hypertension, 192
        myocardial infarction, 191, 191*f*
        thrombosis, 188*f*, 190
    exercises and quiz, 204–210
        answers to, 372–373
    lymphatic system in relation to, 213*f*
    overview of, 180–181, 181*f*
    pharmacology for, 193
    practice and practitioners, 188
    structure and function of, 181–187, 182*f*, 184*f*–187*f*, 188*t*
        blood and blood vessels, 184–187, 187*f*, 188*t*
        heart, 181–184, 182*f*, 184*f*–186*f*
    study table, 194*t*–203*t*
    word elements related to, 180
Cardioversion, 192
Carpals, 81, 82*f*
Carpal tunnel syndrome, 113, 114*f*
Cartilage, 83
Cataract, 341, 341*f*
Catheter, 284, 284*f*
Catheterization, 284, 284*f*
Cavities. *See* Dental caries
Cecum, 258–259, 259*f*
Cell membrane, 38, 40*f*
Cells, 38–39, 39*f*
    elements of, 38–39, 40*f*
Central nervous system (CNS), 128–132, 128*f*–131*f*
Cerebellum, 130, 130*f*
Cerebral cortex, 130
Cerebral vascular accident (CVA), 133
Cerebrum, 130, 130*f*
Cerumen, 339, 341
Cervical vertebrae, 46, 46*f*, 47*t*, 79, 80*f*
Cervix, 305–306
CF. *See* Cystic fibrosis
Chemotherapy, 216
Cheyne-Stokes respiration, 232
CHF. *See* Congestive heart failure
Chlamydia, 309
Cholangiolitis, 263
Cholecystalgia, 281
Cholecystectomy, 281
Cholecystitis, 263
Cholecystopexy, 281
Choledocholithiasis, 263
Cholelithiasis, 263
Cholinergic drugs, 287
Chondrosarcoma, 88
Choroid, 337, 338*f*
Cilia, 227
Ciliary body, 337, 338*f*
Circulation, of heart, 183, 184*f*
Circulatory system, 41
Cirrhosis, 263

Clavicle, 81, 81*f*
Clitoris, 305–306, 305*f*–306*f*
Clotting disorders, 192
CNS. *See* Central nervous system
Coccyx (vertebra), 46, 46*f*, 47*t*, 79, 80*f*
Cochlea, 339, 339*f*
Colon, 259, 259*f*
Colonoscopy, 263
Colposcopy, 313
Combining vowel, 5–6
Common bile duct, 260
Common cold, 232
Concussion, 132, 133*f*
Conductive hearing loss, 341
Cone biopsy, 313, 313*f*
Cones, 337, 338*f*
Congestive heart failure (CHF), 192
Conjunctiva, 337
Conjunctivitis, 341
Constipation, 263
Continuous ambulatory peritoneal dialysis (CAPD),
    285*f*
Corium. *See* Dermis
Cornea, 337, 338*f*
Coronary artery bypass graft (CABG), 189–190, 190*f*
Coronary artery disease (CAD), 188–189, 188*f*–190*f*
Corticosteroids, 166, 216, 237, 342
Costae fluctuantes. *See* Floating ribs
Cowper's glands. *See* Bulbourethral glands
Cranial bones, 77, 78*f*
Cranial cavity, 44, 44*f*
Crohn's disease, 262
Croup, 233
Cryptorchidism, 310
CTD. *See* Cumulative trauma disorders
Cumulative trauma disorders (CTD), 113–114
Cushing's syndrome, 161*t*, 163
Cuticle, 56, 56*f*
CVA. *See* Cerebral vascular accident
Cycloplegics, 342
Cystalgia, 281
Cystectomy, 281
Cystic fibrosis (CF), 234
Cystitis, 284
Cystocele, 310, 311*f*
Cystopexy, 281
Cystoscope, 286
Cytoplasm, 39, 40*f*

D

Dacryocyst, 337, 337*f*
Dacryocystitis, 341
D&C. *See* Dilation and curettage
Deafness, 341
Decongestants, 232, 237
Dendrites, 128, 129*f*
Dental caries, 261
Dermatitis, 57
Dermis, 55, 55*f*
Descending colon, 259, 259*f*

Diabetes insipidus, 161, 161*t*
Diabetes mellitus, 161*t*, 163–164
Diagnostic procedures
    for reproductive system, 311–314, 312*f*–314*f*
    for respiratory system, 236–237, 236*f*–237*f*
Diagnostic terms, suffixes and, 14, 15*t*, 24–25
Dialysis, 285, 285*f*–286*f*
Diaphragm, 228*f*, 230–231
Diarrhea, 263
Diastole, 183, 185*f*
Diastolic pressure, 186
Diencephalon, 130–131, 130*f*
Digestion, 257
Digestive system, 41, 255–279
    abbreviations, 264*t*
    accessory organs of, 257, 257*f*, 259–260, 260*f*
    disorders and treatments of, 261–263, 262*f*
        accessory organ disorders, 263
        lower GI tract disorders, 262–263
        upper GI tract disorders, 261–262, 262*f*
    exercises and quiz, 273–279
        answers to, 376–377
    overview of, 257, 257*f*
    pharmacology for, 264
    structure and function of, 257–259, 258*f*–259*f*
        lower GI tract, 258–259, 259*f*
        summary of, 261*t*
        upper GI tract, 258, 258*f*
    study table, 265*t*–272*t*
    word elements related to, 256
Dilation and curettage (D&C), 313
Direction, prefixes of, 17, 17*t*, 28
Directional terms, 41–42, 42*f*, 43*t*
Disorders and treatments
    of cardiovascular system, 188–192, 188*f*–191*f*
    of digestive system, 261–263, 262*f*
    of ear, 341–342
    of endocrine system, 161–164, 161*t*, 162*f*–163*f*
    of eye, 340–341, 340*f*–341*f*
    of immune and lymphatic system, 215–216
    of integumentary system, 56–59, 57*f*
    of muscular system, 112–115
    of nervous system, 132–135, 133*f*
    of respiratory system, 231–237, 235*f*–237*f*
    of skeletal system, 85–89
    of urinary system, 283–286, 284*f*–287*f*
Disseminated intravascular coagulation, 192
Diuretics, 193, 285–286
Diverticula, 262–263
Diverticulitis, 263
Diverticulosis, 263
Dorsal cavity, 44, 44*f*, 46, 46*f*, 47*t*
Dose designations, error-prone, ISMP list of, 400–403
Ductus deferens, 304
Duodenum, 258, 259*f*
Dura mater, 131, 131*f*
Dwarfism, 161*t*, 162
Dyscrasia, 192
Dyspepsia, 263
Dysphagia, 261
Dysphonia, 233

Dyspnea, 232
Dysuria, 284

E

Ear. *See* Hearing
Earwax. *See* Cerumen
ECG. *See* Electrocardiogram
Echocardiography, 191
Ectopic pregnancy, 309
Ectropion, 341
Eczema, 57, 58*f*
Ejaculation, 304, 304*f*
EKG. *See* Electrocardiogram
Electrocardiogram (ECG, EKG), 184, 186*f*
Elimination, 257
Embryo, 308
Emetics, 264
Emphysema, 234, 235*f*
Endarterectomy, 190
Endocardium, 181, 182*f*
Endocrine system, 41
    abbreviations, 164*t*–165*t*
    disorders and treatments of, 161–164
        adrenal gland, 161*t*, 163, 163*f*
        pancreas, 161*t*, 163–164
        pituitary gland, 161–162, 161*t*, 162*f*
        thyroid gland, 161*t*, 162–163, 163*f*
    exercises and quiz, 172–178
        answers to, 371–372
    overview of, 155
    pharmacology of, 164
    structure and function of, 155–160, 156*f*, 157*t*, 158*f*–160*f*
    study table, 165*t*–171*t*
    word elements related to, 155
Endometriosis, 311, 312*f*
Endometrium, 305
Endoscopy, 261
Epicardium, 182, 182*f*
Epicondylitis, 113–114, 114*f*
Epidermis, 55, 55*f*
Epididymis, 304
Epididymitis, 309
Epidural hematoma, 132, 133*f*
Epigastric pain, 261
Epiglottis, 229–230, 230*f*
Epiglottitis, 233
Epispadias, 309*f*, 310
Epithelial tissue, 55
Error-prone abbreviations, symbols, and dose
        designations, ISMP list of, 400–403
Eructation, 263
Erythrocytes. *See* Red blood cells
Esophagitis, 261
Esophagus, 258
Eupnea, 232
Eustachian tube, 339, 339*f*
Expansion disorders, of respiratory system, 234, 236, 236*f*
    atelectasis, 234, 236
    pneumothorax, 234, 236, 236*f*
Expectorants, 237

External genitalia
    of female reproductive system, 306, 306*f*
    of male reproductive system, 303*f*, 304
External respiration, 227, 231
Eye. *See* Sight
Eyelid, disorders of, 341

F

Facial bones, 77–78, 78*f*
Fallopian tubes, 305–306, 305*f*
    ligation of, 314, 314*f*
Farsightedness. *See* Hyperopia
Feet, bones of, 82*f*–83*f*, 83
Female reproductive system
    external genitalia, 306, 306*f*
    menstrual cycle and fertilization, 306
    pregnancy, 307*f*–308*f*, 308
    structure and function of, 305–308, 305*f*–308*f*
Femur, 81, 82*f*
Fertilization, 302, 306
Fetus, 307*f*, 308
Fibrillation, 191–192
Fibroids, 311
Fibromyalgia, 113
Fibula, 81, 82*f*, 83
Fingers
    bones of, 81, 82*f*
    nails, 56, 56*f*
Fissure, 57, 57*f*
Flatus, 264
Floating ribs, 78, 79*f*
Flu. *See* Influenza
Fovea centralis, 337, 338*f*, 339
Fracture, 85, 86*t*–88*t*
Function. *See* Structure and function
Fundus, 305

G

Gallbladder, 259–260, 260*f*, 281
Gallstones. *See* Cholelithiasis
Gamete, 302
Ganglion, 128
Gastritis, 262
Gastroenterologist, 257
Gastroesophageal reflux disease (GERD), 261
Gastrointestinal (GI) tract, 257, 257*f*
Gastroscopy, 261
Genitalia, external
    of female reproductive system, 306, 306*f*
    of male reproductive system, 303*f*, 304
GERD. *See* Gastroesophageal reflux disease
Gestation, 302, 308
GFR. *See* Glomerular filtration rate
Gigantism, 161*t*, 162
Gingivitis, 261
GI tract. *See* Gastrointestinal tract
Glands
    of endocrine system, 156–160, 156*f*, 157*t*, 158*f*–160*f*
    within skin, 55–56, 55*f*

Glaucoma, 341
Glomerular filtration rate (GFR), 285
Glomerulonephritis, 284
Glomerulus, 282
Glottis, 229, 230*f*
Goiter, 161*t*, 162–163, 163*f*
Gonads, 156*f*, 157*t*, 158*f*, 160
Gonorrhea, 309
Graves' disease, 161*t*, 162
Gravida, 308
Gynecologist, 302

H
H2 blockers, 264
Hair follicles, 55–56, 55*f*
Hand, bones of, 81, 82*f*
Hashimoto thyroiditis, 161*t*, 162
Hb. *See* Hemoglobin
Hearing, 334–360
    abbreviations, 342*t*–343*t*
    disorders and treatments of ear, 341–342
    exercises and quiz, 353–360
        answers to, 380–381
    overview of, 335–337
    pharmacology for, 342
    structure and function of ear, 339, 339*f*
    study table, 343*t*–352*t*
    word elements related to, 336
Heart, 181–184, 182*f*, 184*f*–186*f*
Heart attack. *See* Myocardial infarction
Heartbeat, 183–184, 185*f*–186*f*
Heart rate, 183
Hematologist, 188, 214–215
Hemodialysis, 285, 285*f*
Hemoglobin (Hb), 186–187
Hemophilia, 192
Hemoptysis, 231, 233
Hemorrhage, 192
Hemorrhoids, 263
Hepatitis, 263
Hepatomegaly, 263
Herniated disc, 89
Herniation
    hiatal, 261, 262*f*
    inguinal, 263
    into vagina, 310, 311*f*
Hiatal hernia, 261, 262*f*
Hilum, 282, 283*f*
Hip bone, 81, 82*f*
HIV. *See* Human immunodeficiency virus
Hordeolum, 341
Hormone replacement therapy, 164
Hormones, 155, 157*t*, 158–160, 158*f*–160*f*
HPV. *See* Human papillomavirus
HSG. *See* Hysterosalpingograph
HTN. *See* Hypertension
Human immunodeficiency virus (HIV), 308–309
Human papillomavirus (HPV), 309
Humerus, 81, 81*f*
Hymen, 305–306, 305*f*–306*f*

Hyperemesis, 263
Hyperlipidemia, 189
Hyperopia, 340, 340*f*
Hypertension (HTN), 192
Hyperthyroidism, 161*t*, 162–163, 163*f*
Hypertrophy, 192
Hypophysis. *See* Pituitary gland
Hypospadias, 309*f*, 310
Hypothalamus, 130–131, 130*f*
Hypothyroidism, 161*t*, 162
Hysterectomy, 311, 314
Hysterosalpingograph (HSG), 314

I
Icterus, 263
Ileocecal sphincter, 258, 259*f*
Ileum, 258–259, 259*f*
Immune system, 41. *See also* Lymphatic system
Immunity, 212, 214
Immunization, 214, 216
Immunologist, 215
Immunosuppressants, 216
Impacted cerumen, 341
Impetigo, 58, 58*f*
Incontinence, 283–284
Incus, 339, 339*f*, 340*f*
Infarction, myocardial, 191, 191*f*
Infection
    of ear, 341
    of eye, 341
    of reproductive system, 308–309
    of respiratory system, 232–233
    of skin, 57–59
    of urinary tract, 284
Infectious rhinitis. *See* Common cold
Inflammatory disorders, of integumentary system, 57
Influenza, 233
Inguinal hernia, 263
Institute for Safe Medication Practices (ISMP), list of
        error-prone abbreviations, symbols, and dose
        designations, 400–403
Integumentary system, 41, 53–73
    abbreviations, 61*t*
    disorders and treatments of, 56–60
        burns, 59
        inflammatory disorders, 57
        skin cancer, 59
        skin disorders, 59
        skin infections, 57–59
        skin lesions, 56–57, 57*f*
    exercises and quiz, 67–73
        answers to, 366–367
    overview of, 54
    pharmacology for, 60–61
    structure and function of, 55–56, 55*f*–56*f*
    study table, 62*t*–66*t*
    word elements related to, 54
Internal respiration, 227, 231
Intestinal obstruction, 263
Intussusception, 263

Iris, 337, 338*f*
Ischemia, 188
ISMP. *See* Institute for Safe Medication Practices

J
Jaundice, 263
Jawbones, 77–78, 78*f*
Jejunum, 258, 259*f*
Joints, 83, 84*f*, 84*t*

K
Keratin, 56
Keratitis, 341
Kidneys, 281–282, 282*f*–283*f*
Kidney stones, 286, 287*f*
Kussmaul breathing, 232
Kyphosis, 85–86, 89, 89*f*

L
Labia majora, 305–306, 305*f*–306*f*
Labia minora, 305–306, 305*f*–306*f*
Labyrinth, 339
Labyrinthitis, 341
Lacrimal apparatus, 337
Lacrimal fluid, 337
Lacrimal glands, 337, 337*f*
Lacrimal sac, 337, 337*f*
Lactation, 306
Laparoscopy, 313
Large intestine, 259, 259*f*
Laryngeal pharynx, 228
Laryngitis, 233
Laryngotracheobronchitis, 233
Larynx, 227–229, 228*f*–231*f*
Leg bones, 81, 82*f*, 83
Lesions, of skin, 56–57, 57*f*
Leukemia, 188, 192
Leukocytes. *See* White blood cells
Ligaments, 109
Lingual tonsils, 228, 229*f*
Lipid panel, 189
Liver, 259–260, 260*f*
Lordosis, 89, 89*f*
Lou Gehrig Disease. *See* Amyotrophic lateral sclerosis
Lower esophageal sphincter. *See* Cardiac sphincter
Lower GI tract, 257
    disorders and treatments of, 262–263
    structure and function of, 258–259, 259*f*
LP. *See* Lumbar puncture
Lumbar puncture (LP), 135, 136*f*
Lumbar vertebrae, 46, 46*f*, 47*t*, 79, 80*f*
Lumen, of blood vessels, 186
Lungs, 227, 228*f*, 230–231, 231*f*
Lunula, 56, 56*f*
Lymph, 212–214, 214*f*
Lymphadenitis, 215
Lymphadenopathy, 215

Lymphatic system, 211–225
    abbreviations, 216*t*
    disorders and treatments of, 215–216
    exercises and quiz, 222–225
        answers to, 373–374
    lymphocytes, 212
    overview of, 212
    pharmacology for, 216
    practice and practitioners, 214–215
    structure and function of, 212–214, 213*f*–215*f*
        lymphatic organs, 214, 215*f*
        lymphatic structures, 213–214, 213*f*–214*f*
    study table, 217*t*–221*t*
    word elements related to, 212
Lymphedema, 215
Lymph nodes, 213–214, 215*f*
Lymphocytes, 212

M
Macule, 56, 57*f*
Male reproductive system, 303–304, 303*f*–304*f*
Malleolus, 83, 83*f*, 92*t*
Malleus, 339, 339*f*, 340*f*
Mammary glands, 306
Mammography, 314
Mastectomy, 314
Mastication, 258
Mastitis, 309
Mastoiditis, 341
Mediastinum, 230
Medical conditions, suffixes that signify, 14, 14*t*
Medical specialty/specialists, suffixes associated with, 14–15, 15*t*, 25–26
Medical terms, 3–11
    analyzing, 6
    combining vowel, 5–6
    common elements, 7–8
    exercises and quiz for, 9–11
        answers to, 361
    pronunciation of, 7
    singular and plural endings, 6–7, 7*t*
    word division marks, 6
    word elements, 4–6, 8*t*
Medulla oblongata, 130*f*, 131
Meiosis, 304
Melanin, 55–56
Melanocytes, 55–56
Melena, 262
Ménière's syndrome, 342
Meninges, 131, 131*f*
Menses, 307
Menstrual cycle, 306–307
Menstruation, 305
Mesencephalon, 130*f*, 131
MI. *See* Myocardial infarction
Micturition, 283
Miotics, 342
Mitral valve, 183
MONA, 191
Mood disorders, 135

MS. *See* Multiple sclerosis
Mucolytics, 237
Mucus, 227
Multiple sclerosis (MS), 133–134
Muscle tissue, 40
Muscular dystrophy, 112
Muscular system, 41, 108–125
    abbreviations, 116*t*
    disorders and treatments of, 112–115
        cumulative trauma disorders, 113–114
        muscular system disorders, 112–113
        paralysis, 115
        sports injuries, 115
    exercises and quiz, 120–125
        answers to, 368–369
    overview of, 109
    pharmacology for, 115
    practice and practitioners, 112
    structure and function of, 109–111
        muscle movement, 111, 111*t*
        types of muscle tissue, 109–111, 110*f*
    study table, 116*t*–119*t*
    word elements related to, 109
Myasthenia gravis, 112–113
Mydriatics, 342
Myelin sheath, 128
Myocardial infarction (MI), 191, 191*f*
Myocardium, 181, 182*f*
Myometrium, 305
Myopia, 340, 340*f*
Myringectomy, 342
Myringitis, 341
Myringotomy, 342

N

Nails, 56, 56*f*
Nasal bone, 77–78, 78*f*
Nasal cavity, 227, 228*f*
Nasopharynx, 227–228
Natural immunity, 214
Nearsightedness. *See* Myopia
Necrosis, 191
Neonatologist, 302
Nephritis, 284
Nephrologist, 281
Nephron, 282
Nervous system, 41, 126–153
    abbreviations, 136*t*–137*t*
    disorders of, 132–135
        behavioral disorders, 134–135
        brain trauma, 132, 133*f*
        seizure disorders, 134
        systemic degenerative diseases, 133–134
        tumors, 133
        vascular insults, 132–133, 133*f*
    exercises and quiz, 146–153
        answers to, 369–371
    overview of, 127–128, 128*f*–129*f*
    pharmacology for, 136
    practice and practitioners, 135–136

    structure and function of, 128–132
        central nervous system, 128–132, 128*f*–131*f*
        peripheral nervous system, 128, 128*f*–129*f*, 132
    study table, 137*t*–145*t*
    word elements related to, 127
Nervous tissue, 40
Neurohypophysis, 158
Neurons, 128, 129*f*
Nodule, 56, 57*f*
Normal rhythm, 184, 186*f*
Nose, 227, 228*f*
NPO, 264
Nuclear stress test, 191
Nucleus, 39, 40*f*
Number, prefixes of, 18, 18*t*, 30

O

Obstetrician, 302
Obstruction
    intestinal, 263
    of urinary tract, 286, 287*f*
Obstructive lung diseases, 234, 235*f*
Oliguria, 285
Oncologist, 215
Oophorectomy, 313–314
Oophoritis, 309
Ophthalmologist, 336
Optician, 336
Optometrist, 336
Orbit, 337
Organs, 39*f*, 40
Oropharynx, 227–228
Orthopnea, 232
Os coxae. *See* Hip bone
Ossicles, 339, 339*f*–340*f*
Osteoarthritis, 88
Osteomalacia, 88
Osteomyelitis, 85
Osteoporosis, 85, 88
Osteosarcoma, 88
Otalgia, 341
Otitis, 341
Otodynia, 341
Otologist, 336
Otoplasty, 342
Otorhinolaryngologist, 336
Otosclerosis, 342
Ovary, 305, 305*f*
Ovulation, 307
Ovum, 302, 305
Oxytocin, 157*t*, 158, 158*f*

P

Palpebra, 337
Pancreas, 156*f*, 157*t*, 158*f*, 160, 161*t*, 163–164, 259–260, 260*f*
Papanicolaou test, 313
Pap smear, 313
Papule, 57, 57*f*
Para, 308

Paralysis, 115
Parasympathetic nervous system, 128*f*, 132
Parathyroid gland, 156*f*, 157*t*, 158*f*–159*f*, 159
Parietal layer, of pleura, 230, 231*f*
Parkinson's disease, 133–134, 134*f*
Paronychia, 59, 60*f*
Parotiditis, 261
Patella, 82*f*, 83
Patency, of lungs, 231–232
Pediatrician, 302
Pediculosis, 61
Pelvic cavity, 44, 44*f*–45*f*, 45*t*–46*t*
Pelvic girdle, 81, 82*f*
Pelvic inflammatory disease (PID), 309
Penis, 303, 303*f*, 309, 309*f*
Percutaneous transluminal coronary angioplasty (PTCA),
      189, 189*f*
Pericardium, 182, 182*f*
Perimetrium, 305
Peripheral nervous system (PNS), 128, 128*f*–129*f*, 132
Perirenal fat, 282, 283*f*
Peristalsis, 258
Peritoneal dialysis, 285, 285*f*–286*f*
Peritonitis, 262
Pertussis, 233
Peyer's patches, 214, 215*f*
Phagocytosis, 187, 214
Phalanges
      fingers, 81, 82*f*
      toes, 83, 83*f*
Pharmacology
      for cardiovascular system, 193
      for digestive system, 264
      for endocrine system, 164
      for eyes and ears, 342
      for immune and lymphatic system, 216
      for integumentary system, 60–61
      for muscular system, 115
      for nervous system, 136
      overview of, 60
      for reproductive system, 314
      for respiratory system, 237
      for skeletal system, 89
      for urinary system, 286–287
Pharynx, 227–228, 228*f*–229*f*, 258
Physiology, 38
Pia mater, 131*f*, 132
PID. *See* Pelvic inflammatory disease
Pinna, 339, 339*f*
Pituitary gland, 156, 156*f*, 157*t*–158*t*, 158, 161–162, 161*t*, 162*f*
Placenta, 308
Planes, 43–44, 43*f*
Plantar fasciitis, 114
Plaque, 56, 57*f*
Platelets. *See* Thrombocytes
Pleura, 230, 231*f*
Plural endings, 6–7, 7*t*
Pneumonia, 233
Pneumothorax, 234, 236*f*
PNS. *See* Peripheral nervous system
Polyp, 263

Pons, 130*f*, 131
Position, prefixes of, 18, 18*t*, 29
Practice and practitioners
      cardiovascular system, 188
      immune and lymphatic system, 214–215
      integumentary system, 54
      muscular system, 112
      nervous system, 135–136
      respiratory system, 231
      skeletal system, 85
      suffixes associated with, 14–15, 15*t*, 25–26
Prefixes, 4–6, 8*t*
      categories of, 16–18
      of direction, 17, 17*t*, 28
      exercises and quiz, 28–31, 33
            answers to, 362–365
      list of, 382–386
      of position, 18, 18*t*, 29
      of size or number, 18, 18*t*, 30
      study table, 21*t*–22*t*
      of time or speed, 17, 17*t*, 28
Pregnancy, 307*f*–308*f*, 308
      ectopic, 309
Presbycusis, 341
Presbyopia, 340
Primigravida, 308
Proctologists, 257
Prolapsed uterus, 310
Proliferative phase, of menstrual cycle, 307
Pronunciation, of medical terms, 7
Prostate, 303–304, 303*f*
      transurethral resection of, 312
Prostatectomy, 312–313
Prostatitis, 309
Protective agents, 264
Protein pump inhibitors, 264
Psoriasis, 57, 58*f*
Psychotic disorders, 135
PTCA. *See* Percutaneous transluminal coronary
            angioplasty
Pulmonary circuit, 182
Pulmonary function tests, 237
Pulmonary semilunar valve, 183
Pulse oximetry, 183, 236, 236*f*
Purkinje fibers, 183, 185*f*
Pustule, 57, 57*f*
Pyelonephritis, 284
Pyloric sphincter, 258, 259*f*

R
Radius, 81, 81*f*
Rales, 232
RBCs. *See* Red blood cells
Rectocele, 310–311, 311*f*
Rectum, 259, 259*f*
Red blood cells (RBCs), 186–187, 187*f*
Refractory errors, 340, 340*f*
Renal calculi, 286, 287*f*
Renal failure, 284–285, 285*f*–286*f*
Renal fascia, 282, 283*f*

Reproductive system, 41, 301–333
  abbreviations, 315*t*
  disorders and treatments of, 308–314, 309*f*–314*f*
    diagnostic and surgical procedures, 311–314, 312*f*–314*f*
    other infections, 309
    sexually transmitted diseases, 308–309
    structural abnormalities, 309–311, 309*f*–311*f*
    tumors, 311, 312*f*
  exercises and quiz, 325–333
    answers to, 379–380
  overview of, 302
  pharmacology for, 314
  structure and function of, 303–308, 303*f*–308*f*
    female reproductive system, 305–308, 305*f*–308*f*
    male reproductive system, 303–304, 303*f*–304*f*
  study table, 315*t*–324*t*
  word elements related to, 302
Respiratory system, 41, 226–254
  abbreviations, 237*t*–238*t*
  disorders and treatments of, 231–237, 235*f*–237*f*
    diagnostic procedures and treatments, 236–237, 236*f*–237*f*
    expansion disorders, 234, 236, 236*f*
    infectious disorders, 232–233
    obstructive lung diseases, 234, 235*f*
  exercises and quiz, 247–254
    answers to, 374–375
  overview of, 227, 228*f*
  pharmacology for, 237
  practice and practitioners, 231
  structure and function of, 227–231, 228*f*–231*f*
    bronchi, bronchioles, and alveoli, 228*f*, 229–230
    larynx, 227–229, 229*f*–231*f*
    lungs, 227, 228*f*, 230–231, 231*f*
    nose, 227
    pharynx, 227–228, 228*f*–229*f*, 258
    trachea, 229
  study table, 238*t*–246*t*
  word elements related to, 227
Retention, 283–284
Retina, 337, 338*f*
Retroflexion, of uterus, 310, 310*f*
Retroversion, of uterus, 310, 310*f*
Rheumatoid arthritis, 88–89, 88*f*
Rh factor, 187
Rhinitis. *See* Common cold
Rhonchi, 232
Rib bones, 78, 79*f*
Rickets, 88
Rods, 337, 338*f*
Root words, 4–6, 8*t*
  combining suffixes with, 23–24
  list of, 382–386
Rotator cuff injury, 113

S

Sacrum (vertebra), 46, 46*f*, 47*t*, 79, 80*f*
Salivary glands, 257*f*, 259–260, 260*f*
Salpingitis, 309

Salpingo-oophorectomy, 314
SA node. *See* Sinoatrial node
Scabies, 58, 58*f*
Scapula, 81, 81*f*
Sclera, 337, 338*f*
Scleroderma, 57
Scoliosis, 89, 89*f*
Scrotum, 303, 303*f*
Sebaceous gland, 55–56, 55*f*, 59
Secretory phase, of menstrual cycle, 307
Secundigravida, 308
Seizure disorders, 134
Semilunar valves, 183
Seminal vesicles, 303–304, 303*f*
Sense. *See* Hearing; Sight
Sensorineural hearing loss, 341
Septum, of heart, 182
Sexually transmitted diseases (STDs), 308–309
Shingles, 59
Shin splints, 115
Shoulder bones, 81, 81*f*
Shoulder girdle, 81, 81*f*
Sight, 334–360
  abbreviations, 342*t*–343*t*
  disorders and treatments of eye, 340–341, 340*f*–341*f*
    eyelid disorders, 341
    infection, 341
    refractory errors, 340, 340*f*
  exercises and quiz, 353–360
    answers to, 380–381
  overview of, 335–337
  pharmacology for, 342
  structure and function of eye, 337–339, 337*f*–338*f*
  study table, 343*t*–352*t*
  word elements related to, 335
Sigmoid colon, 259, 259*f*
Singular endings, 6–7, 7*t*
Sinoatrial (SA) node, 183, 185*f*
Sinusitis, 232
Sinus rhythm, 184, 186*f*
Size, prefixes of, 18, 18*t*
Skeletal muscles, 109, 110*f*, 111
Skeletal system, 41, 74–107
  abbreviations, 90*t*
  disorders and treatments of, 85–89
  exercises and quiz, 99–107
    answers to, 367–368
  overview of, 76–77, 76*f*
  pharmacology for, 89
  practice and practitioners, 85
  structure and function of, 77–84
    appendicular skeleton, 76, 76*f*, 81–83, 81*f*–83*f*
    axial skeleton, 76–80, 76*f*–80*f*
    joints, 83, 84*f*, 84*t*
  study table, 90*t*–98*t*
  word elements related to, 75–76
Skin, 54–55, 55*f*
  biopsy of, 59–60
  cancer of, 59
  glands within, 55–56, 55*f*

infections of, 57–59
lesions of, 56–57, 57*f*
other disorders of, 59
Small intestine, 258, 259*f*
Smooth muscles, 109, 110*f*, 111
Somatic nervous system, 128, 128*f*–129*f*, 132
Special senses. *See* Hearing; Sight
Speed, prefixes of, 17, 17*t*, 28
Sperm, 302
Spermatogenesis, 304
Spermatozoon, 302, 304
Sphincters, urethral, 283
Sphygmomanometer, 186
Spinal cavity, 44, 44*f*, 46, 46*f*, 47*t*
Spinal column, 46, 46*f*, 47*t*, 79, 80*f*
Spirometer, 237
Spleen, 214, 215*f*
Sports injuries, 115
Sprain, 85
Sputum, 231
Stapedectomy, 342
Stapes, 339, 339*f*, 340*f*
Statins, 189, 193
STDs. *See* Sexually transmitted diseases
Stent, arterial, 189, 190*f*
Sternum, 78, 79*f*
Stoma, 262
Stomach, 258
Stomatitis, 261
Stridor, 232
Structural abnormalities, of reproductive system, 309*f*–311*f*
Structure and function
    of cardiovascular system, 181–187, 182*f*, 184*f*–187*f*, 188*t*
    of digestive system, 257–259, 258*f*–259*f*, 261*t*
    of ear, 339, 339*f*
    of endocrine system, 155–160, 156*f*, 157*t*, 158*f*–160*f*
    of eye, 337–339, 337*f*–338*f*
    of immune system, 212–214, 213*f*–215*f*
    of integumentary system, 55–56, 55*f*–56*f*
    of muscular system, 109–111, 110*f*, 111*t*
    of nervous system, 128–132, 128*f*–131*f*
    of reproductive system, 303–308, 303*f*–308*f*
    of respiratory system, 227–231, 228*f*–231*f*
    of skeletal system, 77–84
    of urinary system, 282–283, 283*f*
Subcutaneous layer, 55, 55*f*
Subdural hematoma, 132, 133*f*
Sudoriferous (sweat) glands, 55*f*, 56
Suffixes, 4–6, 8*t*
    categories of, 13–16
    combining root words with, 23–24
    exercises and quiz, 23–28, 31–32
        answers to, 362–365
    list of, 382–386
    study table, 19*t*–20*t*
    that denote adjectives, 15–16, 16*t*, 26–27
    that signify diagnostic terms, test information or surgical procedures, 14, 15*t*, 24–25
    that signify medical conditions, 14, 14*t*
    that signify medical specialty/specialists, 14–15, 15*t*, 25–26
Surgical procedures
    for reproductive system, 311–314, 312*f*–314*f*
    suffixes that signify, 14, 15*t*, 24–25
Sweat glands. *See* Sudoriferous glands
Symbols, error-prone, ISMP list of, 400–403
Sympathetic nervous system, 128*f*, 132
Synapses, 128
Synovial joint, 83, 84*f*, 84*t*
Syphilis, 309
Systemic circuit, 182
Systems, 39*f*, 41
Systole, 183, 185*f*
Systolic pressure, 186

T
Tachycardia, 191
Tachypnea, 232
TB. *See* Tuberculosis
T cells, 216
Tendons, 109, 110*f*
Test information, suffixes that signify, 14, 15*t*, 24–25
Testis, 303–304, 303*f*
Testosterone, 304
Thalamus, 130–131, 130*f*
Thoracentesis, 236–237, 237*f*
Thoracic bones, 78, 79*f*
Thoracic cage, 78, 79*f*
Thoracic cavity, 44, 44*f*
Thoracic vertebrae, 46, 46*f*, 47*t*, 79, 80*f*
Throat. *See* Pharynx
Thrombocytes, 187, 187*f*
Thrombocytopenia, 192
Thrombolytic agents, 191
Thrombosis, 188*f*, 191
Thrombus, 191
Thymus, 214, 215*f*
Thyroid gland, 156*f*, 157*t*, 158*f*–159*f*, 159, 161*t*, 162–163, 163*f*
Thyromegaly. *See* Goiter
TIA. *See* Transient ischemic attack
Tibia, 81, 82*f*, 83
Time, prefixes of, 17, 17*t*, 28
Tinea, 58, 59*f*
Tinnitus, 342
Tissues, 39*f*, 40
Toes
    bones of, 83, 83*f*
    nails, 56, 56*f*
Tonsils, 214, 215*f*, 228, 229*f*
Total parenteral nutrition (TPN), 264
TPN. *See* Total parenteral nutrition
Trachea, 229
Tracheostomy, 233
Transient ischemic attack (TIA), 133
Transurethral resection of the prostate (TURP), 311, 312*f*
Transverse colon, 259, 259*f*
Treatments. *See* Disorders and treatments

Tricuspid valve, 183
Tubal ligation, 314, 314f
Tuberculosis (TB), 233
Tumors
    of nervous system, 133
    of reproductive system, 311, 312f
Turgor, 56
TURP. *See* Transurethral resection of the prostate
Tympanectomy, 342
Tympanic membrane, 339, 339f
Tympanoplasty, 342

U

Ulcers, 57, 57f, 59
Ulna, 81, 81f
Upper GI tract, 257
    disorders and treatments of, 261–262, 262f
    structure and function of, 258, 258f
Urea, 282
Uremia, 285
Ureter, 281–282, 282f
Ureteroscope, 286
Urethra, 281, 282f, 283
Urethritis, 284
Uric acid, 282
Urinary bladder, 281–283, 282f
Urinary meatus, 305, 306f
Urinary system, 41, 280–300
    abbreviations, 288t
    disorders and treatment of, 283–286, 284f–287f
        incontinence and retention, 283–284
        renal failure, 284–285, 285f–286f
        urinary tract infections, 284
        urinary tract obstructions, 286, 287f
    exercises and quiz, 293–300
        answers to, 377–378
    overview of, 281, 282f
    pharmacology for, 286–287
    structure and function of, 282–283, 283f
    study table, 288t–292t
    word elements related to, 281
Urinary tract infections (UTIs), 284
Urinary tract obstructions, 286, 287f
Urination, 283
Urine, 282, 282f
Urologist, 281, 302
Uterus, 305, 305f, 310, 310f
UTIs. *See* Urinary tract infections
Uveal tract, 337

V

Vaccinations, 214, 216
Vagina, 305–306, 305f
    herniation into, 310, 311f
Vaginal opening, 305–306, 306f
Vas deferens, 304
Vasectomy, 313, 313f
Vasoconstriction, 186
Vasoconstrictors, 193
Vasodilation, 186
Vasodilators, 193
Veins, 186
Ventral cavity, 44, 44f–45f, 45t–46t
Ventricle, 182
Ventricular fibrillation, 192
Venules, 186
Vermiform appendix. *See* Appendix
Vertebrae, 46, 46f, 47t, 79, 80f
Vertigo, 342
Vesicle, 57, 57f
Viscera, 44
Visceral layer, of pleura, 230, 231f
Vitiligo, 59, 60f
Vitreous humor, 338f, 339
Vocal cords, 229, 230f
Voice box. *See* Larynx
Voiding, 283
Volvulus, 263
Vulva, 305–306, 306f

W

WBCs. *See* White blood cells
Wheal, 57, 57f
Wheezing, 232
White blood cells (WBCs), 186–187, 187f
Whooping cough. *See* Pertussis
Windpipe. *See* Trachea
Word division marks, 6
Word elements, 4–6, 8t
Wrist bones, 81, 82f

X

Xerophthalmia, 341
Xiphoid process, 78, 79f

Z

Zygote, 302